Dizziness and Vertigo Across the Lifespan

Dizziness and Vertigo Across the Lifespan

A. TUCKER GLEASON, PhD
Director of Audiology
Department of Otolaryngology-Head and Neck Surgery
Department of Neurology
University of Virginia School of Medicine
Charlottesville, VA,
United States

BRADLEY W. KESSER, MD
Department of Otolaryngology-Head and Neck Surgery
University of Virginia School of Medicine
Charlottesville, VA,
United States

ELSEVIER

ELSEVIER

3251 Riverport Lane
St. Louis, Missouri 63043

DIZZINESS AND VERTIGO ACROSS THE LIFESPAN   ISBN: 978-0-323-55136-6

Content Strategist: Jessica McCool
Content Development Manager: Taylor Ball
Content Development Specialist: Donald Mumford
Publishing Services Manager: Deepthi Unni
Project Manager: Janish Ashwin Paul
Designer: Gopalakrishnan Venkatraman

Printed in United States of America

Last digit is the print number: 9   8   7   6   5   4   3   2   1

List of Contributors

Yuri Agrawal, MD, MPH, FACS
Associate Professor
Division of Otology, Neurotology and Skull Base
    Surgery
Department of Otolaryngology - Head & Neck Surgery
The Johns Hopkins University School of Medicine
Baltimore, MD, United States

Muhammad Alrwaily, PT, MS, PhD
Division of Physical Therapy
School of Medicine
West Virginia University
Morgantown, WV, United States
Department of Physical Therapy
King Fahad Specialist Hospital
Dammam, Saudi Arabia

Kamran Barin, PhD
Former Assistant Professor of Otolaryngology-Head
    and Neck Surgery and Director
Balance Disorders Clinic
The Ohio State University Medical Center
Columbus, OH, United States

Jamie M. Bogle, PhD
Assistant Professor of Audiology
Mayo Clinic College of Medicine
Department of Otorhinolaryngology
Scottsdale, AZ, United States

Tzu-Pu Chang, MD
Department of Neurology/Neuro-Medical Scientific
    Center
Taichung Tzu Chi Hospital & Tzu Chi University
Buddhist Tzu Chi Medical Foundation
Taichung City, Taiwan

Marcello Cherchi, MD, PhD
Associate Professor
Department of Neurology
Northwestern University Feinberg School of Medicine
Chicago, IL, United States

Edward I. Cho, MD
Associate
House Clinic
Los Angeles, CA, United States
Assistant Clinical Professor
Department of Head and Neck Surgery
David Geffen School of Medicine at UCLA
Los Angeles, CA, United States

Edward E. Dodson, MD
Associate Professor of Otolaryngology-Head and Neck
    Surgery
The Ohio State University Medical Center
Columbus, OH, United States

Jose N. Fayad, MD
ENT Consultant
Otology-Neurotology-Skull Base Surgery
Johns Hopkins Aramco Healthcare Company
Dhahran, Saudi Arabia

Erin Field, PA-C
Department of Otolaryngology
Children's Hospital of Philadelphia
Philadelphia, PA, United States

Gerard J. Gianoli, MD
Clinical Associate Professor
Department of Otolaryngology-Head and Neck Surgery
Tulane University School of Medicine
New Orleans, Louisiana, United States
The Ear and Balance Institute
Covington, LA, United States

John C. Goddard, MD
Division Head of Otology and Neurotology
Physician Director of Audiology
Department of Head and Neck Surgery
Northwest Permanente, PC – Kaiser Permanente
    Northwest
Portland, OR, United States

Howard P. Goodkin, MD, PhD
The Shure Professor of Neurology and Pediatrics
Departments of Neurology and Pediatrics
University of Virginia
Charlottesville, VA, United States

Chris Grindle, MD
Fellow
Department of Otolaryngology
Connecticut Children's Hospital
Hartford, CT, United States

Michael S. Harris, MD
Assistant Professor
Otolaryngology and Communication Sciences
Division of Neuro-Otologic Skull Base Surgery
Medical College of Wisconsin
Milwaukee, WI, United States

Akira Ishiyama, MD
Professor
Head and Neck Surgery Division
David Geffen School of Medicine at UCLA
Los Angeles, CA, United States

Gail Ishiyama, MD
Associate Professor - In Residence
Neurology Department
David Geffen School of Medicine at UCLA
Los Angeles, CA, United States

Gary P. Jacobson, PhD
Director of Audiology and Professor
Vanderbilt Bill Wilkerson Center
Hearing and Speech Sciences
Division of Audiology
Vanderbilt University Medical Center
Nashville, TN, United States

Amir Kheradmand, MD
Assistant Professor
Department of Neurology
Neurovisual and Vestibular Division
Vestibular and Ocular Motor Research (VOR)
    Laboratory
The Johns Hopkins Hospital
Baltimore, MD, United States

David S. Liebeskind, MD
Professor
Neurology Department
David Geffen School of Medicine at UCLA
Los Angeles, CA, United States

Nauman Manzoor, MD
The Ear, Nose, and Throat Institute
University Hospitals Cleveland Medical Center
Case Western Reserve University School of Medicine
Cleveland, OH, United States

Devin L. McCaslin, PhD
Director
Vestibular and Balance Program
Department of Otorhinolaryngology
Mayo Clinic
Rochester, MN, United States

Cliff A. Megerian, MD, FACS
Professor
The Ear, Nose, and Throat Institute
University Hospitals Cleveland Medical Center
Case Western Reserve University School of Medicine
Cleveland, OH, United States

Yaena Min, PhD
Senior Associate
The Moran Company
Arlington, VA, United States

Thierry Morlet, PhD
Head
Auditory Physiology and Psychoacoustics Research
    Laboratory
A.I. duPont Hospital for Children
Wilmington, DE, United States

Sarah E. Mowry, MD, FACS
Assistant Professor
The Ear, Nose, and Throat Institute
University Hospitals Cleveland Medical Center
Case Western Reserve University School of Medicine
Cleveland, OH, United States

Owen Murnane, PhD
Vestibular Research Laboratory
James H. Quillen VA Medical Center
Mountain Home, TN, United States

Robert O'Reilly, MD
Attending Physician
Director, Balance and Vestibular Program
Department of Otolaryngology
Children's Hospital of Philadelphia
Philadelphia, PA, United States

Denia Ramirez-Montealegre, MD, MPH, PhD
Pediatric Neurology
Brain and Spine Institute
The University of Tennessee Medical Center
Knoxville, TN, United States

Kristal Riska, AuD, PhD
Department of Surgery
Division of Head and Neck Surgery & Communication
   Sciences
Duke University School of Medicine
Durham, NC, United States

Maroun T. Semaan, MD, FACS
Assistant Professor
The Ear, Nose, and Throat Institute
University Hospitals Cleveland Medical Center
Case Western Reserve University School of Medicine
Cleveland, OH, United States

Jorge M. Serrador, PhD
Associate Professor
Department of Pharmacology, Physiology and
   Neuroscience
Rutgers Biomedical and Health Sciences
Newark, NJ, United States
War Related Illness & Injury Study Center
Dept of Veteran Affairs
East Orange, NJ
Adjunct Professor of Cardiovascular Electronics
National University of Ireland Galway
Galway, Ireland

Osama A. Shoair, PhD
Clinical Assistant Professor
Ben and Maytee Fisch College of Pharmacy University
   of Texas at Tyler
Tyler, TX, United States

Patricia W. Slattum, PharmD, PhD
Geriatric Pharmacotherapy Program
Department of Pharmacotherapy and Outcomes
   Science
Virginia Commonwealth University
Richmond, VA, United States

James S. Soileau, MD
The Ear and Balance Institute
Covington, LA, United States

Jennie Taylor, MD, MPH
Assistant Professor of Neurology and Neurological
   Surgery
Departments of Neurology and Neurological Surgery
University of California, San Francisco
San Francisco, CA, United States

L. Maureen Valente, PhD
Director of Audiology Studies and Associate Professor
Program in Audiology and Communication Sciences
Washington University School of Medicine
St. Louis, MO, United States

Judith A. White, MD, PhD
Medical Director
Swedish Balance Center
Swedish Neuroscience Institute
Seattle, WA, United States

Susan L. Whitney, DPT, PhD
Department of Physical Therapy
School of Health and Rehabilitation Sciences
University of Pittsburgh
Pittsburgh, PA, United States
King Saud University
Riyadh, Saudi Arabia
Department of Otolaryngology
University of Pittsburgh
Pittsburgh, PA, United States

David S. Zee, MD
Professor
Department of Ophthalmology, Otolaryngology-Head
   and Neck Surgery, Neurology Neuroscience
The Johns Hopkins University School of Medicine
Baltimore, MD, United States

Emily Zwicky, AuD
Pediatric Audiologist
Children's Hospital of Richmond at VCU
Richmond, VA, United States

Preface

The chief complaint of dizziness is one of the hardest complaints we as primary care physicians, family medicine physicians, emergency room physicians, neurologists, otolaryngologists, audiologists, physical therapists, and other healthcare providers face. One reason for this difficulty is that there are just so many darned "things" that can cause dizziness. Central causes, peripheral causes, mixed causes, medications, diseases both physical and psychological—the list is, well, dizzying.

I think we all agree that the best tool in our armamentarium to diagnose dizziness is the history. But in this era of high throughput of patients, declining reimbursement, and tighter schedules, who has the time to take a 45-minute history?

We have compiled this book to help all healthcare professionals who see patients with vertigo and dizziness. Rather than organizing the book by disease, we have chosen to take an age-based approach. There are diagnoses common to children not seen in the elderly, and vice versa. We felt that age was one obvious aspect of the history that could inform further questioning and exploration. Clearly, an organized approach to seeing patients reporting dizziness will help the clinician keep the history focused and directed.

We have included chapters outlining the nature and extent of the problem (Chapter 1) and a few chapters on vestibular testing (Chapters 2, 4, and 8) to help guide the clinician's way. Of course, we have included a number of diagnosis-driven chapters.

As our population ages, we encourage the reader to review the chapters on dizziness in the elderly. Dizziness in this population is generally multifactorial with no easy answers—except fall prevention. We encourage clinicians to develop a fall counseling "talk" to present to their elderly patients, because falls are becoming a leading cause of morbidity and mortality in the United States.

Finally, we hope you enjoy this book. Use it as a reference, as a text for educational purposes, for "light reading," or as a refresher. We hope you enjoy reading it as much as we have enjoyed bringing it to you.

A. Tucker Gleason, PhD
Associate Professor
Director of Audiology
Department of Otolaryngology–Head and
Neck Surgery
Department of Neurology
University of Virginia School of Medicine
Charlottesville, VA, United States

Bradley W. Kesser, MD
Professor
Department of Otolaryngology–Head
and Neck Surgery
Department of Pediatrics
University of Virginia School of Medicine
Charlottesville, VA, United States

Contents

CHAPTER 1

Dizziness Demographics and Population Health

YURI AGRAWAL, MD, MPH, FACS

Dizziness and imbalance are common conditions affecting people of all ages, and particularly the elderly. This chapter begins by defining dizziness, imbalance, and *presbyvestibulopathy*, or age-related vestibular loss, which is of particular interest to the otolaryngologist, the neurologist, and the primary care physician. Then the epidemiology of dizziness, imbalance, and presbyvestibulopathy will be reviewed. Finally, the impacts of these conditions on population health from the perspective of the older adult and the healthcare system will be discussed.

DEFINITIONS OF DIZZINESS, IMBALANCE, AND PRESBYVESTIBULOPATHY

Dizziness connotes a subjective perception of disorientation or involuntary motion, which can occur during movement or at rest.[1] Dizziness can be further characterized as vertigo and/or lightheadedness. Vertigo is the false sensation that either the body or the environment is moving (usually spinning) and may be a symptom of vestibular, visual, or neurologic impairment; psychological factors; or the use of multiple medications ("polypharmacy," see Chapter 18). Lightheadedness is the sensation of impending loss of consciousness associated with transient diffuse cerebral hypoperfusion. Causal factors for lightheadedness typically include cardiovascular disease (e.g., aortic stenosis) and orthostatic hypotension (e.g., resulting from excessive medication use or autonomic instability).

Imbalance connotes disequilibrium or postural instability.[2] Imbalance is usually described either while standing or walking and typically does not occur at rest. Imbalance can result from muscle weakness, arthritis, and/or reduced sensory input (e.g., visual, vestibular, proprioceptive) leading to impaired postural reflexes.

Presbyvestibulopathy refers specifically to aging of the vestibular system, akin to presbycusis (age-related

hearing loss) and presbyopia (age-related vision loss). Numerous lines of evidence demonstrate a progressive decline in vestibular function associated with aging. Histopathologic studies have shown that hair cell populations throughout the vestibular apparatus (including the three semicircular canals and two otolith organs, the saccule and utricle) decline with age. Moreover, declining cell counts have also been observed for vestibular ganglion cells, primary afferents, and vestibular nucleus cell populations.[3–5] Studies that have assessed vestibular physiologic responses have also observed declining semicircular canal and otolith responses associated with age.[6–16]

Presbyvestibulopathy can contribute to symptoms of dizziness and/or imbalance in older individuals. The vestibular system plays an integral role in maintaining the vestibulo-ocular (VOR) and vestibulospinal reflexes (VSR). The VOR is important for stabilizing gaze during head movement, and VOR impairment manifests as dizziness (i.e., abnormal sensation of motion). The VSR is important for trunk and limb stabilization during head movement. VSR dysfunction manifests as imbalance or postural instability. Interestingly, there is increasing recognition of the physiologic importance of vestibulo-autonomic projections (see Chapter 15). Vestibulo-autonomic impairment has been associated with orthostatic hypotension.[17] Thus presbyvestibulopathy may also be a causal factor for the symptom of lightheadedness. An effort is ongoing to establish formal diagnostic criteria for presbyvestibulopathy within the International Classification of Vestibular Disorders, a component of the International Classification of Diseases.[18]

The relationship between dizziness, imbalance, and presbyvestibulopathy is depicted in Fig. 1.1 as a set of overlapping conditions. Emerging evidence suggests that a certain amount of presbyvestibulopathy is present in older individuals but may not manifest

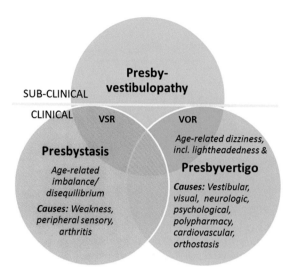

FIG. 1.1 Typology of age-related dizziness, imbalance, and vestibular loss. *VOR*, vestibulo-ocular reflex; *VSR*, vestibulospinal reflex.

symptomatically as dizziness or imbalance.[19,20] This may be because the level of vestibular impairment has not crossed a critical threshold, or because an individual is able to compensate for the presbyvestibulopathy. Presbyvestibulopathy is thus depicted in Fig. 1.1 as asymptomatic or "subclinical" and symptomatic or "clinical." Moreover, it is evident in Fig. 1.1 that multiple factors in addition to reduced vestibular function have been associated with dizziness and imbalance in the geriatric population. It is well known among researchers who study aging that geriatric conditions often result from numerous factors that coexist *at the same time* and that may interact to have nonlinear, synergistic effects. Indeed, Tinetti and colleagues have described dizziness as a "geriatric syndrome," whereby symptoms result not from sole disease entities but from accumulated impairment in multiple systems.[21] As such, presbyvestibulopathy is often not the only contributor to dizziness and imbalance in older adults.

EPIDEMIOLOGY OF DIZZINESS, IMBALANCE, AND PRESBYVESTIBULOPATHY

Prevalence

Estimates of the prevalence of dizziness and imbalance in the geriatric population depend largely on the definitions of dizziness and imbalance used and on the populations surveyed. The populations surveyed can vary with respect to their age ranges, whether they

are population-based or clinic-based, and what types of clinics are being studied (e.g., primary care vs. specialty). Several large population-based studies report a 20%–30% prevalence of dizziness and imbalance in the elderly population (age ≥ 65 years).[22–24] The prevalence of dizziness and imbalance is found to increase steeply with age, with levels over 50% in the community-dwelling population over age 80 years.[25] A study in nursing home residents observes a prevalence of dizziness and vertigo of 68%.[26] Among patients aged ≥65 years presenting to a geriatric primary care clinic, 24% report dizziness and 17% identify dizziness as their major presenting complaint.[27] Within the otolaryngology clinic, one study of 131,000 consecutive patients found that 6% of patients over age 65 years presented with vertigo or a presumed vestibular diagnosis.[28] Interestingly, this large-scale survey of otolaryngology practices found that visits from geriatric patients increased from 14.3% in 2004 to 17.9% in 2010. Moreover, this study noted that the five most common geriatric diagnoses were otologic, including hearing loss, external ear disorders, tinnitus, otitis media/Eustachian tube disorders, and vertigo.

A landmark series of studies based in Germany estimated the population prevalence and incidence more specifically of vestibular vertigo, i.e., vertigo resulting from vestibular impairment. Community-dwelling individuals aged ≥18 years were queried in a national telephone survey regarding symptoms of dizziness and vertigo. Those who reported moderate symptoms were administered a detailed neurotologic interview, from which vestibular vertigo was diagnosed based on symptoms of rotational vertigo, positional vertigo, or recurrent dizziness with nausea and oscillopsia or imbalance. The neurotologic interview was found to have good validity based on a gold standard of neurotology clinic-based diagnoses in establishing a vestibular diagnosis. The lifetime prevalence, 1-year prevalence, and incidence of vestibular vertigo were observed to be 7.8%, 4.9% and 1.5%, respectively.[29] The 1-year prevalence of vestibular vertigo increased with age to 7.2% in 60- to 69-year-olds and 8.8% in individuals over age 80 years. This study was among the first to estimate the population prevalence of presbyvestibulopathy.

A more recent study estimated the prevalence of vestibular impairment in the US population using an objective, rather than subjective (self-report based), test. Data were drawn from the 2001–04 National Health and Nutrition Examination Survey (NHANES). Vestibular function was assessed in NHANES using the modified Romberg test, whereby vestibular impairment was inferred from an inability to stand on a foam pad with eyes closed. About 35% of US adults aged 40 years and older had evidence of balance dysfunction based on this postural metric.[19] The frequency of balance dysfunction increased significantly with age, such that 85% of individuals aged 80 years and above had evidence of balance dysfunction. These estimates are considerably higher than the prevalences of vestibular vertigo reported earlier from the German population. It is possible that the symptom of vestibular vertigo represents *clinical* presbyvestibulopathy, whereas vestibular impairment based on the modified Romberg test encompasses both *clinical* and *subclinical* presbyvestibulopathy.

Of the major vestibular diagnoses, benign paroxysmal positional vertigo (BPPV) is particularly common in older adults and bears special mention (see Chapter 9). Increased BPPV in the elderly may reflect age-related degeneration of the otoconial membrane, leading to abnormal seeding of otoconia in the endolymph.[30] A study of the German population observed a prevalence of 3.4% in individuals over age 60 years and a cumulative lifetime incidence of almost 10% by age 80 years.[31] BPPV accounted for 39% of cases of vertigo in older patients presenting to neurotology clinics.[32] However, older patients do not always experience the classic presentation of BPPV, short episodes of rotatory vertigo associated with changes in head position. A study of 100 older patients presenting to general geriatric practices for chronic medical conditions found that 9% had unrecognized BPPV.[33] Moreover, patients with BPPV had significantly increased fall risk. Another study found that older patients with BPPV were more likely to experience postural instability.[34] This instability could be improved through canalith repositioning maneuvers.

Risk Factors

Epidemiologic analyses of dizziness, imbalance, and presbyvestibulopathy have also investigated risk factors for these conditions. Most studies have observed an increased prevalence of dizziness and imbalance in women.[1] Vestibular vertigo was also more prevalent in women.[35] However, the prevalence of vestibular impairment based on objective modified Romberg testing did not differ by gender.[19] Findings from a review of the most frequently reported causes of dizziness in primary care practice are presented in Table 1.1.[1] The review reported that peripheral vestibular disease was the most common cause of dizziness, observed in 20%–50% of patients.[1] Peripheral vestibular diseases included BPPV, labyrinthitis, and vestibular neuritis. Other common causes of dizziness were cardiovascular disease, systemic infection (leading to orthostatic hypotension), psychiatric disorders, metabolic disturbances, and use of multiple medications. A more recent epidemiologic survey of the elderly population in England found that dizziness was associated with abnormal heart rhythm, hearing loss, vision loss, and low grip strength, whereas imbalance was associated with diabetes, arthritis, low grip strength, and vision loss.[23] With respect to vestibular vertigo, independent risk factors were depression, tinnitus, and cardiovascular risk factors, including hypertension and dyslipidemia.[29] Finally, independent risk factors for vestibular impairment as measured by the modified Romberg test included low socioeconomic status and diabetes mellitus.[19,36]

IMPACTS OF DIZZINESS, IMBALANCE, AND PRESBYVESTIBULOPATHY

Dizziness, imbalance, and presbyvestibulopathy have an immense effect on diverse health and economic

TABLE 1.1
Most Common Causes of Dizziness in Primary Care Practice[1]

Category	Percentage of Patients (%)	Examples
Peripheral vestibular disease	20–50	Benign paroxysmal positional vertigo, labyrinthitis, vestibular neuritis
Cardiovascular disease	10–30	Arrhythmia, congestive heart failure, vasovagal conditions (e.g., carotid sinus hypersensitivity)
Systemic infection	10–20	Systemic viral and bacterial infection
Psychiatric conditions	5–15	Depression, anxiety, hyperventilation
Metabolic disturbances	5–10	Hypoglycemia, hyperglycemia, electrolyte disturbances, thyrotoxicosis, anemia
Medications	5–10	Antihypertensives, psychotropic medications

outcomes that affect the individual and society. In this section, the impact of these conditions on falls, quality of life, activities of daily living, and healthcare utilization are reviewed. Emerging links between presbyvestibulopathy and cognitive decline are also explored.

Falls

Falls are a common and disastrous outcome in older individuals. One in three adults over age 65 years falls each year. About 10% of falls result in hip fracture, and a fall increases the likelihood of nursing home placement 10-fold. Dizziness has been associated with a two- to threefold increased risk of falling.[19,25] Specifically with respect to presbyvestibulopathy, the previously mentioned study from NHANES found that individuals with objective vestibular impairment who were also clinically symptomatic (i.e., reported dizziness) had a 12-fold increase in the odds of falling. In a small pilot study, older fallers were found to have significantly higher rates of peripheral vestibular dysfunction than older non-fallers.[37] A prospective study reported that elderly patients with vestibular asymmetry were significantly more likely to experience an incident fall.[38] Moreover, several studies have observed an association between vestibular asymmetry and fall-related hip and wrist fracture risk.[39–41] One study estimated that ~50,000 excess falls per year in older adults could be attributable to vestibular loss.[10]

Quality of Life

Quality of life measures assess the general quality of life (e.g., the Medical Outcomes Study 36-Item Short Form Health Survey) as well as health-related quality of life (i.e., related to a specific health condition). Dizziness and vestibular vertigo have been associated with significantly poorer quality of life, in both the physical and mental domains. One population-based study in Sweden found that dizziness was one of the most influential symptoms affecting the general quality of life in older individuals.[42] The most widely used measures of dizziness- and imbalance-related quality of life are the Dizziness Handicap Inventory (DHI),[43] the Activities Balance Confidence scale,[44] and the Falls Efficacy scale (which measures fear of falling).[45] Two studies that administered the DHI in patients presenting with dizziness to a primary care clinic and a specialized dizziness clinic found that over 60% of patients reported moderate to severe handicap associated with their dizziness in both clinical contexts.[46,47]

Activities of Daily Living

One measure of the social and economic impact of dizziness, imbalance, and presbyvestibulopathy is the impact on the ability to carry out activities of daily living. Individuals who lose their ability to carry out certain activities of daily living rely more on others and society for daily functioning and in severe cases require placement in a nursing home. In 2008 the US National Health Interview Survey (NHIS) administered a Balance Supplement, and these data were analyzed across several studies to provide numerous insights into the health impacts and economic consequences of dizziness and imbalance in older individuals in the United States. One study considered the impact of dizziness and imbalance in older individuals on the ability to engage in daily activities. This study found that, of the elderly US population who reported dizziness or imbalance (~20% of individuals aged ≥65 years), 52% reported difficulty shopping, 47% reported difficulty driving, and 46% reported difficulty participating in social activities because of their symptoms.[24] Another study using data from NHANES evaluated the impact of vestibular dysfunction (based on the modified Romberg test) on the ability to carry out activities of daily living. Interestingly, when vestibular impairment was considered (rather than the symptoms of dizziness and imbalance), the particular activities that were most affected were managing money, using a fork and knife during eating, and getting in and out of bed.[48]

Healthcare Utilization

With respect to healthcare utilization and economic outcomes, the German population-based study found that vestibular vertigo was more likely than nonvestibular vertigo to be associated with a medical consultation, sick leave, interruption of daily activities, and avoidance of leaving the house.[49] Data from the 2008 NHIS demonstrated that 50% of older individuals with dizziness and balance problems saw at least one medical provider, typically a general practitioner (86% of individuals), a neurologist (24%), or an otolaryngologist (17%). Nearly 35% of older adults with dizziness and balance problems saw three or more providers.[50] About 57% of older individuals with these symptoms obtained an imaging study, and 15% were prescribed a medication, most commonly a diuretic, anxiolytic agent, or meclizine. The study pointed out that despite this high rate of healthcare utilization, >40% of older individuals still did not have a clear diagnosis for their dizziness or balance problem. A single provocative longitudinal study found that patients with disequilibrium at baseline were at a significantly increased risk only for incident cognitive decline compared with controls.[51]

Presbyvestibulopathy and Cognitive Decline

Emerging evidence suggests that vestibular loss associated with presbyvestibulopathy affects not only physical function (e.g., postural/gait abnormality, falls) but also elements of cognitive function. Studies have long documented a link between vestibular loss and cognitive impairment, for instance, memory impairment with perilymph fistulae, and concentration difficulties associated with gentamicin ototoxicity. In 2005 a landmark study reported significant reductions in spatial cognitive skills (spatial memory and spatial navigation) in patients with neurofibromatosis type 2 (NF-2) who had undergone bilateral vestibular schwannoma resection relative to age-matched controls. These patients were also found to have significant reductions in their hippocampal volumes. The hippocampus is known to play a critical role in generating the brain's cognitive map of space, and authors postulated that vestibular loss may have led to hippocampal atrophy and subsequent impairments in spatial cognition.

Cognitive function encompasses multiple domains, including language, attention, memory, executive function, and spatial skills. Evidence suggests that vestibular impairment is most strongly associated with reductions in spatial cognitive function, which follows from the vestibular system's role in sensing head movement and orientation in space. Recent studies have further evaluated the link between vestibular loss and cognition in older adults with presbyvestibulopathy, a far more common condition than NF-2. One study used data from the Baltimore Longitudinal Study of Aging, a cohort of healthy aging adults that has been followed up continuously since 1958. In this study, older adults with reduced vestibular function were found to have significantly poorer spatial cognitive skills relative to older adults with normal vestibular function, although there were no differences in language, memory, attention, or executive function abilities. Similar findings were made using data from NHANES and the NHIS, lending support to the idea that presbyvestibulopathy may increase the risk of spatial cognitive decline in older adults.

A further line of investigation has explored the relationship between vestibular impairment and cognitive decline among individuals with cognitive impairment and dementia, including Alzheimer disease (AD). It has previously been hypothesized that vestibular loss may contribute to the onset of AD, in part owing to the major cholinergic projections that emanate from the vestibular system to the hippocampus, and that are specifically degraded in AD.[52] Recent provocative evidence has shown that patients with AD have significantly poorer vestibular function relative to age-matched controls. AD is a heterogeneous condition, with some patients having greater memory deficits and others having greater spatial or motor deficits. Emerging data suggest that vestibular impairment may be particularly prevalent in patients with a spatial phenotype of AD. These links between presbyvestibulopathy, cognitive decline, and dementia and AD are an area of active, ongoing investigation, and the precise nature of these relationships remains to be further characterized. Patients with AD are twice as likely to fall relative to healthy older adults, and contribute disproportionately to the high rate of falls observed generally in older adults. One in three adults aged 85 years and older will develop AD and dementia, and given the aging population, AD ranks as one of the most significant public health concerns of our time. If vestibular impairment does contribute to the onset or manifestation of AD, this will be critical knowledge to gain.

Finally, dizziness has been associated with a nearly twofold increased risk of mortality relative to older adults without dizziness.[53] This same study, which used NHIS data that were linked to National Death Index data, found that the 5-year mortality rate among individuals with dizziness and imbalance was 9%, which was comparable with the mortality rates observed among individuals with cardiovascular disease (10.5%), cancer (11.6%), and diabetes mellitus (9.8%).

CONCLUSION

The epidemiologic data reviewed in this chapter suggest that dizziness, imbalance, and presbyvestibulopathy are highly prevalent in the population, especially the elderly, and have significant clinical, functional, and economic implications. Several final points deserve mention. First, the use of a common nomenclature to characterize dizziness, imbalance, and presbyvestibulopathy is critically important to advance clinical care and research in this field. Ongoing efforts to codify diagnostic criteria for presbyvestibulopathy are an important first step. Second, although dizziness and imbalance are prevalent in the geriatric population, they are not universal. As one study specifically points out, not all individuals over age 90 years have dizziness.[25] As such, dizziness and imbalance in the geriatric population may be considered "age-concomitant" rather than "age-dependent" conditions.[25] As a corollary, these conditions should be viewed as pathologic, and efforts should be made to treat them. Finally, it follows that the potential scope of managing dizziness and imbalance in the geriatric population is enormous, and these conditions will continue to be a major public health issue as the population ages. There are valuable resources on the Centers for Disease Control website (www.cdc.gov/homeandrecreationalsafety/falls/programs.html). Treatment strategies will be aimed at accurate diagnosis and management of vestibular pathology, vestibular rehabilitation, optimizing vision, and fall prevention.

REFERENCES

1. Sloane PD, Coeytaux RR, Beck RS, Dallara J. Dizziness: state of the science. *Ann Intern Med.* 2001;134(9 Pt 2):823–832.
2. Wetmore SJ, Eibling DE, Goebel JA, et al. Challenges and opportunities in managing the dizzy older adult. *Otolaryngol Head Neck Surg.* 2011;144(5):651–656.
3. Merchant SN, Velazquez-Villasenor L, Tsuji K, Glynn RJ, Wall 3rd C, Rauch SD. Temporal bone studies of the human peripheral vestibular system. Normative vestibular hair cell data. *Ann Otol Rhinol Laryngol Suppl.* 2000;181:3–13.
4. Rauch SD, Velazquez-Villasenor L, Dimitri PS, Merchant SN. Decreasing hair cell counts in aging humans. *Ann N Y Acad Sci.* 2001;942:220–227.
5. Walther L, Westhofen M. Presbyvertigo-aging of otoconia and vestibular sensory cells. *J Vestib Res.* 2007;17(2, 3):89–92.
6. Peterka RJ, Black FO, Schoenhoff MB. Age-related changes in human vestibulo-ocular reflexes: sinusoidal rotation and caloric tests. *J Vestib Res.* 1990;1(1):49–59.
7. Peterka RJ, Black FO, Schoenhoff MB. Age-related changes in human vestibulo-ocular and optokinetic reflexes: pseudorandom rotation tests. *J Vestib Res.* 1990;1(1):61–71.
8. Paige GD. Senescence of human visual-vestibular interactions. 1. Vestibulo-ocular reflex and adaptive plasticity with aging. *J Vestib Res.* 1992;2(2):133–151.
9. Serrador JM, Lipsitz LA, Gopalakrishnan GS, Black FO, Wood SJ. Loss of otolith function with age is associated with increased postural sway measures. *Neurosci Lett.* 2009;465(1):10–15.
10. Rey MCB, Clark TK, Wang W, Leeder T, Bian Y, Merfeld DM. Vestibular perceptual thresholds increase above the age of 40. *Front Neurol.* 2016;7.
11. Maes L, Dhooge I, D'haenens W, et al. The effect of age on the sinusoidal harmonic acceleration test, pseudorandom rotation test, velocity step test, caloric test, and vestibular-evoked myogenic potential test. *Ear Hear.* 2010;31(1):84–94.
12. Tian JR, Shubayev I, Baloh RW, Demer JL. Impairments in the initial horizontal vestibulo-ocular reflex of older humans. *Exp Brain Res.* 2001;137(3–4):309–322.
13. Roditi RE, Crane BT. Directional asymmetries and age effects in human self-motion perception. *J Assoc Res Otolaryngol.* 2012;13(3):381–401.
14. Mossman B, Mossman S, Purdie G, Schneider E. Age dependent normal horizontal VOR gain of head impulse test as measured with video-oculography. *J Otolaryngol Head Neck Surg.* 2015;44(1):29.
15. Li C, Layman AJ, Geary R, et al. Epidemiology of vestibulo-ocular reflex function: data from the Baltimore longitudinal study of aging. *Otol Neurotol.* 2015;36(2):267–272.
16. Matiño-Soler E, Esteller-More E, Martin-Sanchez J-C, Martinez-Sanchez J-M, Perez-Fernandez N. Normative data on angular vestibulo-ocular responses in the yaw axis measured using the video head impulse test. *Otol Neurotol.* 2015;36(3):466–471.
17. Serrador JM, Schlegel TT, Black FO, Wood SJ. Vestibular effects on cerebral blood flow. *BMC Neurosci.* 2009;10:119.
18. Bisdorff A, Von Brevern M, Lempert T, Newman-Toker DE. Classification of vestibular symptoms: towards an international classification of vestibular disorders. *J Vestib Res.* 2009;19(1, 2):1–13.
19. Agrawal Y, Carey JP, Della Santina CC, Schubert MC, Minor LB. Disorders of balance and vestibular function in US adults: data from the national health and nutrition examination survey, 2001–2004. *Arch Intern Med.* 2009;169(10):938–944.
20. Baloh RW, Ying SH, Jacobson KM. A longitudinal study of gait and balance dysfunction in normal older people. *Arch Neurol.* 2003;60(6):835–839.
21. Tinetti ME, Williams CS, Gill TM. Dizziness among older adults: a possible geriatric syndrome. *Ann Intern Med.* 2000;132(5):337–344.
22. Gopinath B, McMahon CM, Rochtchina E, Mitchell P. Dizziness and vertigo in an older population: the blue mountains prospective cross-sectional study. *Clin Otolaryngol.* 2009;34(6):552–556.
23. Stevens KN, Lang IA, Guralnik JM, Melzer D. Epidemiology of balance and dizziness in a national population: findings from the english longitudinal study of ageing. *Age Ageing.* 2008;37(3):300–305.
24. Lin HW, Bhattacharyya N. Balance disorders in the elderly: epidemiology and functional impact. *Laryngoscope.* 2012;122(8):1858–1861.
25. Ekwall A, Lindberg A, Magnusson M. Dizzy – why not take a walk? Low level physical activity improves quality of life among elderly with dizziness. *Gerontology.* 2009;55(6):652–659.
26. Tuunainen E, Poe D, Jantti P, et al. Presbyequilibrium in the oldest old, a combination of vestibular, oculomotor and postural deficits. *Aging Clin Exp Res.* 2011;23(5–6):364–371.
27. Kao AC, Nanda A, Williams CS, Tinetti ME. Validation of dizziness as a possible geriatric syndrome. *J Am Geriatr Soc.* 2001;49(1):72–75.
28. Creighton Jr FX, Poliashenko SM, Statham MM, Abramson P, Johns 3rd MM. The growing geriatric otolaryngology patient population: a study of 131,700 new patient encounters. *Laryngoscope.* 2013;123(1):97–102.
29. Neuhauser HK, von Brevern M, Radtke A, et al. Epidemiology of vestibular vertigo: a neurotologic survey of the general population. *Neurology.* 2005;65(6):898–904.
30. Ishiyama G. Imbalance and vertigo: the aging human vestibular periphery. *Semin Neurol.* 2009;29(5):491–499.
31. von Brevern M, Radtke A, Lezius F, et al. Epidemiology of benign paroxysmal positional vertigo: a population based study. *J Neurol Neurosurg Psychiatry.* 2007;78(7):710–715.

32. Katsarkas A. Dizziness in aging: a retrospective study of 1194 cases. *Otolaryngol Head Neck Surg*. 1994;110(3):296–301.

33. Oghalai JS, Manolidis S, Barth JL, Stewart MG, Jenkins HA. Unrecognized benign paroxysmal positional vertigo in elderly patients. *Otolaryngol Head Neck Surg*. 2000;122(5):630–634.

34. Blatt PJ, Georgakakis GA, Herdman SJ, Clendaniel RA, Tusa RJ. The effect of the canalith repositioning maneuver on resolving postural instability in patients with benign paroxysmal positional vertigo. *Am J Otol*. 2000;21(3): 356–363.

35. Neuhauser HK. Epidemiology of vertigo. *Curr Opin Neurol*. 2007;20(1):40–46.

36. Agrawal Y, Carey JP, Della Santina CC, Schubert MC, Minor LB. Diabetes, vestibular dysfunction, and falls: analyses from the national health and nutrition examination survey. *Otol Neurotol*. 2010;31(9):1445–1450.

37. Liston MB, Bamiou DE, Martin F, et al. Peripheral vestibular dysfunction is prevalent in older adults experiencing multiple non-syncopal falls versus age-matched non-fallers: a pilot study. *Age Ageing*. 2014;43(1):38–43.

38. Ekvall Hansson E, Magnusson M. Vestibular asymmetry predicts falls among elderly patients with multi-sensory dizziness. *BMC Geriatr*. 2013;13(1):77.

39. Kristinsdottir EK, Jarnlo GB, Magnusson M. Asymmetric vestibular function in the elderly might be a significant contributor to hip fractures. *Scand J Rehabil Med*. 2000;32(2):56–60.

40. Kristinsdottir EK, Nordell E, Jarnlo GB, Tjader A, Thorngren KG, Magnusson M. Observation of vestibular asymmetry in a majority of patients over 50 years with fall-related wrist fractures. *Acta Otolaryngol*. 2001;121(4):481–485.

41. Nordell E, Kristinsdottir EK, Jarnlo GB, Magnusson M, Thorngren KG. Older patients with distal forearm fracture. A challenge to future fall and fracture prevention. *Aging Clin Exp Res*. 2005;17(2):90–95.

42. Grimby A, Rosenhall U. Health-related quality of life and dizziness in old age. *Gerontology*. 1995;41(5):286–298.

43. Jacobson GP, Newman CW. The development of the dizziness handicap inventory. *Arch Otolaryngol Head Neck Surg*. 1990;116(4):424–427.

44. Powell LE, Myers AM. The activities-specific balance confidence (ABC) scale. *J Gerontol A Biol Sci Med Sci*. 1995;50A(1):M28–M34.

45. Tinetti ME, Richman D, Powell L. Falls efficacy as a measure of fear of falling. *J Gerontol*. 1990;45(6):P239–P243.

46. Dros J, Maarsingh OR, Beem L, et al. Impact of dizziness on everyday life in older primary care patients: a cross-sectional study. *Health Qual Life Outcomes*. 2011;9:44.

47. Ten Voorde M, van der Zaag-Loonen HJ, van Leeuwen RB. Dizziness impairs health-related quality of life. *Qual Life Res*. 2012;21(6):961–966.

48. Harun A, Semenov YR, Agrawal Y. Vestibular function and activities of daily living: analysis of the 1999 to 2004 national health and nutrition examination surveys. *Gerontol Geriatr Med*. 2015;1. http://dx.doi.org/10.1177/2333721415607124.

49. Neuhauser HK, Radtke A, von Brevern M, Lezius F, Feldmann M, Lempert T. Burden of dizziness and vertigo in the community. *Arch Intern Med*. 2008;168(19): 2118–2124.

50. Roberts DS, Lin HW, Bhattacharyya N. Health care practice patterns for balance disorders in the elderly. *Laryngoscope*. 2013;123(10):2539–2543.

51. Kerber KA, Enrietto JA, Jacobson KM, Baloh RW. Disequilibrium in older people: a prospective study. *Neurology*. 1998;51(2):574–580.

52. Previc FH. Vestibular loss as a contributor to Alzheimer's disease. *Med Hypotheses*. 2013;80(4):360–367.

53. Corrales CE, Bhattacharyya N. Dizziness and death: an imbalance in mortality. *Laryngoscope*. 2016;126(9):2134–2136.

CHAPTER 2

Technological Advances in Testing the Dizzy Patient: The Bedside Examination Is Still the Key to Successful Diagnosis

TZU-PU CHANG, MD • DAVID S. ZEE, MD • AMIR KHERADMAND, MD

INTRODUCTION

Dizziness is a common complaint across many clinical settings and often an intimidating challenge for physicians to diagnose despite modern advances in medical technology and imaging. Lack of a systematic approach to examination of the vestibular system is often to blame for unnecessary tests and incorrect diagnoses. However, an understanding of basic vestibular and ocular motor physiology, when applied with targeted history taking and proper examination techniques, can usually steer clinicians to the correct diagnosis at the bedside. This is particularly important when evaluating patients with acute vestibular symptoms because the pressing question in such cases is whether the underlying cause is anatomically "peripheral" (affecting the labyrinth or the vestibular nerve) or "central" (affecting the vestibular projections or brain networks involved in ocular motor function, postural control, or perception of spatial orientation). Such a diagnostic challenge translates to whether the patient has a relatively benign, usually self-limited condition or a serious and potentially life-threatening injury. The suspicion of a central lesion should initiate emergency procedures including evaluation and treatment for stroke (see Chapter 16). On the other hand, peripheral vertigo is not life threatening, even though it can be severely disabling. Usually in patients with peripheral vestibular disorders, timely rehabilitation and proper therapeutic maneuvers enhance recovery and assure an optimal clinical outcome.

In this chapter we first outline physiologic principles underlying the evaluation of the vestibular system and then review the key elements of examination in the context of recent technical advances in video-oculography (VOG) and mobile devices, such as tablet computers and smartphones. Using these portable technologies, the vestibular examination can now be quantified at the bedside to improve diagnostic accuracy and clinical management. In this process, a careful and thorough evaluation of eye movements is critical for diagnosis because of the close anatomic and physiologic connections between the vestibular and ocular motor systems. Clinical or "bedside" vestibular and ocular motor evaluations must always be put into the context of a thorough history and general neurologic examination, and when needed, other neurootologic laboratory testing, including formal tests of hearing and vestibular and balance function.

PHYSIOLOGIC PRINCIPLES FOR VESTIBULAR EXAMINATION

In normal individuals, when the head is still, both vestibular nerves and the vestibular nuclei on either side of the brainstem have equal resting discharge and thus there is no perception of head motion or need for any vestibulo-ocular compensation. Movement of the head toward one side excites the labyrinth on that side and inhibits the labyrinth on the other side, e.g., right head rotation stimulates the right lateral semicircular canal and inhibits the left. Such a change in the balance of activity between the vestibular nuclei leads to the perception of head motion and also activates the vestibulo-ocular reflex (VOR) in the opposite direction of the head movement so that the eyes can maintain fixation on the intended visual target. The slow-phase eye movements during the VOR compensate for horizontal (yaw), vertical (pitch), or torsional (roll) head rotations. Normally, the VOR matches the direction and speed of the head movement during yaw and pitch rotations. In contrast, during rotation around the roll axis, the VOR is less than compensatory, but this apparently is of less functional importance for central vision because images still remain on or close to the fovea.

A knowledge of the geometric arrangement of the semicircular canals aids accurate interpretation of VOR function. The lateral (horizontal) canal lies orthogonal to the sagittal plane and makes a 30-degree angle with the true horizontal plane. The anterior (superior) and posterior canals are oriented roughly vertically, almost orthogonal to each other, and each makes a roughly 45-degree angle with the sagittal plane. During rotation around the roll axis, eye movements are aligned with head movements, but the gain (eye movement/head movement) is lower (dynamic roll VOR gain is roughly 50%).

Following a unilateral vestibular injury, the balance in the levels of tonic activity between the vestibular nuclei must be restored to eliminate spontaneous nystagmus and postural imbalance, a process that may take days to complete. With a complete unilateral peripheral vestibular loss, the nystagmus is unidirectional, with the fast component beating away from the side of the lesion irrespective of the gaze position. There is often a torsional component with the top pole of the eyes beating away from the side of the lesion. With partial lesions the patterns of nystagmus vary depending on how vestibular inputs from the semicircular canals are affected, but a pure vertical or a pure torsional spontaneous nystagmus usually points to a central lesion (Table 2.1). If nystagmus is peripheral in origin, the horizontal component is more intense when the gaze is pointed in the direction of the fast phase; i.e., opposite, or away from the side of the lesion (Alexander's law; Fig. 2.1). With central lesions in the cerebellum or brainstem, the nystagmus does not always follow Alexander's law and can be more intense when looking in the direction of the slow phase. In patients with central disorders, there may be a superimposed component of nystagmus related to impaired eccentric gaze holding in which there is right-beating nystagmus upon right gaze and left-beating nystagmus upon left gaze.

Patients with loss of vestibular function, especially in cases with bilateral loss, often have difficulty with tasks during head movements, for example, reading street signs while driving or reading labels on items while walking down the aisles in the grocery store. Such a "dynamic" vestibular imbalance can be brought out during the bedside examination, especially in response to high-acceleration or high-frequency stimuli such as head impulses. These stimuli normally rely mostly on excitation rather than inhibition of the labyrinths. Therefore, in patients with a unilateral loss the abnormality is most apparent when the head is rotated toward the side of the

TABLE 2.1
Pattern of Nystagmus in Peripheral Vestibular Lesion Based on Affected Semicircular Canals (SCCs)

Peripheral Vestibular Lesion	Nystagmus/Direction
Horizontal SCC	Horizontal/beating away from the side of the lesion
Anterior SCC	Upbeat and torsional/top pole beating away from the side of the lesion
Posterior SCC	Downbeat and torsional/top pole beating away from the side of the lesion
Anterior + Horizontal SCCs	Horizontal, upbeat, and torsional/all beating away from the side of the lesion
Posterior + Horizontal SCCs	Horizontal, downbeat, and torsional/all beating away from the side of the lesion
Anterior + Horizontal + Posterior SCCs	Horizontal and torsional/both beating away from the side of the lesion

impaired labyrinth. Head shaking and vibration over the skull are other maneuvers that can bring out a vestibular deficit, which manifests as a nystagmus with a slow phase toward the side of the vestibular deficit. These provocative stimuli are especially important when examining patients with chronic unilateral vestibular loss in whom naturally occurring central repair mechanisms have already compensated for the static vestibular tone asymmetry and eliminated the spontaneous nystagmus. In such cases, if the level of activity from the paretic side is suddenly restored after central adaptation has taken place, an excessive vestibular tone may arise on the paretic side and result in a new imbalance in the levels of tonic activity between the vestibular nuclei. This new imbalance can lead to "recovery" nystagmus in which slow phases are directed *toward* the intact ear.

The central vestibular system within the brainstem and cerebellum also has an important role in improving low-frequency sustained responses of the VOR, for example, during prolonged, constant-velocity head movements. This mechanism is called "velocity storage," important for understanding the pathophysiology of head shaking–induced nystagmus and the changes in the time constant of vestibular responses, as reflected in the duration of the VOR response to a constant-velocity rotation.[1]

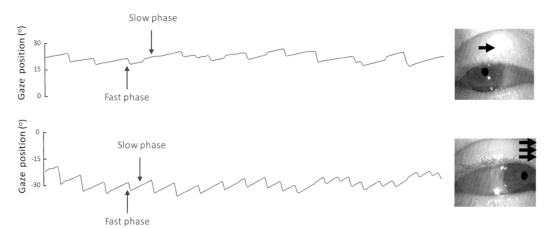

FIG. 2.1 Alexander's law from a bedside video-oculography recording in a patient with right-sided vestibular loss and "peripheral" nystagmus. Horizontal traces show left-beating nystagmus that is weaker in the right gaze (positive gaze positions) and stronger in the left gaze (negative gaze positions). Above the image of the eye, the *black arrows* show the direction of the fast phase of the nystagmus and the number of *arrows* represents the intensity of the nystagmus (slow phase velocity).

Just as a tone imbalance in the semicircular canals causes spontaneous nystagmus, imbalance in the otolith and especially utricular pathways can induce the ocular tilt reaction (OTR). The OTR consists of a lateral head tilt (ear to shoulder), vertical misalignment of the eyes (skew deviation with the eye on the side of the higher ear being relatively higher in its orbit than the eye on the side of the lower ear), and a torsional deviation of both eyes with the top poles rotating toward the side of the lower eye (ocular counter-roll or OCR). There is often an associated perceptual tilt of the visual world toward the side of the lower ear. As mentioned, the OTR reflects a vestibular tone imbalance from the otolith organs analogous to the spontaneous nystagmus that occurs with a tone imbalance from the semicircular canals.

VESTIBULAR EXAMINATION IN ACUTE-ONSET DIZZINESS, VERTIGO, AND IMBALANCE

Patients with acute vertigo often have nausea or vomiting, unstable gait, nystagmus, and are intolerant of head motion. With such a clinical presentation, called the *acute vestibular syndrome*, the vital question at the bedside is to correctly distinguish benign, usually peripheral dizziness (e.g., vestibular neuritis) from more serious and potentially life-threatening "central" dizziness (e.g., brain infarction).[2] Overall, approximately 25% of patients presenting to the emergency department with acute vestibular syndrome are found to have posterior circulation strokes.[3] Traditionally, clinicians rely on

the general, non-ocular-motor neurologic examination to distinguish central and peripheral causes of vertigo. However, only a small fraction of stroke patients presenting with dizziness present with such focal neurologic signs (roughly 19% of patients with stroke, excluding those with truncal ataxia).[4] Examination of the VOR and evaluation of eye movements, posture, and balance are the most sensitive and accurate approach to the correct diagnosis in patients with acute-onset vertigo.[5,6] In the following section we review the key parts of the bedside examination that can distinguish between peripheral and central lesions and help diagnose the cause of dizziness in these patients.

Vestibulo-ocular Examination
Head impulse test, evaluation of nystagmus, and test of skew deviation

A battery of ocular motor examinations including <u>H</u>ead <u>I</u>mpulse test, evaluation of <u>N</u>ystagmus, and <u>T</u>est of <u>S</u>kew deviation (HINTS) helps distinguish between peripheral and central causes in patients with the acute vestibular syndrome.[4] HINTS is highly sensitive in detecting central lesions (sensitivity, 96.8%; specificity, 98.5%)[4] with a diagnostic accuracy higher than that of the diffusion brain MRI within the first 48 hours from the onset of symptoms.[7] The components of the HINTS examination—nystagmus, head impulse test, and skew deviation—are discussed in more detail later in this chapter. Using this bedside battery, one should suspect **central** lesions in patients with an *intact* head impulse test (indicating normal peripheral vestibular function), *direction-changing nystagmus* (i.e., right beating on right gaze and left beating on left gaze), or *skew deviation* of the eyes. On the other hand, the combination of abnormal head impulse test, direction-fixed, primarily horizontal nystagmus (obeying Alexander's law) and absence of skew deviation usually suggests a peripheral vestibular lesion (Table 2.3).

Peripheral versus central nystagmus (Table 2.2)
In patients with acute vestibular syndrome, spontaneous nystagmus is often observed at the bedside. As mentioned earlier, nystagmus caused by a peripheral

vestibular lesion is mainly horizontal and often mixed with a torsional component. The slow phase of the nystagmus is directed toward the side of the lesion (i.e., the side of vestibular weakness), and the fast phase is away from the side of the lesion. This peripheral nystagmus does not change direction; however, the intensity of nystagmus increases at gaze positions in the direction of the fast phase, away from the side of the lesion (i.e., the nystagmus conforms to Alexander's law) (Fig. 2.1).[8] In addition, peripheral nystagmus is often weakened or suppressed by visual fixation and is enhanced or brought out by removing visual fixation using Frenzel goggles, VOG, occlusive ophthalmoscopy, or simply by looking at the movement of the corneal bulge under the closed eyes. Visual suppression of the torsional component of nystagmus is relatively poor compared with that of the horizontal or vertical component in humans. Thus the true direction of the nystagmus is best evaluated in the absence of visual fixation.

Central lesions, too, may lead to horizontal, vertical, or torsional nystagmus. Spontaneous pure vertical or pure torsional nystagmus is often associated with central lesions, but it is not a sensitive sign because only about 9% of patients with central lesions present with pure vertical or torsional nystagmus.[4] Peripheral nystagmus is usually suppressed by visual fixation. This finding is not highly specific for peripheral lesions, as visual fixation may still weaken or suppress nystagmus in patients with small cerebellar or brainstem infarcts.[9-11]

TABLE 2.2
Key Features of Peripheral Vestibular Nystagmus Versus Central Nystagmus

Peripheral Vestibular Nystagmus	Central Nystagmus
Mixed, horizontal torsional beating away from the lesion	Mixed, pure torsional, or pure vertical
Increase with gaze toward the fast phase (Alexander's law)	May increase with gaze away from the fast phase (anti-Alexander's law)
Strongly suppressed by visual fixation	May be suppressed by visual fixation
Does not change direction with change in gaze position	May change direction (e.g., gaze-evoked or rebound nystagmus)

TABLE 2.3
HINTS Findings in Acute Peripheral Vestibular and Central Lesions

Lesion Site	Spontaneous Nystagmus	Direction-Changing Nystagmus	Head Impulse Test	Ocular Tilt Reaction
Labyrinth or vestibular nerve	Contralesional	None	Positive HIT, ipsilesional	Ipsiversive (skew is rare)
Vestibular nucleus[14]	Contralesional	contra > ipsi	Positive HIT, ipsilesional	Ipsiversive
Nucleus prepositus hypoglossi[14]	Ipsilesional	ipsi > contra	Positive HIT, contralesional	Ipsiversive
Inferior cerebellar peduncle[30]	Ipsilesional	None	Negative HIT	Contraversive
Flocculus[10,11a]	Ipsilesional	ipsi > contra (weak)	Positive HIT, contralesional	Contraversive
Tonsil[11]	Ipsilesional (weak)	ipsi > contra	Negative HIT	Contraversive
Nodulus[31]	Ipsilesional	None	Negative HIT	Contraversive

Contra, contralesional; *HINTS*, head impulse test, evaluation of nystagmus, and test of skew deviation; *HIT*, head impulse test; *Ipsi*, ipsilesional; *OTR*, ocular tilt reaction.

The effect of gaze position on nystagmus can help distinguish between central and peripheral causes. This can be simply evaluated by having the patient change the position of their eyes in the orbit to the far gaze positions. Nystagmus from peripheral causes is usually unidirectional (i.e., right or left beating) and conforms to Alexander's law. Nystagmus from central causes, on the other hand, may not remain unidirectional or may not conform to Alexander's law and thus can become more intense at gaze positions in the **opposite** direction of the fast phase. Patients with central lesions also often have nystagmus that changes direction with gaze position. This "gaze-evoked" nystagmus beats in the same direction as the eccentric position of the eyes in the orbit (e.g., right beating in right gaze and left beating in left gaze) (Fig. 2.2). Such "direction-changing" nystagmus, primarily caused by lesions involving the gaze-holding networks within the brainstem or cerebellum, is an important sign of central lesions in the acute vestibular syndrome (sensitivity of approximately 21% and specificity of 100%).[4] Note that low-velocity spontaneous nystagmus from peripheral vestibular lesions might appear only at gaze positions in the direction of the fast phase because of Alexander's law. This unidirectional peripheral nystagmus should not be confused as direction-changing central nystagmus.

In addition, in some patients with central lesions, the velocity of direction-changing nystagmus may differ considerably depending on the gaze position.[12,13] Such nystagmus has been reported in cerebellopontine angle tumors (affecting both the cerebellum and the vestibular nerve) as well as in acute cerebellar and brainstem strokes with a combined peripheral vestibular and central involvement.[11,14] This type of nystagmus, known as Bruns nystagmus, reflects the combination of a vestibular imbalance and a disturbed gaze-holding network. Bruns nystagmus is of low frequency and large amplitude in gaze positions toward the side of the lesion and is of high frequency and small amplitude in gaze positions away from the side of the lesion.[15,16]

Sometimes patients with gaze-evoked nystagmus on eccentric gaze may have transient nystagmus when the eyes return to the straight-ahead (i.e., central) position. This "rebound" nystagmus has a fast phase beating opposite to the previous gaze direction.[17] Rebound nystagmus is often encountered in patients with cerebellar or brainstem dysfunction and is likely related to a bias caused by adaptive mechanisms counteracting the centripetal drift during the gaze-evoked nystagmus.[18-20] Transient physiologic nystagmus may occur at extreme eccentric gaze positions in normal individuals. This physiologic, end-gaze nystagmus is different from the pathologic, gaze-evoked nystagmus, which usually is sustained and triggered at relatively modest eccentric gaze positions (e.g., 25 degrees away from the central position), and in addition may be followed by rebound nystagmus when the eyes return to the central position. Strong downbeat nystagmus in the straight ahead position or even only on lateral gaze is also pathologic and implies a central origin, especially with lesions involving the vestibulocerebellar pathways. Combined downbeat and horizontal gaze-evoked nystagmus is known as "side-pocket nystagmus."[21]

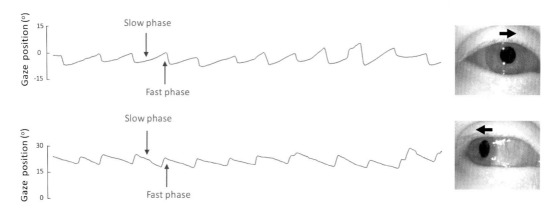

FIG. 2.2 Direction-changing nystagmus from a bedside video-oculography recording in a patient with a pontine infarct. Horizontal traces show left-beating nystagmus in the straight-ahead position. The nystagmus becomes right beating in right gaze. The *black arrows* above the eye show the direction of the fast phase of the nystagmus.

Head impulse test

The bedside head impulse maneuver can detect peripheral vestibular loss involving the function of the semicircular canals and the cranial nerve VIII.[22] The patient is instructed to look at a visual target, and the examiner quickly turns the head with brief, high-acceleration rotations of approximately 10 degrees excursion (peak velocity of at least 150 degrees/second). Head rotation normally generates an imbalance in the resting vestibular tone by affecting the level of activity from the semicircular canals, which depends on the direction and velocity of head rotation. At high velocities, the vestibular input from the side opposite to the direction of rotation is fully inhibited and the VOR depends primarily upon excitatory inputs from the labyrinth on the side of rotation. Accordingly, a vestibular loss on the side of rotation results in a VOR that does not match the high-velocity head movement and thus a corrective "catch-up" or "refixation" saccade must be triggered during or after head rotation to keep the eyes on the visual target. Usually patients with central lesions that spare vestibular pathways have a normal head impulse response.[23,24] On the other hand, an abnormal head impulse response can be seen with lesions involving the vestibular nucleus, nucleus prepositus hypoglossi, CN VIII fascicles in the brainstem, cerebellar flocculus, or the vascular territory of the anterior inferior cerebellar artery (AICA) that includes both labyrinth and vestibulocerebellum.[10,14,24,25] Therefore, although seemingly counterintuitive, a **normal** head impulse test points to a central lesion in patients with the acute vestibular syndrome (sensitivity of 93% and specificity of 100%).[4]

Head impulses are performed horizontally with right and left rapid head rotations to examine the function of the lateral semicircular canals. For examination of the vertical canals, head impulses are performed in the coplanar canal orientations: right anterior/left posterior and left anterior/right posterior planes. In some patients after recovery from vestibular loss, preprogrammed "covert" saccades are generated during head impulses that compensate for the defective VOR. Covert saccades are difficult to detect with the naked eye, and VOR function may seem intact in these patients.[26] These covert saccades may be converted to more easily seen, "overt" saccades (that occur *after* the head movement is completed) by making the direction and amplitude of the head movement unpredictable during the head impulse testing.[27]

Test of skew deviation

Skew deviation is a sign of static imbalance in the otolith-ocular inputs with a vertical misalignment of eyes that is relatively "concomitant," i.e., the degree of misalignment changes little with gaze position. Skew deviation can usually be detected using the alternate cover test while the patient is looking at a visual target.[1] During this test, the examiner covers the eyes alternately while looking for the corrective vertical eye movement in the uncovered eye. The corrective movement of the uncovered eye indicates that it was not visualizing the target and hence there is an underlying vertical misalignment. Skew is more common in central lesions involving the otolith-ocular pathways and overall is more enduring and larger compared with skew caused by peripheral vestibular lesions.[4,28] Thus skew deviation is a valuable sign to detect central lesions in the acute vestibular syndrome (sensitivity of 25% and specificity of 96%).[4] Skew can also help localize central lesions in combination with other neurologic or ocular motor findings. Because fibers of the otolith-ocular pathways cross at the mid-pons, skew often presents with the lower eye on the side of the lesion in caudal pontomedullary lesions and with the higher eye on the side of the lesion in rostral pontomesencephalic lesions.[29]

HINTS plus hearing loss

Hearing loss is often thought to point to a peripheral labyrinthine lesion in patients with acute vestibular syndrome. However, new-onset hearing loss with vertigo should always raise suspicion for central lesions and specifically infarcts within the AICA distribution that supplies the cerebellum and brainstem as well as the labyrinth.[32,33] Accordingly, HINTS plus acute hearing loss has a better sensitivity for detecting a central etiology in patients with acute vestibular syndrome (96.5% HINTS vs. 99.1% HINTS plus).[4]

Vestibulo-ocular Examination and Video-oculography

With the advent of the new-generation, light-weight VOG goggles, examination of the vestibular system can be easily quantified and analyzed at the bedside. Using this technology, the video head impulse test (vHIT) can provide quantitative assessments of VOR function for individual horizontal and vertical semicircular canal planes (see Chapter 8).[33a,34,35] The head sensor on the VOG goggles can measure head velocity, and the video cameras on the goggles can track eye movement by detecting the pupil or iris pattern. The eye and head recordings can then be used to measure VOR gain,

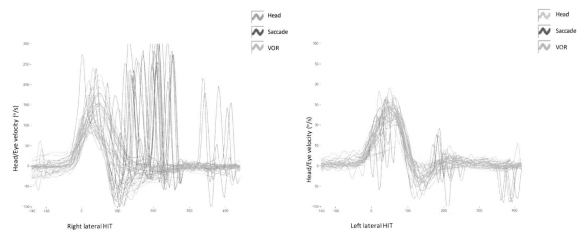

FIG. 2.3 Video head impulse test in a patient with a right-sided peripheral vestibular loss. The superimposed velocity traces of head and eye movements are shown for lateral head impulses (vestibulo-ocular reflex [VOR] traces are in green, head traces to the right are in orange, head traces to the left are in blue, and saccade traces are in red). With head impulses to the right side there are delayed, catch-up saccades (red), and the VOR gain (eye velocity/head velocity) is reduced to 0.4 compared with the normal gain of 0.87 on the left side.

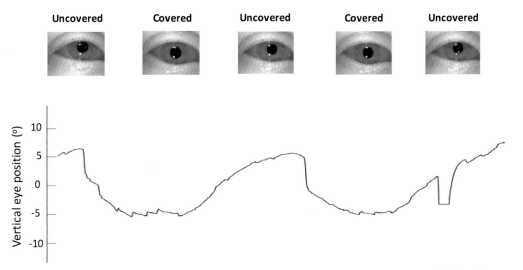

FIG. 2.4 Skew deviation from a bedside video-oculography recording in a patient with right-sided pontine infarct. The eye position trace shows the vertical movement of the right eye during the alternate cover test. When the right eye is covered, it goes down as the left eye is taking up the visual fixation. When the right eye is uncovered (and the left eye is covered), the right eye goes back up during refixation on the visual target.

although one must always be aware of artifacts induced by slippage of the goggles, or when the recordings are unreliable because a sick patient cannot cooperate with the examination. Because the eye and head movements are recorded simultaneously, vHIT traces can detect covert saccades during head impulses, which may be hard to see with the naked eye (Fig. 2.3).[36] VOG can also be used to quantify spontaneous nystagmus or positional nystagmus and the ocular motor components of the OTR, such as skew deviation (Fig. 2.4). Such a quantitative VOG examination makes a "telemedicine" approach possible, enabling remote consultation for dizzy patients seen in outpatient settings (e.g., HINTS examination using VOG).[37,38]

Balance and Gait Evaluation

Evaluation of balance is an essential part of the vestibular examination. Patients with acute-onset vertigo, however, are highly sensitive to motion and often cannot tolerate standing or walking. The severity of vertigo affects postural control and can cause imbalance irrespective of the cause of dizziness. Thus in patients with acute vestibular syndrome it is often not possible to perform a thorough balance evaluation. Nevertheless, simple tests such as sitting or standing up can still be useful to screen for severe truncal ataxia. Patients with peripheral vestibular loss can still rely on their visual and somatosensory inputs to stand and walk with slight assistance despite ongoing vestibular symptoms. If they cannot do so, one must suspect a central etiology.[5,39]

VESTIBULAR EXAMINATIONS IN CHRONIC DIZZINESS

Static Vestibular Evaluation

Spontaneous nystagmus from unilateral peripheral vestibular loss weakens over time and may not be observed at the bedside, as the central vestibular tone is rebalanced between the vestibular nuclei in the process of recovery. However, if this central rebalancing is incomplete, an underlying peripheral vestibular imbalance can often be brought out by removing visual fixation or using provoking maneuvers that can unmask the persisting asymmetry in the peripheral vestibular inputs. Frenzel goggles are used traditionally for removing visual fixation during vestibular examination. The goggles are fitted with magnifying lenses (+20 diopters) and internal lighting to illuminate the patient's eyes so the examiner can see any spontaneous nystagmus when the patient has no visual fixation. Frenzel goggles are best applied in an otherwise dark room. VOG goggles equipped with infrared cameras are also useful for bedside vestibular examination. They allow magnified viewing of the eyes on a television or computer screen while visual fixation is removed with a cover occluder. In addition, the ocular motor findings can be viewed and recorded at the bedside. Another method for removing visual fixation is with an ophthalmoscope, as subtle nystagmus can be detected by looking at the fundus. Here the examiner can remove visual fixation by covering the other eye and asking the patient to keep the eyes straight ahead while the examiner looks at the fundus (i.e., occlusive ophthalmoscopy). The optic disk is then observed for abnormal movements. During ophthalmoscopy the direction of horizontal and vertical movements of the fundus are **opposite** to the direction of the globe, as the optic disc is behind the axis around which the eye

is rotating. Also, magnifying cardboard goggles that are now widely available for virtual reality applications can be used for removing visual fixation and simultaneously recording eye movements via smartphones. Another less expensive method is to use a magnifying glass or a plastic sheet magnifier to remove visual fixation and examine one eye while covering the other eye.[40] A penlight-cover test can also be used during which visual fixation is removed by shining a "blinding" penlight in one eye while the other eye is covered.[41]

Provoking Maneuvers
Head shaking

In patients with unilateral vestibular loss, an asymmetry in vestibular inputs during high-velocity head rotations leads to an asymmetric accumulation of activity in the central velocity-storage mechanism within the vestibular nuclei. As a result, a vigorous nystagmus appears immediately following head shaking with slow phases directed toward the affected side, which sometimes is followed by a less intense reversal phase with slow phases directed toward the intact side. This reversal phase reflects the effect of short-term central adaptation mechanisms.[42,43] In patients with Ménière's disease, however, the direction of head shaking–induced nystagmus does not have a localizing value as the nystagmus can be related to increase or decrease of vestibular function or central vestibular adaptation related to recovery. The head shaking test is also performed with removing visual fixation. The head is rotated repeatedly within the patient's comfortable range of motion at a frequency of 3 cycles/second for approximately 15 seconds.

The head shaking–induced nystagmus may also occur in central disorders.[44] For example, vertical nystagmus after horizontal head shaking, known as "perverted" or "cross-coupled" nystagmus, indicates a central disorder.[44–46] Head shaking–induced nystagmus from central causes is usually due to lesions involving the vestibulocerebellum (i.e., within the flocculus/paraflocculus, nodulus, or ventral uvula), vestibular nuclear complex, or its connections within the brainstem involved in the velocity-storage mechanism.[47] Head shaking–induced nystagmus may also occur in the lateral medullary (Wallenberg) syndrome, beating in the opposite direction of the spontaneous nystagmus.[48] These findings are related to unilateral loss of cerebellar inhibition over the velocity-storage mechanism within the vestibular nucleus. Head shaking–induced nystagmus is usually suppressed by pitching the head forward in peripheral vestibular lesions but not in patients with central vestibular lesions.[49]

With vertical head shaking, vertical nystagmus is rarely seen, as the velocity storage for the vertical VOR is weaker than for the horizontal VOR.[50] However, because the orientation of the posterior semicircular canal is tilted toward the horizontal plane, activation of the posterior canals also contributes to the horizontal VOR. Thus an asymmetric contribution to the velocity-storage mechanism during vertical head shaking may produce a horizontal nystagmus. Vertical semicircular canal function can also be examined with circular head shaking, i.e., circular rotation of the head in a clockwise or counterclockwise direction.[51] With circular head shaking, the anterior and posterior canals are stimulated together, which results in torsional nystagmus. The absence of nystagmus after circular head shaking implies loss of function in the vertical semicircular canals.

Skull vibration

The vibration test is performed with removing visual fixation while a small handheld muscle massager is applied over each of the mastoid bones and then the vertex. Vibration (e.g., 60–100 Hz) over the mastoid bones can induce robust nystagmus in patients with an underlying vestibular imbalance. In normal individuals, however, there is often either no nystagmus or provoked nystagmus beating to the side of the vibration (i.e., right beating with vibration over the right mastoid and left beating with vibration over the left mastoid).[1] With unilateral peripheral vestibular loss, the vibration-induced nystagmus beats away from the side of the lesion irrespective of the side of vibration on the skull (i.e., slow phase toward the side of the lesion). In these patients, nystagmus is provoked in at least two of the three vibration sites (i.e., mastoids and the vertex) and the slow-phase velocity correlates with the unilateral canal weakness in the caloric test.[52,53] Spontaneous nystagmus from peripheral vestibular loss is often intensified with skull vibration. On the other hand, vibration-induced nystagmus beating in the opposite direction of spontaneous nystagmus has been reported with lateral medullary infarction.[54] When vertical nystagmus is triggered by vibration over the skull, a central lesion should be suspected, for example, in patients with Wernicke disease.[1] Unlike head shaking, vibration-induced nystagmus is not mediated through the velocity-storage mechanism because it ceases as soon as the vibration ends.

Hyperventilation

The hyperventilation test is also performed with removing visual fixation while the patient repetitively breathes deeply through the mouth for about 40 seconds. With peripheral vestibular injuries such as vestibular schwannoma or neurovascular compression, the alkalosis and consequent changes in calcium currents can improve conduction on demyelinated nerves, resulting in a transient increase of neural activity on the side of the lesion. This new imbalance provokes nystagmus with the slow phase directed toward the intact ear.[55,56] In patients with vestibular neuritis, however, such nystagmus can be contralesional or ipsilesional depending on when the patient is tested in the course of recovery (see recovery nystagmus discussed earlier in the section on the physiologic principles).[57,58] In the chronic stage, the slow phase of the nystagmus is often directed toward the side of the vestibular loss. Hyperventilation can also enhance or induce downbeat nystagmus in cerebellar disorders, craniocervical junction anomalies, or in patients with perilymph fistula.[59-61] Also, in superior canal dehiscence, hyperventilation can excite the dehiscent superior canal and provoke downbeating, torsional nysgamus.[61]

Dynamic Vestibular Evaluation

Dynamic visual acuity

Patients with vestibular loss often have oscillopsia that is brought on or exacerbated by head movement. Dynamic visual acuity can be used to evaluate such visual symptoms. First, visual acuity is measured with the head motionless in the upright position. The head is then rotated repeatedly at a high frequency (2 cycles/second) in the horizontal or vertical plane while the patient reads a visual acuity chart. Dynamic visual acuity is abnormal if there is a loss of more than two lines on the visual acuity chart compared with the measurement with the head stationary. In patients with bilateral vestibular loss, there is often a loss of more than four lines. Dynamic visual acuity can also be used to assess VOR recovery and track the effect of vestibular rehabilitation.[62-64]

Slow and fast head rotations

In addition to the head impulse test, VOR can be evaluated with slow head rotations. During slow head rotations, both low-frequency VOR and smooth pursuit maintain the eyes on a visual target. Therefore, catch-up saccades during slow head rotation are the sign of peripheral vestibular loss combined with central ocular motor dysfunction; for example, in patients with spinocerebellar ataxia type 3 (SCA-3), or patients with cerebellar ataxia, neuropathy, and vestibular areflexia syndrome (CANVAS).[65-67] The VOR can also be examined during ophthalmoscopy while the patient

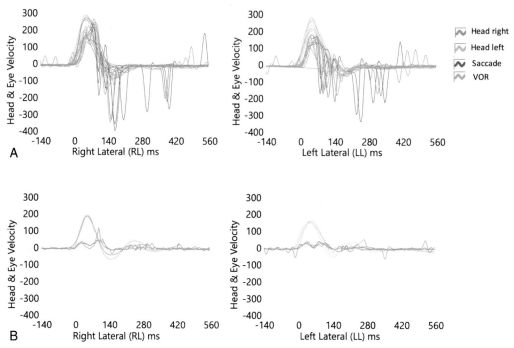

FIG. 2.5 During "suppression" head impulse paradigm (SHIMP), a normal individual **(A)** has to make catch-up saccades to regain visual fixation on the target after the head rotation, as the intact vestibulo-ocular reflex (VOR) drives the eyes off the head-mounted target during the fast rotation. A patient with vestibular loss **(B)**, on the other hand, does not show corrective saccades, as the eyes do not move during the head rotation because of the defective VOR.

is looking at a distant target using the other eye. The examiner gently shakes the head horizontally or vertically (2 cycles/second) while looking at the optic disc. With normal vestibular function the optic disc remains steady, but in patients with vestibular loss it oscillates during the head shaking.

Another useful test of VOR function at the bedside is the modified "suppression" head impulse paradigm (SHIMP; Fig. 2.5).[68] Here, the examiner quickly turns the head while the patient is looking at a head-mounted target (i.e., the visual target moves with the head as opposed to a stationary target fixed with respect to the patient during the head impulse test). Patients with vestibular loss are able to maintain visual fixation on the head-mounted target without corrective saccades, as the eyes do not move in the opposite direction of the head rotation due to the defective VOR. Healthy individuals, however, have to make catch-up saccades to regain the target after the head turn, as the intact VOR drives the eyes off the head-mounted target during the fast head rotation. Thus, in contrast to vHIT in which the compensatory saccades indicate vestibular loss, the catch-up "anticompensatory" saccade in the

direction of the head movement is the sign of a normal VOR during SHIMP. In addition, unlike HIT, corrective saccades in SHIMP usually appear after the end of the head movement (i.e., no covert saccades). Therefore, when covert saccades contaminate VOR traces during HIT, SHIMP can be used to eliminate them and allow accurate measurement of the gain of the slow phases of the VOR. Likewise, SHIMP can be used to measure VOR gain in patients with spontaneous nystagmus. In these patients, with head rotation toward the side of the vestibular loss, the fast phase of the spontaneous nystagmus is in the opposite direction of the corrective saccades during SHIMP. In contrast, during HIT the fast phase of nystagmus and corrective saccades occur in the same direction and are difficult to distinguish. Therefore, SHIMP can be used to overcome measurement error of VOR gain resulting from covert saccades and spontaneous nystagmus.

Evaluation of Otolith Function
Ocular tilt reaction (OTR)
Patients with otolith imbalance show an OTR with skew deviation (vertical misalignment of the eyes not

TABLE 2.4
Components of Ocular Tilt Reaction and Their Localizations Within the Otolith-Ocular Pathways

	LOCALIZATION	
Ocular Tilt Reaction	**Peripheral Vestibular and Caudal Brainstem**	**Rostral Brainstem**
Skew deviation	Vertical misalignment of the eyes with the lower eye on the side of the lesion	Vertical misalignment of the eyes with the higher eye on the side of the lesion
Ocular counter-roll deviation	Torsional deviation of both eyes with the top poles rotating toward the side of the lesion	Torsional deviation of both eyes with the top poles rotating away from the side of the lesion
Head tilt	Toward the side of the lesion	Away from the side of the lesion
Tilt of upright perception	Toward the side of the lesion	Away from the side of the lesion

due to ocular muscle palsy), torsional deviation of the eyes (OCR deviation), and head tilt.[29] In these patients, the skew deviation is such that the lower eye is usually on the side toward which the head is tilted (Table 2.4). The lower eye is extorted, and the higher eye is intorted (i.e., OCR deviation). The OTR is usually compensated quickly after peripheral lesions but tends to be more enduring after central lesions and often with all components present, for example, with lesions affecting the vestibular nucleus or the medial longitudinal fasciculus pathway.[69–71] The abnormal OCR deviation can be detected using fundus photos, in which torsional eye position is measured as the angle between a horizontal line and the line connecting the optic disc to the fovea.[72] Other methods include using visual field perimetry to measure the torsional deviation by plotting a line connecting the fixation point (fovea) and the blind spot with respect to a horizontal line.[73]

OCR occurs as a normal physiologic response to lateral head tilt. This physiologic response to head tilt is different from OCR deviation from otolith-ocular imbalance, which is often accompanied by a head tilt to compensate for the torsional deviation of the eyes. Normally, during head tilt, activity from both semicircular canals and otoliths results in a dynamic OCR response, which consists of torsional nystagmus with slow phases away and fast phases toward the side of the head tilt. With sustained lateral head tilt, however, the OCR is primarily driven by inputs from the otolith organs (mainly utricles), which consists of ocular torsion about 10%–25% of the head tilt. Thus otolith-ocular function can be evaluated by measuring OCR during static head tilt. Such measurement can use real-time VOG tracking of torsional eye position at the bedside.[74] In this test, OCR values less than 10% of the head tilt indicate vestibular loss, although there is often a symmetric reduction even with unilateral vestibular loss, especially in patients with chronic loss of vestibular function (Fig. 2.6). Therefore, to detect the side of the loss of otolith function, one must infer from the results of other vestibular bedside tests, such as vHIT. With such an approach, video-OCR (vOCR) can detect loss of otolith function, whereas vHIT detects loss of semicircular canal function, which points to the side of vestibular loss.

Skew deviation
Skew deviation can be detected using the alternate cover test while the patient is fixating on a visual target. When skew deviation is subtle, subjective tests of diplopia using the red glass or Maddox rod are helpful. In the red glass test, the patient focuses on a penlight while a red lens is placed by convention in front of the right eye. With vertical misalignment, the red and white lights are seen apart one above the other, with the higher light pointing to the lower eye and vice versa. The Maddox rod test is similar, except that it converts a point light into a thin line, making it easier to report the relative locations of the two separate images. When the parallel lines on the Maddox rod are oriented vertically before the eye, a horizontal red line is seen by the patient, which can be compared with the position of the point light (seen by the other eye) to detect vertical misalignment. Unlike trochlear palsy or oculomotor palsy, skew deviation is usually a concomitant deviation, as the vertical misalignment changes little with gaze position. Skew deviation, however, may lessen when the patient lies supine.[75] Alternating skew deviation, which changes direction on lateral gaze, is usually seen in patients with cerebellar dysfunction (the right eye is usually higher than the left eye in right gaze and the left eye is higher than the right eye in left gaze).[76,77]

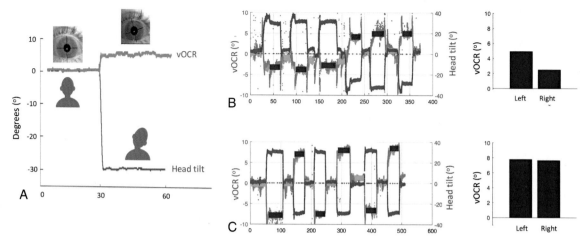

FIG. 2.6 Bedside video ocular counter-roll (vOCR) test as a measure of otolith-ocular function. The OCR (blue trace) response is normally in the opposite direction of the head tilt (brown trace) **(A)**. An example of vOCR recording with 30-degree head tilts (three head tilts in each direction) is shown in a patient with acute right-side vestibular hypofunction **(B)** and a healthy individual **(C)**. The vOCR is calculated as the average difference between the ocular torsion in the upright position (*green lines*) and during 30-degree head tilts (*red lines*). The patient shows reduced OCR with head tilts to the right (2.7 degrees; gain 9%), whereas the OCR is normal with head tilts to the left (4.8 degrees, gain 16%) **(B)**. In the healthy individual the vOCR values are normal during head tilts in both directions (right 7.5 degrees, gain 25%; left 7.6 degrees, gain 25%) **(C)**.

Subjective visual vertical

Because otolith organs encode the orientation of the head with respect to gravity, lesions involving the otolith pathways can distort the perception of upright.[78] Perception of upright orientation is typically studied by means of a task known as the subjective visual vertical (SVV). In this task, what the patient reports as the orientation of a visual line (in absence of additional visual cues), is used to determine their perceived earth-vertical. SVV can be measured at the bedside using the "bucket test" or, with recent advances in mobile devices, using software applications on tablet computers (Fig. 2.7). The bucket test is performed while the patient is sitting upright looking into an opaque bucket.[79,79a] The rim of the bucket removes any visual cues to upright orientation. Inside the bucket, there is a line at the bottom that is set to the 90-degree mark on a protractor attached to the exterior of the bucket. A plumb line is connected to the base of the protractor so that when the bucket is rotated the plumb line indicates deviation from the true vertical (Fig. 2.7A). For SVV measurement, the examiner rotates the bucket clockwise or counterclockwise from random starting points and stops when the patient perceives the inside line as vertical (e.g., 10 measurements in each direction). With tablet or smartphone applications, SVV is also measured with a visual

line presented on the screen in a completely dark room (Fig. 2.7B). In each trial, the task is either to report the visual line orientation or alternatively to adjust the line into vertical position based on perceived upright orientation. SVV can then be calculated after probing various line orientations in multiple trials (Fig. 2.7C).

SVV is a sensitive test for detecting loss of otolith function in both central and peripheral lesions. The normal range of SVV deviation with the head upright is within 2 degrees of the true vertical.[79] With lateral head tilts, however, normally there are systematic errors in perceived upright orientation. The SVV errors occur in the direction of the tilt at large tilt angles (i.e., greater than 60 degrees), which reflects underestimation of upright orientation. At small tilt angles (i.e., less than 60 degrees), on the other hand, SVV errors occur in the opposite direction of the head tilt, which reflects overestimation of upright orientation. Patients with peripheral vestibular loss often show underestimation of upright perception during static head tilt even at small tilt angles.[80–83] With lesions involving the otolith-ocular pathways before crossing the midline in the brainstem (i.e., the lower pons and medulla, vestibular nerve, and labyrinth), the SVV deviates toward the side of the lesion. With lesions that involve pathways after crossing the midline in the brainstem (i.e., within the

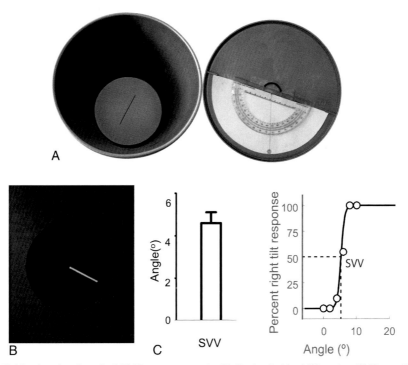

FIG. 2.7 Subjective visual vertical (SVV) measurement with the bucket test **(A)** and an SVV paradigm on a tablet computer **(B)**. In the bucket test, the examiner rotates the bucket clockwise or counterclockwise from random starting points and stops when the patient perceives the inside line as vertical (e.g., 10 measurements in each direction). The line inside the bucket is set to the 90-degree mark on a protractor attached to the exterior of the bucket. A plumb line is connected to the base of the protractor so that when the bucket is rotated the *plumb line* indicates deviation from the true vertical. Using a tablet application, SVV can be measured with a visual line presented on the screen in a completely dark room. In each trial, the task is either to report the visual line orientation or alternatively to adjust the line into the vertical position based on perceived upright orientation. Depending on the method of measurement, SVV can be calculated as the average of multiple adjustments to perceived upright orientation (**C**, left graph) or by calculating the 50% probability of right and left tilt responses (**C**, right graph).

upper pons and midbrain), the SVV deviates opposite to the side of the lesion.[72] Thus, in patients with OTR, SVV deviation is in the same direction as the head tilt. With cerebellar lesions, SVV deviation can be ipsilesional (e.g., with lesions involving the cerebellar hemispheres, middle cerebellar peduncle, or the cerebellar tonsil) or contralesional (e.g., with lesions involving the dentate nucleus, nodulus, or uvula).[84–86] SVV may also deviate with supratentorial lesions, particularly lesions within the thalamus and the cerebral cortex involving the temporoparietal junction. These patients mostly have contralesional SVV deviations; however, roughly 10% of patients may show ipsilesional SVV deviations.[87] Supratentorial lesions are not accompanied by ocular torsion or skew deviation, and in such cases the abnormal SVV represents disruption in neural

networks that integrate sensory inputs encoding eye, head, and body orientations.

Ocular Motor Examination

In addition to evaluation of the vestibular system, a complete ocular motor examination is essential to correctly differentiate between central and peripheral vestibular lesions. The ocular motor evaluation should include examination of eccentric gaze holding (looking for gaze-evoked nystagmus), saccades, pursuit, VOR cancellation, optokinetic nystagmus, and convergence.

Saccades

Saccades are examined by instructing the patient to change visual fixation between two visual targets on command (e.g., a hand-held pen and examiner's nose). The examination should be performed in both directions horizontally and vertically. The examiner observes the eye movements for latency, speed, trajectory, and also the accuracy with which the eyes land on the target. These parameters help localize central lesions; for example, lesions in the paramedian pontine reticular formation cause slow horizontal saccades, and lesions in the midbrain involving the rostral interstitial nucleus of the medial longitudinal fasciculus cause slow vertical saccades.[88,89] Lesions in the dorsolateral medulla affecting the olivocerebellar pathway after it crosses the midline of the brainstem cause saccadic hypermetria toward the side of the lesion and saccadic hypometria away from the side of the lesion.[90] Lesions involving the dorsal vermis (lobule VI, VII) cause saccadic hypometria toward the side of the lesion, whereas involvement of the fastigial nucleus usually causes hypermetria in both directions, as the fastigial projections course through the contralateral fastigial nucleus before exiting the cerebellum through pathways along the superior cerebellar peduncle.[91] Lesions in the cerebral cortex, on the other hand, can delay the initiation of saccades or cause them to be hypometric when directed opposite to the side of the lesion.[92]

Smooth pursuit and VOR cancellation

For evaluation of horizontal and vertical smooth pursuit, a visual target (e.g., a hand-held pen) is moved at approximately 5–10 degrees/second in front of the patient. If smooth pursuit is intact, eye movements match the speed of the target, but if abnormal, visual tracking is punctuated by corrective saccades, needed to catch up to the target. Many patients with peripheral vestibular loss and spontaneous nystagmus seem to have disrupted smooth pursuit, especially in the direction of the fast phases of the nystagmus. Lesions affecting the ocular motor networks involving the vestibular nuclei, cerebellar flocculus, paraflocculus, nucleus prepositus hypoglossi, dorsal vermis, and fastigial nucleus can cause pursuit deficits, as they share much circuitry within the brainstem and cerebellum.[10,11,14,25,93] Pursuit is also commonly impaired in the elderly and by medications acting on the central nervous system. Thus pursuit deficits should always be interpreted in the context of other ocular motor findings.[1]

Combined eye-head tracking of a moving visual target requires cancellation of the VOR, which can be examined by instructing the patient to track a head-fixed, slowly moving target (e.g., a long pointer held on the patient's head). VOR cancellation is intact if the eyes remain fixed on the visual target during head movement. It is impaired if the eyes are taken off the target by a still functioning VOR, which then requires catch-up saccades to the visual target to maintain visual fixation. Smooth pursuit and VOR cancellation share similar mechanisms. Thus patients with impaired pursuit often have impaired VOR cancellation. However, VOR cancellation seems to be intact in patients with no VOR function, as there is no eye movement to be suppressed during the head movement.[94] For example, cancellation of the VOR seems to be normal in a patient with CANVAS because of the peripheral vestibular loss, but smooth pursuit tested with the head stationary is abnormal because of cerebellar dysfunction.[65,66]

Optokinetic reflex

Optokinetic nystagmus can be induced with an optokinetic drum, a banded cloth, a tablet application, or simply with the examiner moving the outstretched fingers in front of the patient. Looking at these moving visual patterns normally induces nystagmus with the slow phase in the direction of the pattern movement. Central lesions involving pursuit, vestibular, and saccadic pathways can cause reduction or elimination of optokinetic nystagmus. Peripheral vestibular loss also produces asymmetries of optokinetic nystagmus, particularly during the acute phase, which can result in directional preponderance of optokinetic responses toward the side of the lesion.[95]

Balance and Gait Examination

Maintaining balance reflects complex interactions between multiple sensory and motor neural mechanisms. Although balance problems are not specific to vestibular dysfunction, evaluation of balance often helps to (1) assess the severity of postural imbalance and gait disturbance in vestibular dysfunction, (2) differentiate between central and peripheral vestibular lesions, and (3) track recovery from vestibular loss.

Romberg test

In this test the patient stands with heels touching and then closes the eyes. Normal individuals with eyes closed can maintain balance without difficulty. There are, however, different variations and levels of difficulty to the Romberg test: standing with feet next to each other, standing one foot in front of the other (tandem Romberg), or standing on one foot. Each variation is performed with eyes open and closed. Usually patients with vestibular or proprioceptive loss have an obvious increase in the swaying or may have a fall, or an unintended step with eyes closed, especially under more difficult conditions.[96,97] This pattern is different from cerebellar dysfunction whereby patients often have difficulty with balance and may fall even with eyes open. Generally, distraction (i.e., mental

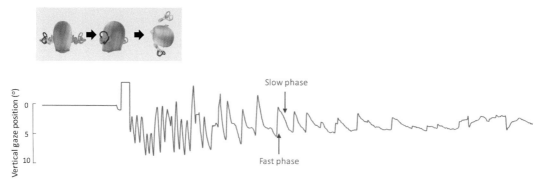

FIG. 2.8 Positional nystagmus from a bedside video-oculography recording during the Dix-Hallpike test in a patient with left posterior canal benign paroxysmal positional vertigo. The vertical eye position trace shows an upbeating nystagmus (i.e., slow phases directed toward the feet [inferiorly]), which is paroxysmal and gradually dissipates in a few seconds.

alerting tasks) can reduce the swaying in cases of psycho-genic disorders, whereas in other pathologies distraction can actually worsen the balance problem.

Modified clinical test of sensory interaction and balance

Modified clinical test of sensory interaction and balance (mCTSIB)[98,99] is a quantitative method based on Romberg tests and is a simplified form of the clinical test of sensory interaction and balance (CTSIB).[100] During the test, the patient stands with feet together and arms crossed in front of the chest. The balance is evaluated by watching for falls or unintended steps under four conditions, each lasting 20 seconds: (1) standing on a firm surface with eyes open; (2) standing on a firm surface with eyes closed; (3) standing on foam with eyes open; (4) standing on foam with eyes closed. mCTSIB can be used to measure imbalance from vestibular dysfunction or track recovery in these patients.[101,102]

Gait

During gait evaluation, one has to look for the step length and stance width, variability in cadence (steps per minute), as well as path deviation to the sides while taking steps. In bilateral vestibulopathy, gait tends to be broad-based and often becomes worse with the eyes closed. In a unilateral peripheral vestibular loss, patients may have a path deviation toward the side of the vestibular loss. In these patients, however, gait improves with increasing speed.

Stepping tests

Unterberger or Fukuda's stepping test is helpful to detect vestibular imbalance.[103,104] The patient is asked to march in place with the eyes closed. Patients with unilateral vestibular loss tend to rotate toward the side of vestibular loss. Such rotations can be quantified at the bedside using smartphone applications.[105]

Positional Vertigo

Benign paroxysmal positional vertigo (BPPV) is an exceedingly common cause of vertigo and should be sought in all patients with acute or chronic dizziness or imbalance (see Chapter 9).[106,107] It is caused by dislodged otoconia (calcium carbonate crystals normally located on the maculae of the utricle), which may slough off spontaneously or as a result of trauma and fall into the semicircular canals. Thus positional symptoms and signs depend on the position of the head with respect to gravity and the free-floating otoconia that abnormally stimulate the semicircular canals (canalolithiasis). Rolling over, getting in or out of bed, or looking up when standing are common triggers for the positional symptoms. Less commonly, the otoconial debris adhere to the cupula of the semicircular canals (cupulolithiasis) and cause less intense but more persistent positional vertigo. The diagnosis of BPPV and its localization can be made quickly using positioning maneuvers, particularly the Dix-Hallpike test for the most common variant, the posterior canal BPPV.

Dix-Hallpike test

The patient first sits upright in bed with the legs extended. The head is turned 45 degrees to one side, and the patient is then brought down into the supine position while the head is kept hyperextended about 30 degrees below the bed (Fig. 2.10A–C). The examiner observes for paroxysmal nystagmus that develops seconds after the head is brought down and is usually transient, lasting less than 30 seconds (Fig. 2.8). The

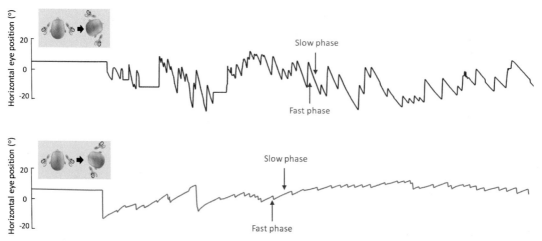

FIG. 2.9 Positional nystagmus from a bedside video-oculography recording during the supine roll maneuver in a patient with right horizontal canalolithiasis. The horizontal eye position trace shows geotropic nystagmus with fast phases toward the ground (i.e., right beating with the head roll to the right shown in red and left beating with the head roll to the left shown in blue). The nystagmus is stronger on the right side, which is where the lowermost ear is on the side of the canalolithiasis.

patient is then brought back into the sitting position, and the procedure is repeated in the same order for the other side. Usually, symptoms develop only in the right or left ear down positions, although bilateral cases may also occur, especially after trauma. Nystagmus from posterior canal BPPV is upbeating and torsional (top pole beating toward the ground and the lower ear). The positional nystagmus in BPPV is best seen if the effect of visual fixation is eliminated (e.g., with Frenzel goggles). The positional nystagmus of BPPV can also be easily recorded and analyzed at the bedside using VOG goggles (Fig. 2.8). Thus, using the Dix-Hallpike test, posterior canal BPPV is diagnosed when: (1) the positional nystagmus is elicited with the appropriate head orientation, (2) the direction of the nystagmus matches the predicted semicircular canal stimulation in that head position, (3) there is a latency before the onset of the nystagmus (i.e., paroxysmal nystagmus), and (4) nystagmus is transient and not persistent (usually less than one minute). Patients with central lesions may also have positional nystagmus that is typically persistent without a latency, and rarely shows mixed torsional and vertical components as seen in BPPV. For example, patients with cerebellar lesions may present with persistent positional downbeat nystagmus,[108,109] and patients with vestibular migraine may have positional nystagmus, which is usually weak but sustained.[110–112]

Horizontal canal BPPV is relatively less common and often presents with pure horizontal nystagmus that changes direction when the head is turned from one side to the other in the supine position. In such cases, canalolithiasis often produces nystagmus with the fast phase toward the ground (geotropic nystagmus) (Fig. 2.9), whereas cupulolithiasis leads to rather persistent nystagmus, with the fast phase away from the ground (apogeotropic nystagmus).[112] Central positional nystagmus, for example, with lesions involving the cerebellar nodulus, may also cause apogeotropic nystagmus, but often, it has associated vertical and torsional components and there is usually a spontaneous nystagmus in the upright head position.[113]

Epley maneuver

Treatment of posterior canal BPPV is extremely effective and can be performed readily at the bedside using a canalith repositioning procedure, most commonly the Epley maneuver.[114] This can be done as soon as BPPV is detected during Dix-Hallpike testing by keeping the neck extended while the patient is lying supine (Fig. 2.10D–F). The following steps are then taken: (1) the head is rotated 90 degrees so that the unaffected ear is brought about 45 degrees downward, (2) the patient's head is then rotated another 90 degrees so that the nose is brought 45 degrees toward the ground and at the same time the patient is asked to move into the left lateral decubitus position, (3) the patient drops the legs over the edge of the table while the head is kept in the nose-down position, and then the patient sits up while the head is kept rotated 45 degrees before it is slowly moved back to the neutral straight ahead position.

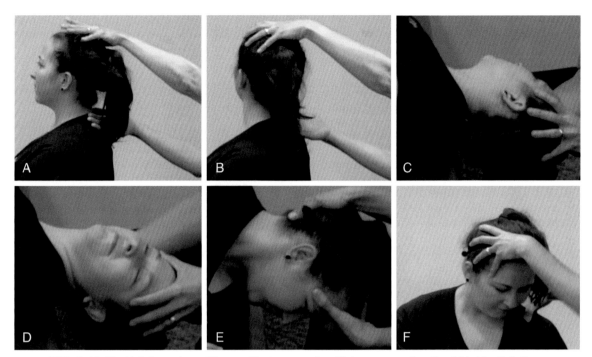

FIG. 2.10 Dix-Hallpike and canalith repositioning procedure (Epley maneuver) on the right side. Both the Dix-Hallpike test and Epley maneuver start with the patient sitting upright with legs extended **(A)**. The head is then rotated by approximately 45 degrees to the right side **(B)**. The examiner helps the patient to lie down backward quickly, maintaining the head turn in approximately 30 degrees of extension (right ear is below the right shoulder) **(C)**. The Epley maneuver continues with rotating the head 90 degrees so that the unaffected ear is brought about 45 degrees downward **(D)**. The patient's head is then rotated another 90 degrees so the nose is brought 45 degrees toward the ground **(E)**. The head is kept in the nose-down position, and then the patient sits up while the head is kept rotated 45 degrees before it is slowly moved back to the neutral straight ahead position **(F)**.

The head position in each step is usually held for one minute or so until the positional nystagmus and symptoms abate. The entire maneuver may be repeated as necessary until no nystagmus or symptoms are present. The Semont maneuver is another canalith repositioning procedure for treatment of posterior canal BPPV in which the patient is moved quickly from lying on the side of the affected ear to lying on the other side.[115]

CONCLUSIONS

When evaluating patients with dizziness, understanding basic vestibular and ocular motor physiology along with proper examination techniques are critical for reaching the correct diagnosis. With the use of portable technologies, the vestibular examination can now be quantified at the bedside to improve diagnostic accuracy and clinical management. During the examination, clinicians should look for signs of static and dynamic vestibular imbalance. Patients with vestibular loss often have spontaneous nystagmus as a sign of static vestibular imbalance affecting the function of the semicircular canals. Spontaneous nystagmus from peripheral vestibular loss usually weakens over time and may not be observed directly at the bedside after recovery. Thus one must remove visual fixation to detect vestibular nystagmus (e.g., using Frenzel goggles or VOG). Nystagmus from vestibular imbalance can also be brought out using provoking maneuvers such as head shaking or vibration over the mastoids. As a sign of dynamic vestibular imbalance, the head impulse maneuver can detect loss of vestibular function involving the semicircular canals. A static otolith-ocular imbalance can induce an OTR, which consists of a lateral head tilt, skew, and OCR deviation. Also, there is often an associated tilt of SVV related to the OCR deviation, which can be measured at the bedside using the bucket test or SVV paradigms on tablet computers. The OTR is more common in central than in peripheral lesions involving otolith-ocular pathways. As a bedside test of otolith-ocular function, VOG can be used to measure OCR induced by a sustained lateral head tilt (vOCR). In this test, vOCR values less than 10% of the head tilt indicate vestibular loss. The vOCR can be combined with the vHIT for a bedside evaluation of vestibular function. In this approach, vOCR can detect loss of otolith function, whereas vHIT detects loss of semicircular canal function as well as the side of vestibular loss.

In sum, the combination of bedside findings from static and dynamic vestibular imbalance can correctly identify central and peripheral vestibular dysfunctions. This is especially important when evaluating patients with an acute vestibular syndrome, as the suspicion of a central lesion requires emergency procedures, including stroke treatment, whereas a peripheral lesion requires mainly symptomatic and supportive management in the acute stage. In these patients, the HINTS battery is useful to correctly distinguish between peripheral and central etiologies. Using HINTS, one should suspect central lesions in patients with an intact head impulse test (i.e., no catch-up saccades), direction-changing nystagmus (i.e., right beating on right gaze and left beating on left gaze), or skew deviation, whereas an abnormal head impulse test, direction-fixed nystagmus, and absence of skew deviation usually suggests a peripheral vestibular lesion. Finally, positional testing and evaluation of balance should always be part of the bedside vestibular examination. The diagnosis of BPPV can be made swiftly using positioning tests (e.g., Dix-Hallpike test), and it can be treated promptly using repositioning maneuvers (e.g., Epley or Semont maneuver).

ACKNOWLEDGMENTS

The recordings in Figures 2.1–2.9 were performed as part of the AVERT clinical trial (NIH/NIDCD U01 DC013778). We thank the study's Principal Investigator, Dr. David Newman-Toker and the rest of the AVERT team for providing these resources.

REFERENCES

1. Leigh R, Zee D. *The Neurology of Eye Movements*. 5th ed. New York: Oxford University Press; 2015.
2. Hotson JR, Baloh RW. Acute vestibular syndrome. *N Engl J Med*. 1998;339(10):680–685. http://dx.doi.org/10.1056/NEJM199809033391007.
3. Norrving B, Magnusson M, Holtås S. Isolated acute vertigo in the elderly; vestibular or vascular disease? *Acta Neurol Scand*. 1995;91(1):43–48. http://dx.doi.org/10.1111/j.1600-0404.1995.tb05841.x.
4. Kattah JC, Talkad AV, Wang DZ, Hsieh Y-H, Newman-Toker DE. HINTS to diagnose stroke in the acute vestibular syndrome: three-step bedside oculomotor examination more sensitive than early MRI diffusion-weighted imaging. *Stroke J Cereb Circ*. 2009;40(11):3504–3510. http://dx.doi.org/10.1161/STROKEAHA.109.551234.
5. Carmona S, Martínez C, Zalazar G, et al. The diagnostic accuracy of truncal ataxia and HINTS as cardinal signs for acute vestibular syndrome. *Front Neurol*. 2016;7. http://dx.doi.org/10.3389/fneur.2016.00125.
6. Vanni S, Pecci R, Casati C, et al. STANDING, a four-step bedside algorithm for differential diagnosis of acute vertigo in the Emergency Department. *Acta Otorhinolaryngol Ital*. 2014;34(6):419–426.
7. Newman-Toker DE, Kerber KA, Hsieh Y-H, et al. HINTS outperforms ABCD2 to screen for stroke in acute continuous vertigo and dizziness. *Acad Emerg Med*. 2013;20(10):986–996. http://dx.doi.org/10.1111/acem.12223.
8. Robinson DA, Zee DS, Hain TC, Holmes A, Rosenberg LF. Alexander's law: its behavior and origin in the human vestibulo-ocular reflex. *Ann Neurol*. 1984;16(6):714–722. http://dx.doi.org/10.1002/ana.410160614.
9. Kim H-A, Lee H. Isolated vestibular nucleus infarction mimicking acute peripheral vestibulopathy. *Stroke*. 2010;41(7):1558–1560. http://dx.doi.org/10.1161/STROKEAHA.110.582783.
10. Park H-K, Kim J-S, Strupp M, Zee DS. Isolated floccular infarction: impaired vestibular responses to horizontal head impulse. *J Neurol*. 2013;260(6):1576–1582. http://dx.doi.org/10.1007/s00415-013-6837-y.
11. Lee S-H, Park S-H, Kim J-S, Kim H-J, Yunusov F, Zee DS. Isolated unilateral infarction of the cerebellar tonsil: ocular motor findings. *Ann Neurol*. 2014;75(3):429–434.
11a. Yacovino DA, Akly MP, Luis L, Zee DS. The floccular syndrome: dynamic changes in eye movements and vestibulo-ocular reflex in isolated infarction of the cerebellar flocculus. *Cerebellum Lond Engl*. August 2017. http://dx.doi.org/10.1007/s12311-017-0878-1.
12. Lloyd SKW, Baguley DM, Butler K, Donnelly N, Moffat DA. Bruns' nystagmus in patients with vestibular schwannoma. *Otol Neurotol*. 2009;30(5):625–628. http://dx.doi.org/10.1097/MAO.0b013e3181a32bec.
13. Venkateswaran R, Gupta R, Swaminathan RP. Bruns nystagmus in cerebellopontine angle tumor. *JAMA Neurol*. 2013;70(5):646. http://dx.doi.org/10.1001/jamaneurol.2013.619.
14. Lee S-U, Park S-H, Park J-J, et al. Dorsal medullary infarction. *Stroke*. 2015;46(11):3081–3087. http://dx.doi.org/10.1161/STROKEAHA.115.010972.
15. Croxson GR, Moffat DA, Baguley D. Bruns bidirectional nystagmus in cerebellopontine angle tumours. *Clin Otolaryngol Allied Sci*. 1988;13(2):153–157. http://dx.doi.org/10.1111/j.1365-2273.1988.tb00756.x.
16. Nedzelski JM. Cerebellopontine angle tumors: bilateral flocculus compression as cause of associated oculomotor abnormalities. *Laryngoscope*. 1983;93(10):1251–1260. http://dx.doi.org/10.1002/lary.1983.93.10.1251.

17. Hood JD, Kayan A, Leech J, et al. Rebound nystagmus. *Brain*. 1973;96(3):507–526.

18. Yamazaki A, Zee DS. Rebound nystagmus: EOG analysis of a case with a floccular tumour. *Br J Ophthalmol*. 1979;63(11):782–786.

19. Bondar RL, Sharpe JA, Lewis AJ. Rebound nystagmus in olivocerebellar atrophy: a clinicopathological correlation. *Ann Neurol*. 1984;15(5):474–477. http://dx.doi.org/10.1002/ana.410150512.

20. Hashimoto T, Sasaki O, Yoshida K, Takei Y, Ikeda S. Periodic alternating nystagmus and rebound nystagmus in spinocerebellar ataxia type 6. *Mov Disord*. 2003;18(10):1201–1204. http://dx.doi.org/10.1002/mds.10511.

21. Wagner JN, Glaser M, Brandt T, Strupp M. Downbeat nystagmus: aetiology and comorbidity in 117 patients. *J Neurol Neurosurg Psychiatry*. 2008;79(6):672–677. http://dx.doi.org/10.1136/jnnp.2007.126284.

22. Halmagyi GM, Curthoys IS. A clinical sign of canal paresis. *Arch Neurol*. 1988;45(7):737–739. http://dx.doi.org/10.1001/archneur.1988.00520310043015.

23. Newman-Toker DE, Kattah JC, Alvernia JE, Wang DZ. Normal head impulse test differentiates acute cerebellar strokes from vestibular neuritis. *Neurology*. 2008;70(24 Part 2):2378–2385. http://dx.doi.org/10.1212/01.wnl.0000314685.01433.0d.

24. Mantokoudis G, Tehrani ASS, Wozniak A, et al. VOR gain by head impulse video-oculography differentiates acute vestibular neuritis from stroke. *Otol Neurotol*. 2015;36(3):457–465. http://dx.doi.org/10.1097/MAO.0000000000000638.

25. Kim S-H, Zee DS, du Lac S, Kim HJ, Kim J-S. Nucleus prepositus hypoglossi lesions produce a unique ocular motor syndrome. *Neurology*. 2016;87(19):2026–2033. http://dx.doi.org/10.1212/WNL.0000000000003316.

26. Weber KP, Aw ST, Todd MJ, McGarvie LA, Curthoys IS, Halmagyi GM. Head impulse test in unilateral vestibular loss: vestibulo-ocular reflex and catch-up saccades. *Neurology*. 2008;70(6):454–463. http://dx.doi.org/10.1212/01.wnl.0000299117.48935.2e.

27. Tjernström F, Nyström A, Magnusson M. How to uncover the covert saccade during the head impulse test. *Otol Neurotol*. 2012;33(9):1583–1585. http://dx.doi.org/10.1097/MAO.0b013e318268d32f.

28. Brandt TH, Dieterich M. Different types of skew deviation. *J Neurol Neurosurg Psychiatry*. 1991;54(6):549–550.

29. Brodsky MC, Donahue SP, Vaphiades M, Brandt T. Skew deviation revisited. *Surv Ophthalmol*. 2006;51(2):105–128. http://dx.doi.org/10.1016/j.survophthal.2005.12.008.

30. Choi J-H, Seo J-D, Choi YR, et al. Inferior cerebellar peduncular lesion causes a distinct vestibular syndrome. *Eur J Neurol*. 2015;22(7):1062–1067. http://dx.doi.org/10.1111/ene.12705.

31. Moon IS, Kim JS, Choi KD, et al. Isolated nodular infarction. *Stroke*. 2009;40(2):487–491. http://dx.doi.org/10.1161/STROKEAHA.108.527762.

32. Lee H, Kim JS, Chung E-J, et al. Infarction in the territory of anterior inferior cerebellar artery: spectrum of audiovestibular loss. *Stroke*. 2009;40(12):3745–3751. http://dx.doi.org/10.1161/STROKEAHA.109.564682.

33. Kim H-A, Lee H. Recent advances in central acute vestibular syndrome of a vascular cause. *J Neurol Sci*. 2012;321(1-2):17–22. http://dx.doi.org/10.1016/j.jns.2012.07.055.

33a. Chang T-P, Wang Z, Winnick AA, et al. Sudden hearing loss with vertigo portends greater stroke risk than sudden hearing loss or vertigo alone. *J Stroke Cerebrovasc Dis Off J Natl Stroke Assoc*. November 2017. http://dx.doi.org/10.1016/j.jstrokecerebrovasdis.2017.09.033.

34. Bartl K, Lehnen N, Kohlbecher S, Schneider E. Head impulse testing using video-oculography. *Ann N Y Acad Sci*. 2009;1164(1):331–333. http://dx.doi.org/10.1111/j.1749-6632.2009.03850.x.

35. MacDougall HG, Weber KP, McGarvie LA, Halmagyi GM, Curthoys IS. The video head impulse test: diagnostic accuracy in peripheral vestibulopathy. *Neurology*. 2009;73(14):1134–1141. http://dx.doi.org/10.1212/WNL.0b013e3181bacf85.

36. Blödow A, Pannasch S, Walther LE. Detection of isolated covert saccades with the video head impulse test in peripheral vestibular disorders. *Auris Nasus Larynx*. 2013;40(4):348–351. http://dx.doi.org/10.1016/j.anl.2012.11.002.

37. Newman-Toker DE, Tehrani ASS, Mantokoudis G, et al. Quantitative video-oculography to help diagnose stroke in acute vertigo and dizziness toward an ECG for the eyes. *Stroke*. 2013;44(4):1158–1161.

38. Newman-Toker DE, Curthoys IS, Halmagyi GM. Diagnosing stroke in acute vertigo: the HINTS family of eye movement tests and the future of the "eye ECG". *Semin Neurol*. 2015;35(5):506–521. http://dx.doi.org/10.1055/s-0035-1564298.

39. Kim J-H, Kim S, Lee DH, Lee T-K, Sung K-B. Isolated axial lateropulsion with ipsilesional subjective visual vertical tilt in caudal lateral medullary infarction. *J Vestib Res Equilib Orientat*. 2015;25(1):41–45. http://dx.doi.org/10.3233/VES-150543.

40. Strupp M, Fischer C, Hanß L, Bayer O. The takeaway Frenzel goggles: a Fresnel-based device. *Neurology*. 2014;83(14):1241–1245. http://dx.doi.org/10.1212/WNL.0000000000000838.

41. Newman-Toker DE, Sharma P, Chowdhury M, Clemons TM, Zee DS, Santina CCD. Penlight-cover test: a new bedside method to unmask nystagmus. *J Neurol Neurosurg Psychiatry*. 2009;80(8):900–903. http://dx.doi.org/10.1136/jnnp.2009.174128.

42. Kim M-B, Huh SH, Ban JH. Diversity of head shaking nystagmus in peripheral vestibular disease. *Otol Neurotol*. 2012;33(4):634–639. http://dx.doi.org/10.1097/MAO.0b013e31824950c7.

43. Lee YJ, Shin JE, Park MS, et al. Comprehensive analysis of head-shaking nystagmus in patients with vestibular neuritis. *Audiol Neurotol*. 2012;17(4):228–234. http://dx.doi.org/10.1159/000336958.

44. Huh YE, Kim JS. Patterns of spontaneous and head-shaking nystagmus in cerebellar infarction: imaging correlations. *Brain J Neurol.* 2011;134(Pt 12):3662–3671. http://dx.doi.org/10.1093/brain/awr269.

45. Minagar A, Sheremata WA, Tusa RJ. Perverted head-shaking nystagmus: a possible mechanism. *Neurology.* 2001;57(5):887–889.

46. Choi J-Y, Jung I, Jung J-M, et al. Characteristics and mechanism of perverted head-shaking nystagmus in central lesions: video-oculography analysis. *Clin Neurophysiol.* 2016;127(9):2973–2978. http://dx.doi.org/10.1016/j.clinph.2016.07.003.

47. Raphan DT, Matsuo V, Cohen B. Velocity storage in the vestibulo-ocular reflex arc (VOR). *Exp Brain Res.* 1979;35(2):229–248. http://dx.doi.org/10.1007/BF00236613.

48. Choi K-D, Oh S-Y, Park S-H, Kim J-H, Koo J-W, Kim JS. Head-shaking nystagmus in lateral medullary infarction: patterns and possible mechanisms. *Neurology.* 2007;68(17):1337–1344. http://dx.doi.org/10.1212/01.wnl.0000260224.60943.c2.

49. Zuma E, Maia FC, Cal R, D'Albora R, Carmona S, Schubert MC. Head-shaking tilt suppression: a clinical test to discern central from peripheral causes of vertigo. *J Neurol.* 2017;264(6):1264–1270. http://dx.doi.org/10.1007/s00415-017-8524-x.

50. Bertolini G, Bockisch CJ, Straumann D, Zee DS, Ramat S. Do humans show velocity-storage in the vertical rVOR? In: *Progress in Brain Research.* vol. 171. Elsevier; 2008:207–210. http://linkinghub.elsevier.com/retrieve/pii/S0079612308000628.

51. Haslwanter T, Minor LB. Nystagmus induced by circular head shaking in normal human subjects. *Exp Brain Res.* 1999;124(1):25–32.

52. Koo J-W, Kim J-S, Hong SK. Vibration-induced nystagmus after acute peripheral vestibular loss: comparative study with other vestibule-ocular reflex tests in the yaw plane. *Otol Neurotol.* 2011;32(3):466–471.

53. Dumas G, Perrin P, Schmerber S. Nystagmus induced by high frequency vibrations of the skull in total unilateral peripheral vestibular lesions. *Acta Otolaryngol (Stockh).* 2008;128(3):255–262. http://dx.doi.org/10.1080/00016480701477677.

54. Chang T-P, Wu Y-C. Vibration-induced reversal of spontaneous nystagmus in lateral medullary infarction. *Neurology.* 2013;80(14):1353. http://dx.doi.org/10.1212/WNL.0b013e31828ab336.

55. Minor LB, Haslwanter T, Straumann D, Zee DS. Hyperventilation-induced nystagmus in patients with vestibular schwannoma. *Neurology.* 1999;53(9):2158.

56. Hüfner K, Barresi D, Glaser M, et al. Vestibular paroxysmia diagnostic features and medical treatment. *Neurology.* 2008;71(13):1006–1014.

57. Park HJ, Shin JE, Lee YJ, Park MS, Kim JM, Na BR. Hyperventilation-induced nystagmus in patients with vestibular neuritis in the acute and follow-up stages. *Audiol Neurotol.* 2011;16(4):248–253. http://dx.doi.org/10.1159/000320841.

58. Hong J-H, Yang J-G, Kim H-A, Yi H-A, Le H. Hyperventilation-induced nystagmus in vestibular neuritis: pattern and clinical implication. *Eur Neurol.* 2013;69(4):213–220. http://dx.doi.org/10.1159/000345802.

59. Walker MF, Zee DS. The effect of hyperventilation on downbeat nystagmus in cerebellar disorders. *Neurology.* 1999;53(7):1576.

60. Kheradmand A, Zee DS. The bedside examination of the vestibulo-ocular reflex (VOR): an update. *Rev Neurol (Paris).* 2012;168(10):710–719. http://dx.doi.org/10.1016/j.neurol.2012.07.011.

61. Minor LB, Carey JP, Cremer PD, Lustig LR, Streubel S-O. Dehiscence of bone overlying the superior canal as a cause of apparent conductive hearing loss. *Otol Neurotol.* 2003;24(2):270–278.

62. Schubert MC, Herdman SJ, Tusa RJ. Vertical dynamic visual acuity in normal subjects and patients with vestibular hypofunction. *Otol Neurotol.* 2002;23(3):372–377.

63. Herdman SJ, Hall CD, Schubert MC, Das VE, Tusa RJ. Recovery of dynamic visual acuity in bilateral vestibular hypofunction. *Arch Otolaryngol Neck Surg.* 2007;133(4):383–389.

64. Schubert MC, Migliaccio AA, Clendaniel RA, Allak A, Carey JP. Mechanism of dynamic visual acuity recovery with vestibular rehabilitation. *Arch Phys Med Rehabil.* 2008;89(3):500–507.

65. Petersen JA, Wichmann WW, Weber KP. The pivotal sign of CANVAS. *Neurology.* 2013;81(18):1642–1643. http://dx.doi.org/10.1212/WNL.0b013e3182a9f435.

66. Szmulewicz DJ, Waterston JA, MacDougall HG, et al. Cerebellar ataxia, neuropathy, vestibular areflexia syndrome (CANVAS): a review of the clinical features and video-oculographic diagnosis: Szmulewicz et al. *Ann N Y Acad Sci.* 2011;1233(1):139–147. http://dx.doi.org/10.1111/j.1749-6632.2011.06158.x.

67. Gordon CR, Joffe V, Vainstein G, Gadoth N. Vestibulo-ocular arreflexia in families with spinocerebellar ataxia type 3 (Machado-Joseph disease). *J Neurol Neurosurg Psychiatry.* 2003;74(10):1403–1406.

68. MacDougall HG, McGarvie LA, Halmagyi GM, et al. A new saccadic indicator of peripheral vestibular function based on the video head impulse test. *Neurology.* 2016;87(4):410–418. http://dx.doi.org/10.1212/WNL.0000000000002827.

69. Böhmer A, Rickenmann J. The subjective visual vertical as a clinical parameter of vestibular function in peripheral vestibular diseases. *J Vestib Res.* 1995;5(1):35–45.

70. Choi JW, Kang SI, Rhee JH, Choi BY, Kim J-S, Koo J-W. Clinical implication of ocular torsion in peripheral vestibulopathy. *Eur Arch Otorhinolaryngol.* 2015;272(7):1613–1617. http://dx.doi.org/10.1007/s00405-014-2952-3.

71. Brandt T, Dieterich M. Pathological eye-head coordination in roll: tonic ocular tilt reaction in mesencephalic and medullary lesions. *Brain.* 1987;110(3):649–666.

72. Dieterich M, Brandt T. Ocular torsion and tilt of subjective visual vertical are sensitive brainstem signs. *Ann Neurol.* 1993;33(3):292–299. http://dx.doi.org/10.1002/ana.410330311.

73. Versino M, Newman-Toker DE. Blind spot heterotopia by automated static perimetry to assess static ocular torsion: centro-cecal axis rotation in normals. *J Neurol*. 2010;257(2):291–293. http://dx.doi.org/10.1007/s00415-009-5341-x.

74. Otero-Millan J, Treviño C, Winnick A, Zee DS, Carey JP, Kheradmand A. The video ocular counter-roll (vOCR): a clinical test to detect loss ofotolith-ocular function. *Acta Otolaryngol (Stockh)*. 2017:1–8.

75. Wong AMF. Understanding skew deviation and a new clinical test to differentiate it from trochlear nerve palsy. *J Am Assoc Pediatr Ophthalmol Strabismus*. 2010;14(1):61–67. http://dx.doi.org/10.1016/j.jaapos.2009.11.019.

76. Tsuda H, Nagamata M, Tanaka K. Alternating skew deviation due to hemorrhage in the cerebellar vermis. *Intern Med*. 2012;51(19):2793–2796.

77. Colen CB, Ketko A, George E, Van Stavern GP. Periodic alternating nystagmus and periodic alternating skew deviation in spinocerebellar ataxia type 6. *J Neuroophthalmol*. 2008;28(4):287–288.

78. Friedmann G. The judgement of the visual vertical and horizontal with peripheral and central vestibular lesions. *Brain*. 1970;93(2):313–328.

79. Zwergal A, Rettinger N, Frenzel C, Dieterich M, Brandt T, Strupp M. A bucket of static vestibular function. *Neurology*. 2009;72(19):1689–1692.http://dx.doi.org/10.1212/WNL.0b013e3181a55ecf.

79a. Frisén L. Practical estimation of ocular torsion and the subjective vertical. *Neuro-ophthalmology*. 2000;23:195.

80. Aubert H. Eine scheinbare bedeutende Drehung von Objecten bei Neigung des Kopfes nach rechts oder links. *Arch Für Pathol Anat Physiol Für Klin Med*. 1861;20(3–4):381–393.

81. Müller G. Über das Aubertsche Phänomen. *Z Sinnesphysiol*. 1916;49:109–246.

82. Tarnutzer AA, Bockisch C, Straumann D, Olasagasti I. Gravity dependence of subjective visual vertical variability. *J Neurophysiol*. 2009;102(3):1657–1671. http://dx.doi.org/10.1152/jn.00007.2008.

83. Bronstein AM. The interaction of otolith and proprioceptive information in the perception of verticality. The effects of labyrinthine and CNS disease. *Ann N Y Acad Sci*. 1999;871:324–333.

84. Baier B, Dieterich M. Ocular tilt reaction: a clinical sign of cerebellar infarctions? *Neurology*. 2009;72(6):572–573. http://dx.doi.org/10.1212/01.wnl.0000342123.39308.32.

85. Baier B, Bense S, Dieterich M. Are signs of ocular tilt reaction in patients with cerebellar lesions mediated by the dentate nucleus? *Brain*. 2008;131(6):1445–1454. http://dx.doi.org/10.1093/brain/awn086.

86. Kim H-A, Lee H, Yi H-A, Lee S-R, Lee S-Y, Baloh RW. Pattern of otolith dysfunction in posterior inferior cerebellar artery territory cerebellar infarction. *J Neurol Sci*. 2009;280(1-2):65–70. http://dx.doi.org/10.1016/j.jns.2009.02.002.

87. Brandt T, Dieterich M, Danek A. Vestibular cortex lesions affect the perception of verticality. *Ann Neurol*. 1994;35(4):403–412. http://dx.doi.org/10.1002/ana.410350406.

88. Barton EJ. Effects of partial lidocaine inactivation of the paramedian pontine reticular formation on saccades of macaques. *J Neurophysiol*. 2003;90(1):372–386. http://dx.doi.org/10.1152/jn.01041.2002.

89. Bhidayasiri R, Riley DE, Somers JT, Lerner AJ, Büttner-Ennever JA, Leigh RJ. Pathophysiology of slow vertical saccades in progressive supranuclear palsy. *Neurology*. 2001;57(11):2070–2077.

90. Kommerell G, Hoyt WF. Lateropulsion of saccadic eye movements: electro-oculographic studies in a patient with Wallenberg's syndrome. *Arch Neurol*. 1973;28(5):313–318.

91. Kheradmand A, Zee DS. Cerebellum and ocular motor control. *Front Neurol*. 2011;2(53):1–15.

92. Genc B, Genc E, Acik L, Ilhan S, Paksoy Y. Acquired ocular motor apraxia from bilateral frontoparietal infarcts associated with Takayasu arteritis. *J Neurol Neurosurg Psychiatry*. 2004;75(11):1651–1652. http://dx.doi.org/10.1136/jnnp.2004.036525.

93. Robinson FR, Straube A, Fuchs AF. Participation of caudal fastigial nucleus in smooth pursuit eye movements. II. Effects of muscimol inactivation. *J Neurophysiol*. 1997;78(2):848–859.

94. Leigh RJ, Sharpe JA, Ranalli PJ, Thurston SE, Hamid MA. Comparison of smooth pursuit and combined eye-head tracking in human subjects with deficient labyrinthine function. *Exp Brain Res*. 1987;66(3):458–464.

95. Lopez C, Borel L, Magnan J, Lacour M. Torsional optokinetic nystagmus after unilateral vestibular loss: asymmetry and compensation. *Brain*. 2005;128(7):1511–1524. http://dx.doi.org/10.1093/brain/awh504.

96. Lanska DJ, Goetz CG. Romberg's sign development, adoption, and adaptation in the 19th century. *Neurology*. 2000;55(8):1201–1206.

97. Fitzgerald B. A review of the sharpened Romberg test in diving medicine. *SPUMS J*. 1996;26(3):142–146.

98. Whitney SL, Wrisley DM. The influence of footwear on timed balance scores of the modified clinical test of sensory interaction and balance. *Arch Phys Med Rehabil*. 2004;85(3):439–443.

99. Wrisley DM, Whitney SL. The effect of foot position on the modified clinical test of sensory interaction and balance. *Arch Phys Med Rehabil*. 2004;85(2):335–338.

100. Cohen H, Blatchly CA, Gombash LL. A study of the clinical test of sensory interaction and balance. *Phys Ther*. 1993;73(6):346–351; discussion 351–354.

101. Agrawal Y, Carey JP, Hoffman HJ, Sklare DA, Schubert MC. The modified Romberg balance test: normative data in US adults. *Otol Neurotol*. 2011;32(8):1309–1311. http://dx.doi.org/10.1097/MAO.0b013e31822e5bee.

102. Jacobson GP, McCaslin DL, Piker EG, Gruenwald J, Grantham S, Tegel L. Insensitivity of the "Romberg test of standing balance on firm and compliant support surfaces" to the results of caloric and VEMP tests. *Ear Hear*. 2011;32(6):e1–e5. http://dx.doi.org/10.1097/AUD.0b013e31822802bb.

103. Moffat DA, Harries MLL, Baguley DM, Hardy DG. Unterberger's stepping test in acoustic neuroma. *J Laryngol Otol.* 1989;103(9):840–841. http://dx.doi.org/10.1017/S0022215100110254.

104. Fukuda T. The stepping test: two phases of the labyrinthine reflex. *Acta Otolaryngol (Stockh).* 1959;50(1-2):95–108.

105. Whittaker M, Mathew A, Kanani R, Kanegaonkar RG. Assessing the Unterberger test: introduction of a novel smartphone application. *J Laryngol Otol.* 2014;128(11):958–960. http://dx.doi.org/10.1017/S0022215114002539.

106. von Brevern M, Radtke A, Lezius F, et al. Epidemiology of benign paroxysmal positional vertigo: a population based study. *J Neurol Neurosurg Psychiatry.* 2007;78(7):710–715. http://dx.doi.org/10.1136/jnnp.2006.100420.

107. Gold DR, Morris L, Kheradmand A, Schubert MC. Repositioning maneuvers for benign paroxysmal positional vertigo. *Curr Treat Options Neurol.* 2014;16(8):307. http://dx.doi.org/10.1007/s11940-014-0307-4.

108. Yabe I, Sasaki H, Takeichi N, et al. Positional vertigo and macroscopic downbeat positioning nystagmus in spinocerebellar ataxia type 6 (SCA6). *J Neurol.* 2003;250(4):440–443. http://dx.doi.org/10.1007/s00415-003-1020-5.

109. Lee J-Y, Lee W-W, Kim JS, Kim HJ, Kim J-K, Jeon BS. Perverted head-shaking and positional downbeat nystagmus in patients with multiple system atrophy. *Mov Disord.* 2009;24(9):1290–1295. http://dx.doi.org/10.1002/mds.22559.

110. von Brevern M, Radtke A, Clarke AH, Lempert T. Migrainous vertigo presenting as episodic positional vertigo. *Neurology.* 2004;62(3):469–472.

111. von Brevern M. Acute migrainous vertigo: clinical and oculographic findings. *Brain.* 2004;128(2):365–374. http://dx.doi.org/10.1093/brain/awh351.

112. Lechner C, Taylor RL, Todd C, et al. Causes and characteristics of horizontal positional nystagmus. *J Neurol.* 2014; 261(5):1009–1017. http://dx.doi.org/10.1007/s00415-013-7223-5.

113. Kim H-A, Yi H-A, Lee H. Apogeotropic central positional nystagmus as a sole sign of nodular infarction. *Neurol Sci.* 2012;33(5):1189–1191. http://dx.doi.org/10.1007/s10072-011-0884-x.

114. Epley JM. The canalith repositioning procedure: for treatment of benign paroxysmal positional vertigo. *Otolaryngol Head Neck Surg.* 1992;107(3):399–404. http://dx.doi.org/10.1177/019459989210700310.

115. Semont A, Freyss G, Vitte E. Curing the BPPV with a liberatory maneuver. *Adv Otorhinolaryngol.* 1988;42:290–293.

CHAPTER 3

Development of the Vestibular System and of Balance Function: Differential Diagnosis in the Pediatric Population

ROBERT O'REILLY, MD • THIERRY MORLET, PHD • CHRIS GRINDLE, MD • EMILY ZWICKY, AUD • ERIN FIELD, PA-C

Clinicians are just beginning to adequately recognize pediatric vestibular disorders as an area of significant importance in the overall well-being of children. Mandates for universal newborn hearing screening have resulted in an early focus on auditory function in infants, facilitating the early identification and management of children with auditory pathology. This has vastly improved outcomes for children with hearing loss and has resulted in a welcomed spillover of increased awareness that auditory *and* vestibular pathology frequently co-occur.

From the day we are born until we reach old age, we are profoundly dependent on our sense of balance for our well-being and survival. Balance competence relies on complex interactions and central mediation of three important sensory systems: vision, vestibular function, and proprioception. Structurally, sensory systems related to balance are fully developed at birth. From infancy, balance function continues to mature with a sequential acquisition of motor milestones, including head control, sitting, standing, and walking, and develops thereafter through experiential learning and adaptation until adolescence. Changes in balance function are most rapid and pronounced during infancy and in preschool years when motor milestones needed for walking are realized, and as postural control and coordinated movements are refined. Nevertheless, changes in balance function continue to be evident as a function of aging throughout the human lifespan.[1]

OVERVIEW OF THE VESTIBULAR SYSTEM

The vestibular system is comprised of two otolith organs (the saccule and utricle), which sense linear acceleration (i.e., gravity and translational movements), and three semicircular canals, orthogonal with respect to each other, which are responsive to angular acceleration. The sensory hair cells of the otolith organs are located in the maculae and ampullae of the semicircular canals. Hair cell activation resulting from endolymphatic fluid flow (from head or body movement relative to gravity or a stationary position) generates afferent impulses that are transmitted to bipolar cells of the vestibular (Scarpa) ganglion, which houses cell bodies of vestibular afferent neurons. The axons of bipolar cells pass through the internal auditory canal (IAC) as separate superior and inferior divisions that come together as a single vestibular nerve. The superior vestibular nerve innervates the superior and lateral semicircular canals as well as the utricle. The inferior vestibular nerve innervates the posterior semicircular canal and the saccule. The vestibular nerve joins the cochlear nerve at the porus acusticus of the IAC, and together they travel through the cerebellopontine angle to the brainstem. These first-order neurons terminate in vestibular nuclei in the floor of the fourth ventricle without crossing the midline. The four major vestibular nuclei include the superior, lateral, medial, and descending vestibular nuclei. From the vestibular nuclei, axons project to the cerebellum, extraocular motor nuclei, antigravity muscles, and contralateral vestibular nuclei. Cortical representation of the vestibular system is at the level of parietal and insular regions of the cortex.[2]

EMBRYOLOGY
Inner Ear
Ongoing research and technological advances have significantly improved our understanding of the cellular differentiation and morphogenesis of the human vestibular labyrinth.[3] The first stages of inner ear

development begin as diffuse thickenings of surface ectoderm on either side of the embryonic (rhombencephalon) hindbrain. During the third week of embryonic development, the thickened surface ectoderm from either side of the embryonic hindbrain begins to invaginate, forming the otic placodes.

During week 4, the otic placodes are surrounded by proliferating embryonic mesoderm, creating otic pits. The otic pits subsequently pinch off from the surface ectoderm to form the closed, rounded structures of the otic vesicles. The otic vesicles further differentiate into upper and lower portions, forming the membranous cochlea and the vestibular apparatus. Different rates of growth among the semicircular canals, vestibular aqueduct, oval window, round window, and cochlea have been observed, suggesting that each part of the inner ear follows distinct trajectories during development.[4] The vestibular apparatus, located superiorly in relation to the cochlea, develops earlier and grows at a faster rate than the cochlea. The otic vesicle elongates and differentiates to form a dorsal utricular portion and a ventral saccular portion. The utricular portion becomes the semicircular canals and the utricle. Superior semicircular canals form first, followed by posterior and then lateral canals. The saccular portion becomes the saccule and the cochlear duct. The communication between the saccule and membranous cochlea narrows to form the ductus reuniens.

The bone that encapsulates the membranous labyrinth forms rapidly from the embryonic mesoderm over a period of approximately 5 weeks, between gestational weeks 19 and 23. Ossification of the otic capsule and encapsulation first occur in the area of the cochlea and superior semicircular canal at approximately 19 weeks' gestation. Encapsulation then appears to progress in an outward fashion from areas surrounding the vestibule to the canal vertices, with the last area of encapsulation being the posterolateral area of the horizontal semicircular canal at approximately 21–23 weeks' gestation.[3] Current consensus is that the vestibule is adultlike in form and size by 25 weeks of gestation; however, recent findings suggest that some parts of the labyrinth only reach the final size after birth. This seems to be the case for the internal aperture of the vestibular aqueduct, which is still growing and smaller than adult size at 39 weeks' gestation.[4]

Maturation of Vestibular Receptors

Around the third week of gestation, sensory epithelia develop from the ectoderm in the cristae of the forming semicircular canals and in the maculae of the forming otolith organs. By 7 weeks of gestation, small quantities of otoconia are present in the utricle. Thereafter, development proceeds quite rapidly, and within 1 week more otoconia are present in both the utricle and saccule, and cellular differentiation of the macular neural substrate is readily evident. Observations during the period of 7–12 weeks' gestation show that the calcium content of otoconia increases markedly in both the utricle and saccule; however, comparisons along the entire continuum of macular development reveal that the otoconia of the utricle appear to be more mature and varied in size and shape than saccular otoconia.[5] Vestibular hair cells first appear at approximately 7 weeks' gestation. Although vestibular hair cells are not fully differentiated, the beginnings of synapse formation in vestibular hair cells are observed in the human fetus at approximately 9–10 weeks' gestation. Differentiation of type I and type II hair cells begins between 11 and 13 weeks' gestation. In general, the morphologic sequence is from apex to base in the cristae and from center to periphery in the maculae. Significant numbers of fully formed calyx nerve endings are observed at 20 weeks' gestation. The maturing ampullary cristae become active as early as the eighth or ninth week of fetal life.[6] Reflexogenically, vestibular receptors become fully active by the 32nd week of gestation, at which time a fully developed Moro reflex can be elicited.[7] These observations suggest that vestibular afferents are mature and functional in the early stages of human development.

Development of vestibular pathways

Vestibular ganglion cells are of various shapes until the 21st week of gestation and become uniform in shape around the 24th week of gestation when development of the inner ear is complete. Morphometric studies show that ganglion cells grow until the 39th week, reaching maturity around the time of birth.[8] Neuronal connections between the labyrinths and the oculomotor nuclei in the brainstem occur between the 12th and 24th weeks of gestation. Myelination of the vestibular nerve begins around the 20th fetal week; it is the first cranial nerve to complete myelination.[9] The vestibular nuclear complex is functional at 21 weeks' gestation.

DEVELOPMENTAL REFLEXES

With the maturation of physiologic processes and anatomical structures, certain developmental reflexes can be elicited at birth or soon thereafter. These are primitive in nature, usually disappear as the child matures, and primarily reflect integrity of the brainstem and spinal cord.[10] Their persistence beyond the normally expected age of dissipation indicates delayed maturation or impaired nervous system function. Asymmetry of these reflexes suggests either a central or a peripheral nervous system disorder.

The *Moro reflex* is elicited by holding the child supine and allowing the head to drop approximately 30 degrees in relation to the trunk. Extension and abduction of the arms with fanning out of the fingers, followed by adduction of the arms at the shoulder, takes place as a normal response. This reflex normally disappears by age 5–6 months.

The *tonic neck reflex* is tested by turning the head of the child to one side while the child is lying supine with shoulders fixed. The arm and leg toward the side that the head is turned extend, whereas the arm and leg on the opposite side flex. This reflex normally disappears by the age of 6 months.

The *head righting reflex* develops by the age of 4–6 months. To test this reflex, the child's trunk is held 30 degrees from the vertical. A normally responding infant will then tilt the head so that it remains vertical. At approximately 5 months, the child will additionally move the lower limbs away from the side to which they have been tilted, thereby signaling functional integration of visual, vestibular, and proprioceptive stimuli.[9]

The *parachute reaction* can be elicited in infants over the age of 5 months with a sudden downward movement of a vertically held child, which causes the lower limbs to extend and abduct. This reflex is considered to represent visual-vestibular interaction[9] with the otolith organs presumably involved.

The *Doll's eye response* is found normally in full-term babies within 2 weeks of birth. When the baby (facing the examiner) is held at arm's length and rotated in one direction around the examiner, a deviation of the eyes and head opposite to the direction of the rotation is produced, representing vestibular activity. Owing to an immature saccadic system at this stage, the fast component of a normal nystagmic response is not seen. Later, however, nystagmus is apparent, with the fast component in the direction of rotation.[11]

Development of Vestibular-Induced Reflexes

Balance and equilibrium are maintained through a series of events triggered by sensory stimulation. Incoming sensory inputs received from vestibular, visual and somatosensory/proprioceptive systems are directed to the vestibular nuclei and cerebellum for processing and calibration. In response to afferent inputs, the vestibular nuclear complex creates direct and remarkably rapid efferent connections to muscles controlling eye movement, as well as the neck and spinal cord. These motor outputs stimulate three vestibular reflexes (vestibulo-ocular vestibulospinal, and vestibulocollic), which allow us to maintain control of our gaze, postural stability, and our balance and equilibrium. It is through examination of these reflexes that we are provided a window for

uncovering vestibular dysfunction. Understanding how vestibular responses differ among infants, children, adolescents, and adults is crucial when attempting to evaluate and diagnose vestibular pathology.

Vestibulo-ocular reflex

The purpose of the vestibulo-ocular reflex (VOR) is to stabilize gaze and maintain clear vision when the body or head is in motion. Objects of visual interest are maintained on the fovea of the retina through inputs from semicircular canals and otolith organs.

Historically, data regarding VOR function in infants and children have been somewhat limited owing to technical difficulties inherent in achieving compliance and obtaining accurate recordings. The VOR is also subject to alteration from a variety of nonvestibular influences, including subject attention and state of arousal, unintended ocular fixation due to light leaks, inadequate calibration, and insufficient head stabilization during testing. In several decades of research with children, many techniques have been used to explore and record the pediatric VOR. These include caloric stimulation, rotational (torsion swing) stimulation, and passive whole body (en bloc) rotation techniques. Depending on the technique used, parameters such as the speed of the slow component of eye movement (expressed in degrees per second), amplitude of nystagmus beat, and latency and duration of response have been recorded.[12] Researchers using en bloc rotational techniques have explored factors such as gain (the ratio of peak eye velocity to peak head velocity), phase (the timing difference between head and eye velocities), symmetry (the comparison of rightward and leftward eye velocities), and vestibular time constant (the number of seconds required for the slow-phase eye velocity to decline by two-thirds of its maximum value).

The VOR is present at birth; however, vestibular time constants are approximately one-half of normal adult values in neonates aged 24–120 hours. Vestibular time constants appear to approach adult values by 2 months of age.[13] These differences are a reflection of the immaturity of visual pathways at birth, which indicates that maturation of visual pathways is a necessary precursor for adequate calibration of the VOR and for competent function of velocity storage mechanisms necessary for stable vision. Reflexive slow component nystagmus of the VOR generated by vestibular stimulation is routinely observed at birth; however, the centrally mediated fast component, which returns and maintains the eyes within the physical confines of the orbits, is variably present.[14] Infants demonstrate inaccurate saccades, frequently requiring more than one saccade to reach the target. The saccadic system is immature at birth, continuing to develop up to the age of 2 years.[15] The velocity of the VOR slow component as well as the frequency of nystagmic beats increase as a function of age until age 6–12 months, after which values reach a plateau and stabilize.[12] Smooth pursuit is also only possible at very low frequencies in neonates because of foveal immaturity. A higher gain of the VOR in response to sinusoidal rotation is observed in children compared with adults and is due to immature visual-vestibular interaction, with poorer suppression of the VOR response. VOR gain and vestibular time constants in response to sustained angular acceleration reveal that vestibular time constants increase, whereas VOR gain shows small but significant decreases as a function of age from 2 months to 11 years.[16] In a recent large longitudinal study, Casselbrant et al.[17] observed that, in response to both sinusoidal and constant velocity rotations on an earth vertical axis, VOR gain increases linearly (ratio of peak eye velocity to peak head velocity) as a function of age from 3 to 9 years but phase differences appear to remain stable. These findings are in contrast to several other studies that have shown a decreased or stable VOR gain as a function of a child's increasing age.

In summary, the human VOR goes through several developmental stages, with a healthy response developing by several months beyond full term,[18] and absence of the VOR by the age of 10 months should be considered an abnormal finding.[12,19] It is evident that regardless of the parameter explored, the underlying prevailing motif across all studies of pediatric VOR is that qualitative differences exist between the VOR function of children and adults[20-24] and that these differences seem to persist until preadolescence.

Vestibulospinal reflex

Whether the body is stationary or in motion, continuous afferent signals from vision and vestibular inputs detect the body's orientation and relationship to gravity. These inputs combine with touch receptors of the skin as well as proprioceptors on the soles of the feet, the hands, and torso to detect the body's contact with the environment. The sum of these inputs provides the information needed to generate the vestibulospinal reflex (VSR), which stabilizes the body and maintains postural control. VSR signals travel along three major pathways, including the lateral, medial, and reticulospinal tracts. When activated, these neural tracts impact anterior horn cells of the spinal cord and generate myotactic, deep tendon reflexes in antigravity skeletal muscles of the limbs and trunk.

The VSR has more numerous and complex innervations than the VOR, but just as the VOR works to contract and relax paired ocular muscles, the VSR works to create a push-pull arrangement of agonist and antagonist muscle groups firing across the neural axis. A variety of diagnostic tests exploring aspects of VSR function have been developed for use with both children and adults. In general, when comparing the VSR function of children with that of adults, as noted by Rine,[25] the postural control of these groups varies significantly. As detailed later in this chapter, the vestibulospinal mechanism and effectiveness of the vestibular system in postural control continues to develop until at least 15 years of age.

Vestibulocollic reflex

The vestibulocollic reflex (VCR) plays an important role in stabilizing vision by compensating for head movements when the body is in motion. Through patterned contractions of neck muscles, the VCR stabilizes the bobbing of the head caused by vibrations transmitted from the heels as they strike the ground during walking and running. Thus the VCR assists in stabilizing the head on the neck and in keeping the head still and level, especially during ambulation. As we walk, vestibular signals caused by linear translations stimulate nerve receptors of the saccule. In response, the saccule transmits afferent signals along the inferior vestibular nerve and ganglion to the vestibular nuclear complex in the brainstem. From vestibular nuclei, efferent signals are sent via the medial vestibulospinal tract and spinal accessory nerve to neck muscles, including the sternocleidomastoid muscle, one of the long neck muscles extending from the thorax to the base of the skull behind the ear.

In the last decade, VCR function has become routinely explored through recordings of vestibular evoked myogenic potentials (VEMPs). VEMPs have become an increasingly popular clinical technique because, unlike other tests of vestibular function, VEMPs provide information regarding saccular and inferior vestibular nerve function. This is a significant benefit because otolith organs and anterior and posterior semicircular canals may be more instrumental in locomotion and posture control than horizontal semicircular canals explored by the VOR.[26] In addition, the VEMP test is an objective measure that can be reliably recorded from surface electrodes in a wide variety of patients, including infants and young children. VEMPs are stimulated by high-intensity auditory stimuli that cause robust vibration of the ossicular chain and stimulate the saccule, which rests in close proximity. Neural impulses traveling along the VEMP neural pathway stimulate the VCR, creating an efferent inhibitory release of the tonically contracted sternocleidomastoid muscle. VEMP recordings appear as a biphasic EMG potential, with an initial positive deflection at 13 ms post stimulus onset (P13) and a negative deflection at 23 ms (N23). A word of caution is required regarding high stimulus intensities necessary to elicit VEMPs. When a stimulus is delivered to the small ear canal of a pediatric patient, stimulus intensity can reach 130–135 dB, which can be painful and potentially damaging to hearing.

Studies recording VEMPs in preterm neonates, infants, and young children have confirmed the efficacy of VEMP recordings in the pediatric population. These studies have pointed out differences between VEMP responses of children and adults, suggesting again maturational effects from preschool age through adolescence.[24,27]

BALANCE AND MOTOR DEVELOPMENT

Maintenance of postural balance requires an active sensorimotor control system. In adults, the sensory systems are well organized and act in a context-specific way.[28] Postural control involves sensory feedback,[29] and visual and proprioceptive inputs need to be integrated in order for the center of foot pressure to move in phase with the body's center of mass. In children, the sensory systems are not completely developed, although their anatomic structures are mature early in life.[30] Proprioceptive, visual, and vestibular systems develop more slowly than the hierarchically lower automatic motor processes that mature early in childhood.[31] The importance of visual cues in maintaining static posture has been well demonstrated, particularly in children who are accustomed to visually monitoring the body during postural adjustments.[32,33] As important are cognitive functions for organization and integration of available sensory information under both static and dynamic conditions, and this has also been well documented.[34] Hence, selection of the appropriate balance strategy not only depends on environmental demands but also is a function of neuromaturation and experience.

In typically developing children, postural stability proceeds in a cephalocaudal fashion, with the infant first achieving control of the head, then the trunk, and finally postural stability in standing.[35,36] The newborn infant, when held ventrally with a hand under the abdomen, cannot hold up the head. By 6 weeks of age the head is held in the plane of the body and by 12 weeks, above this level. Head control, allowing the baby to look around in a horizontal plane, is achieved by 16 weeks of age, and by the 36th week, the infant is

able to sit unsupported for a few minutes. By the age of 1 year, the child is able to crawl on hands and knees and stand up holding on to furniture. At approximately 15–16 months of age the child is normally able to start walking.[37]

Coordination of postural responses develops until at least 10[28,31] to 15 years of age.[24,26,38,39] In balance control, somatosensory inputs receive priority in adults, whereas children prefer visual inputs to vestibular information in achieving their postural equilibrium.[40] Infants and young children (aged 4 months to 2 years) are dependent on the visual system to maintain balance.[41,42] At 3–6 years of age, children begin to use somatosensory information appropriately,[31,40,43,44] although some studies indicate that development continues until the age of 9–11 years.[45] In the case of an intersensory conflict, the vestibular system provides a referential function by suppressing any input that is not congruent with vestibular information.[43] Owing to presumably mature vestibular function, even with misleading visual information, adults are able improve their postural control. Children by age 12 years are still not able to select and process misleading visual information.[46] Among the three sensory inputs in children, the vestibular system seems to be the least effective in postural control,[40,47–49] and functional efficiency of the vestibular system in children of 10–15 years of age is still developing.[43,44,48] Development of several visual functions, such as saccade latency, contrast sensitivity, or chromatic sensitivity, does not approach adult levels until approximately 12 years of age.[50] The visual influence on standing stability is reported to be established at adult levels around the age of 15 years.[43,44] Adult-like postural stability resulting from complete maturation of the three integral sensory systems and the ability to solve intersensory conflict situations can thus be assumed in adolescents around 15 years of age.[24,26,43,44,48,51]

In summary, vestibular function is present at birth but continues to mature so that it is most responsive between 6 and 12 months of age. Subsequently, vestibular responses are gradually modulated and refined by developing central inhibitory influences, cerebellar control, visual development, and central vestibular adaptation[9,15,16] and reach adultlike maturity around 15 years of age.

INCIDENCE OF VESTIBULAR DISORDERS IN THE PEDIATRIC POPULATION

The general prevalence of pediatric vestibular dysfunction is estimated between 8% and 18%, although the incidence of vertigo as a primary complaint in a review of hospital records was less than 1%.[52]

The Differential Diagnosis

Children do not complain about vestibular dysfunction, and therefore the diagnosis relies on careful questioning of the child (if applicable) and parents, targeted imaging/testing, and an astute clinician to synthesize the findings into a cohesive diagnosis. Abnormal responses in children need further clarification to distinguish whether the problem rests primarily with the vestibular system and vestibular pathways or with abnormalities in visual, motor, or proprioceptive systems, which jointly contribute to acquisition of motor milestones.

Patient History

Vertigo, defined as the subjective sensation of movement, can be difficult for many patients to describe. This is intrinsically the case because central vestibular projections to the cerebral cortex are diffuse. This challenge is even more apparent in the pediatric population where children do not have the breadth of experience or vocabulary to describe this sensation. As such, vestibular disorders in children can be difficult to recognize. Children with vestibular disorders are often written off as clumsy or uncoordinated, or dysfunction is misjudged to be secondary to a behavioral abnormality. Children may present with complaints of abdominal pain, ataxia, headache, visual disturbance, hearing loss, otalgia, or otorrhea. On the other hand, children with vestibular disorders may have no complaints. In a study of 62 children with basilar skull fracture, 34% of whom had sensorineural hearing loss (SNHL), "few" of the children had vestibular complaints.[53]

It is frequently possible with a careful history, engaging both the child and caregiver, to identify the likely cause of the balance disorder even in the most complex patients. A series of focused questions, based on the excellent work by G. Michael Halmagyi,[54] helps differentiate the nature of the pathology in most patients (Table 3.1).

Care should be given to note any symptoms that may be related to vestibular dysfunction, such as vertigo, oscillopsia, drop attacks without loss of consciousness, lateropulsion, and vegetative symptoms (e.g., nausea, emesis, malaise). Of particular importance in children is to determine if there is any history of delayed motor development (e.g., rolling over, sitting, crawling, walking, or running), frequent falls, and even learning disabilities, which may result from poor dynamic visual acuity due to deficiency of the VOR.

"What Does It Feel like?"

This question is the first step in differentiating a true illusion of movement (vertigo) that is indicative of abnormality in the vestibular end organ or pathways from some other unrelated sensation, such as a pre-syncopal feeling. This is particularly important in early teenage females who can develop orthostatic hypotension. One must elicit any evidence of anxiety with hyperventilation, which will produce a light-headed feeling. Vestibular disorders will almost always produce some sense of vertigo, which is exacerbated by movement. Central vestibular pathway disorders tend not to produce as large a degree of vegetative symptoms or exacerbation by movement as is common with peripheral disorders. Any change in sensorium, particularly with a history of seizure disorder, should prompt consideration of temporal lobe seizures.

"What Other Symptoms Are Associated With It?"

It is important to ascertain any evidence of aural symptoms (i.e., hearing loss, aural fullness, tinnitus, and fluctuation in hearing) that might be related to vestibulopathy. Evidence of neurologic symptoms or cranial nerve weakness needs to be investigated. A history of headache or paroxysmal torticollis is important to ascertain if the patient has migraine-related vertigo or benign recurrent vertigo of childhood. The clinician should also inquire about palpitations, dyspnea, or feelings of anxiety.

"How Long Do the Symptoms Typically Last and How Many Have Occurred?"

This is a key question that helps differentiate the nature of vestibulopathy. Very brief, recurrent episodes are generally indicative of benign paroxysmal positional vertigo (BPPV). This is important to consider in the setting of head trauma, particularly in children who participate in contact sports. Episodes lasting hours at a time may indicate attacks of hydrops, migraine, or posterior circulation compromise (which is extremely rare in children). One long episode generally indicates an insult to the vestibular apparatus such as might result from vestibular neuritis or labyrinthitis. In contradistinction to adults, most children with a normal central nervous system (CNS) attain central compensation for this type of lesion much more rapidly than adults (days vs. weeks to months).

"What Makes It Worse or Better?"

Onset with rolling over, bending over, or looking up is typical of posterior semicircular canal BPPV. Worsening of vertigo with Valsalva maneuver or straining may be seen with perilymph fistula, particularly if there is a history of head or ear trauma or known middle or inner ear malformation.

TABLE 3.1

Clinical Information Regarding the Patient History Obtained From a Series of Focused Questions

Question	Clinical Information
What does it feel like?	• Is this vestibular/labyrinthine (vertigo) or something else (presyncope, syncope, seizure)
What other symptoms are associated with it?	• Declining hearing after head trauma (EVA) • Tinnitus, hearing loss (hydrops) • Dysarthria, diplopia, paresthesias (vertebrobasilar disease) • Cranial nerve weakness (skull base, intracranial lesions) • Headache, paroxysmal torticollis (migraine, BPVC) • Sweating, palpitations, dyspnea (orthostasis, panic attacks)
How long do the symptoms last and how many have occurred?	• Seconds to minutes (BPPV) • Hours (TIA, migraine, hydrops) • Days to weeks (labyrinthitis, vestibular neuritis)
What makes it better or worse?	• Vestibular generated vertigo always worse with movement • Rolling, bending (BPPV) • Valsalva (PLF)
What is the background history?	• Otologic disease (PLF, labyrinthitis, BPPV) • SNHL (syndromic/nonsyndromic/congenital vs. acquired), ototoxic medications, congenital or acquired vestibular hypofunction • Neuropathies (peripheral neuropathy) • Vascular disease (congenital cardiopulmonary disease, von Hippel-Lindau with intracranial vascular lesions) • Family history neoplasms (NF-2, Gorlin syndrome, Costello syndrome) (acoustic neuroma, medulloblastoma) • Anxiety/depression (panic attacks) • Motion intolerance (migraine) • Family history of balance disorders (periodic ataxias, migraine, hereditary vestibulopathy) • Autoimmune disease (autoimmune inner ear disease) • Seizure history (temporal lobe seizures) • Ophthalmologic disease (oculomotor anomaly, amblyopia, disorders of acuity, depth perception) • Trauma

BPPV, benign paroxysmal positional vertigo; *BPVC*, benign paroxysmal vertigo of childhood; *EVA*, enlarged vestibular aqueduct; *PLF*, perilymphatic fistula; *SNHL*, sensorineural hearing loss; *TIA*, transient ischemic attack.

"What is the Background History?"

It is of vital importance to elicit any history of otologic disease or surgery (cochlear implant, chronic ear or cholesteatoma surgery), exposure to ototoxic medications, head or ear trauma, autoimmune disease, seizure disorder, ophthalmologic disease, hearing loss of any type, vascular or cardiac disease, and family history of neoplasm, as these may guide the differential diagnosis and workup.

Physical Examination

The physical examination should include the standard ear, nose, and throat examination and neurologic examination, including cranial nerve examination, muscle strength, reflexes, and cerebellar testing. In addition, a test of visual acuity and dynamic visual acuity should be

considered. Next the clinician should search for evidence of static and dynamic imbalance of vestibular function.

Static Imbalance

In infants and young children who cannot cooperate with many parts of the examination, the presence of a functional VOR can be assessed by looking for per-rotation and post-rotation nystagmus while accelerating in a circle. To asses this, the clinician sits on a rotating stool, occupies the child's gaze with an interesting object attached to the clinician, and accelerates briefly in alternating directions. With an intact VOR, fast-phase nystagmus toward the direction of acceleration can be observed. Older children are instructed to look at a finger or some interesting object that will hold

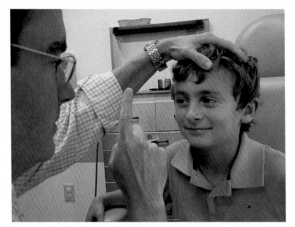

FIG. 3.1 Search for spontaneous and gaze-evoked nystagmus.

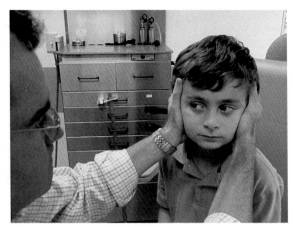

FIG. 3.3 Head thrust maneuver to test the vestibular ocular reflex.

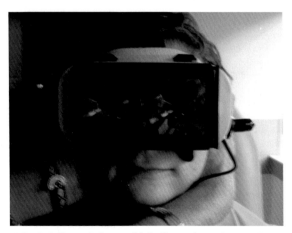

FIG. 3.2 Frenzel glasses (high-diopter lenses) prevent fixation and aid in identification of nystagmus.

their attention to search for spontaneous nystagmus or gaze-evoked nystagmus, the former indicative of active asymmetry in vestibular function and the latter indicative of a CNS disorder (Fig. 3.1). Spontaneous nystagmus is most easily seen when fixation is removed with Frenzel glasses (Fig. 3.2).

This should be done in all cardinal gaze positions but not the extremes of gaze (>30 degrees) to prevent physiologic nystagmus from extraocular muscle elasticity. In patients recovering from acute peripheral vestibular injury, the progression of central compensation can be observed as they progress from third degree, to second degree, to first degree, to no spontaneous nystagmus.

Vertical nystagmus indicates either a pontine lesion (up-beating nystagmus) or cranial cervical junction lesion (down-beating nystagmus). The latter is very important to note in children, as it may be seen in association with ataxia in children with large compressing Chiari malformations. This may be magnified by asking the patient to perform the Valsalva maneuver. Having the patient slightly hyperventilate may unmask nystagmus produced by demyelinating lesions of the brain parenchyma or from eighth nerve compression. Tragal compression may produce predominantly horizontal nystagmus seen in perilymph fistula. Neck rotation with the head stable is said to produce nystagmus related to "cervicogenic vertigo."

Dynamic Imbalance

Tests of dynamic imbalance include the "head thrust maneuver" or "head impulse test." The patient is asked to fixate on a stationary target and the head rapidly moved left, right, up, or down (Fig. 3.3). If the VOR is deficient, a stationary gaze cannot be maintained and corrective "refixation" saccades are evident. This may be followed by a test to observe post-headshake nystagmus. With Frenzel glasses in place, the head is oscillated from side to side symmetrically then stopped. Vestibular asymmetry leads to several easily observable beats of nystagmus, with the fast phase directed toward the side of the intact horizontal semicircular canal. The Dix-Hallpike maneuver can be performed to search for evidence of BPPV (Fig. 3.4). Right, left, and center head hanging positions are tested. This can be followed by particle repositioning maneuvers if necessary.

Vestibulospinal Testing

The clinician can assess the Romberg, sharpened Romberg, and tests of past pointing. The Fukuda stepping

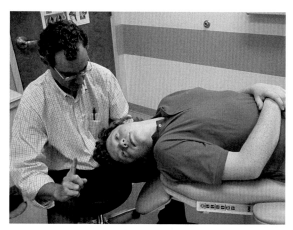

FIG. 3.4 Dix-Hallpike maneuver.

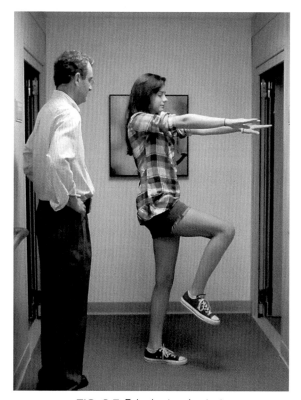

FIG. 3.5 Fukuda stepping test.

test is easily performed by asking the child to march in place with eyes closed to look for abnormal rotation (Fig. 3.5).

Gait and Gross Motor Assessment

Subjective evaluation of age-appropriate gait can be tested in the clinic to look for gait asymmetry and

ataxia. Age-appropriate gross motor assessments are also available, such as the Peabody test of gross motor development (15 days–71 months of age) and the Bruininks-Oseretsky test of motor performance (4–21 years of age). Such testing may be important to complete the picture in children with imbalance, as hypotonia and delayed motor development significantly affect balance performance.

CHARACTERISTICS OF VESTIBULAR DISORDERS IN THE PEDIATRIC POPULATION

To help pare down the differential diagnosis of balance disorders in children, various authors have subcategorized disorders based on the site of origin (i.e., peripheral or central), frequency of symptoms (i.e., acute nonrecurring, recurrent, or chronic), or nonvertiginous dizziness, disequilibrium, or ataxia.[55,56] When considering that balance is maintained by visual, proprioceptive, and vestibular systems and that a dysfunction in any one of these areas could manifest as a balance disorder, it is understandable that the differential diagnosis would be broad. In a review of all pediatric patients complaining of dizziness or with vestibular dysfunction who presented to our clinics over a 4-year period, patients could be broadly categorized into three groups. Peripheral vestibulopathy was found in 29.5% (39 of 132) of patients, migraine/benign recurrent vertigo of childhood was found in 24.2% (32 of 132) of patients, and the remaining 45% were divided into several groups, each comprising fewer than 10% of the total patient population. Diagnoses in this group included motor/developmental delay, traumatic brain injury, CNS structural lesion, behavioral disorders, idiopathic imbalance, neurodegenerative disease, encephalopathy, vascular lesions, peripheral neuropathy, and oculomotor disorders. These findings are consistent with other large series that have looked at pediatric vestibular dysfunction.[52,55–59]

More recently, we have reviewed our last 472 patients who were evaluated in a multidisciplinary vestibular and balance clinic (Table 3.2). Most of the patients were found to have a central cause of their vertigo, with migraine affecting 46%. Many patients with peripheral vestibular disorders also had SNHL and/or inner ear malformations. Almost 13% of patients had a mixed central and peripheral injury, presenting a significant therapeutic challenge.

SNHL is reported to be associated with vestibular dysfunction in 20%–70% of pediatric patients.[60] On analysis of children with profound SNHL, Cushing

TABLE 3.2
Diagnosis of Vestibular Disorders in the Pediatric Population

Diagnosis (% Total)		N	Age at Diagnosis (years ± SD)	Gender (% Females)
Central (45.13%)		**213**	**10.3 ± 4.8**	**57.7**
	Migraine	98	12.1 ± 4.0	64.3
	BPVC/Paroxysmal Torticollis	17	3.2 ± 2.4	70.6
	Structural	66	10.0 ± 4.3	45.4
	Vascular	13	11.5 ± 3.3	69.2
	Other (ataxia, neurodegeneration)	12	10.7 ± 6.3	58.3
	Inflammatory	7	3.1 ± 2.0	42.8
Peripheral (25.85%)		**122**	**10.0 ± 5.0**	**54.1**
	SNHL, OM	34	6.8 ± 4.3	47.0
	Inner ear malformation/Erosion	32	9.2 ± 4.7	46.9
	Vestibular hypofunction	21	10.3 ± 4.7	66.7
	Inflammatory (vestibular neuritis/labyrinthitis)	20	13.7 ± 4.3	70
	Endolymphatic hydrops	8	12.7 ± 3.8	25
	BPPV	7	14 ± 3.3	71.4
Central and Peripheral (12.92%)		**61**	**12.5 ± 4.1**	**44.3**
	TBI/Temporal bone fracture	54	13.2 ± 3.5	38.9
	CMV	6	6.3 ± 4.2	83.3
	Other	1	15	100
Miscellaneous (16.1%)		**76**	**8 ± 4.7**	**47.4**
	Developmental delays	50	6.1 ± 4.1	44
	Other	10	10 ± 4.2	40
	Anxiety	10	12.6 ± 1.9	70
	Psychiatric	6	13.2 ± 2.9	50

BPPV, benign paroxysmal positional vertigo; *BPVC*, benign paroxysmal vertigo of childhood; *CMV*, cytomegalovirus; *SNHL*, sensorineural hearing loss; *TBI*, traumatic brain injury; *OM*, otitis media.

et al.[61] showed that there was a 50% incidence of horizontal semicircular canal dysfunction and a 38% incidence of saccular dysfunction. Identification of these concomitant vestibular impairments is of critical importance, as therapies can be tailored to adequately deal with multiple sensory deficits.

Otitis media can be a significant contributor to balance disorders in children. This is thought to be due to either pressure changes within the middle ear or toxins secreted into the middle ear that leak into the inner ear and directly affect the vestibule.[62,63] When tested, children often have abnormalities present in electronystagmography and motor proficiency tests. Myringotomy with tympanostomy tube insertion has been reported to mitigate balance disorders associated with otitis media.[64] In the case of chronic otitis media with cholesteatoma formation, there may be direct involvement of the vestibule by the cholesteatoma. Typically this occurs in lateral and posterior semicircular canals. There may be erosion of bone, leading to perilymphatic (semicircular canal) fistula or labyrinthitis. In some cases, vertigo may be the presenting symptom of chronic otitis media. Children with otitis media with effusion rely more on vision than those without effusion. These children also have demonstrated increased postural sway with moving visual scenes.[65]

Congenital vestibular hypofunction can be associated with syndromic or non-syndromic causes. Usher syndrome is the most common autosomal recessive cause of SNHL associated with vestibular dysfunction. There are three major types. Type I includes profound hearing loss, retinitis pigmentosa, and vestibular hypofunction. Type II has less hearing loss and normal vestibular function. Type III is characterized by progressive SNHL and progressive vestibular dysfunction. It is important to differentiate among the types of this syndrome, as this can have profound effects on targeted therapy for patients with multiple sensory losses. Genetic testing is available for Usher syndrome.

Pendred syndrome is another autosomal recessive cause of vestibular dysfunction. This is a constellation of Mondini malformation (incomplete partition of the cochlea), dilated vestibule, and enlarged vestibular aqueduct (EVA). Vestibular dysfunction may be present in up to one-third of patients.[66] Nonsyndromic, congenital malformations of the inner ear, such as Mondini malformation, Scheibe aplasia (cochleosaccular dysplasia), and EVA may have vestibular manifestations.

CHARGE syndrome (coloboma, heart defects, choanal atresia, retardation of growth and development, genital anomalies, and ear abnormalities) has variable degrees of ear abnormalities, although almost all patients have congenital absence of semicircular canals.

BPPV is the most common cause of vertigo in the adult population (see Chapter 9). This phenomenon of brief periods of motion-provoked, position-dependent vertigo is thought to arise from displaced otoconia in the semicircular canals or on the cupula of the semicircular canals (typically, the posterior semicircular canal). This pathology is rare in children. For those children affected, there is often a history of trauma or vestibular neuritis. Symptoms typically resolve over time, but patients may benefit from canalith repositioning exercises (e.g., Epley maneuver).

Vestibular neuritis is presumed to result from viral infection of the vestibular nerve or labyrinthine end organ (see Chapter 10). Children with vestibular neuritis experience severe, sudden onset of vertigo and spontaneous nystagmus without hearing loss. The onset of symptoms is typically abrupt and is caused by sudden loss of vestibular function on the affected side. These symptoms may last for weeks to months in adults, but in children, symptoms are typically resolved completely by 2–4 weeks. This may reflect the increased plasticity of central compensation mechanisms in children.[67]

Meniere's disease is an idiopathic condition of the labyrinth associated with endolymphatic hydrops. The complete pathophysiology of Meniere's disease is poorly understood. Symptoms in children are the same as those in adults: tinnitus, fluctuating hearing loss, especially in low frequencies, and episodic vertigo. Meniere's disease is exceedingly rare in children, responsible for less than 4% of children with balance disorders.[68] Because of its rarity in children, care must be taken to rule out other inner ear anomalies (e.g., EVA syndrome) and autoimmune inner ear disease, which may present with a "hydropic" clinical picture.

Congenital cytomegalovirus (CMV) infection is estimated to affect 0.4%–2.3% of live births in the United States, and up to 90% of those are asymptomatic at birth. About 8%–15% of asymptomatic patients will present with SNHL later in life. Symptomatic CMV infection leads to SNHL in 30%–65% of patients. Vestibular insult can be expected in patients who are severely affected. The dual CNS and inner ear insult resulting from congenital CMV may be very difficult to rehabilitate. Fluctuation and deterioration in hearing typically parallels spells of vertigo in this population.[69]

The surgical trauma of cochlear implantation can cause vestibular symptoms. The standard placement of the implant electrode array within the scala tympani of the cochlea is purported to cause alterations in normal inner ear fluid composition, inflammation, and fibrosis with hair cell loss.[70] Transient dizziness is common after cochlear implantation but typically resolves rapidly. It has been noted that up to 50% of cochlear implant candidates have a preexisting vestibular deficit and that those with normal vestibular function will have alteration of vestibular function after implant.[71] Clinically, this appears to be of limited consequence in most of the pediatric patients, as they achieve rapid vestibular compensation in the face of a normal CNS.

Trauma of the temporal bone can precipitate vertigo. Temporal bone fractures occur in approximately 10% of pediatric patients with blunt head trauma.[66] Fracture can be longitudinal (i.e., along the axis of the petrous bone; 70%–80%) or transverse (i.e., perpendicular to the axis of the petrous bone; 20%–30%). Transverse fracture is most likely to involve the otic capsule, with resultant vestibular injury and SNHL.[55] In addition to the injury from the trauma itself, the insult can predispose the patient to BPPV later in life. Compensation for the consequent loss of vestibular function is generally rapid in children.

Head trauma and direct trauma of the tympanic membrane or middle ear may result in acquired perilymphatic fistula. Typical of this would be stapes subluxation from "Q-tip" injury to the tympanic membrane. Typical symptoms of perilymph fistula include hearing loss and vertigo, particularly after straining. In patients with suspected perilymph fistula, surgical repair may be considered to control vertigo symptoms when conservative management is unsuccessful.

Cogan syndrome is an autoimmune process that presents with nonsyphilitic interstitial keratitis, acute SNHL, and vestibulopathy. The hearing loss may be progressive. The timing and association of symptoms of Cogan syndrome can be highly variable, making diagnosis difficult.[72] Despite this, an accurate and prompt diagnosis is essential, as high-dose steroids may help to limit the degree of SNHL and vestibulopathy.

Labyrinthitis is an acute inflammatory process of the labyrinth. Typically, symptoms are both auditory and vestibular and may range from minor to severe. Bacterial labyrinthitis is usually the result of bacterial invasion of the inner ear through the cochlear aqueduct in patients with bacterial meningitis. The labyrinth may also be infected from a middle ear source. Both medical and surgical intervention may be required to control this process, and the vestibular insult is often complete and profound. In addition, several viruses are known to cause labyrinthitis, including those viruses causing mumps, measles, influenza, and infectious mononucleosis.

Congenital and acquired "third windows" of the labyrinth may result in vestibular symptoms through the "Tullio" effect. Semicircular canal dehiscence is readily diagnosed by appropriate imaging (computed tomography [CT]) and a characteristically abnormally low VEMP threshold with a very large amplitude response.[73]

Unlike the typical presentation of throbbing unilateral frontal head pain in adults, children often manifest migraine with other symptoms. Disequilibrium and vertigo are very common migraine equivalents in children. In our series, migraine was the underlying diagnosis in 24.2% of patients. Vertigo and disequilibrium may precede headache; however, vertigo may occur in isolation separate from the headache. Symptoms may be severe and may last for several hours. Patients may have associated nausea, vomiting, photophobia, phonophobia, and sensitivity to odors. Symptoms may be worsened by fatigue.[56]

Diagnosis of migraine-related vertigo requires a careful and detailed history and physical examination. The otologic examination typically is normal in these patients, but there may be subtle abnormalities in audiometric and vestibular testing, including pathologic nystagmus during an acute attack[74] and reduced otoacoustic emission suppression.[75] Basic audiometry is usually normal[76]; thus the lack of objective findings does not preclude the diagnosis. Imaging is often obtained to rule out intracranial masses or lesions, and findings on CT and MRI are normal. Migraine-related vertigo is most common in teenage females.

Benign paroxysmal vertigo of childhood (BPVC) is a unique migraine variant that was first described by Basser in 1964.[77] BPVC typically occurs in children 3–8 years old. Attacks are sudden in onset, may occur in any position (i.e., sitting, standing, moving, stationary), and are typically brief, lasting only a few seconds to minutes. The affected child may remain still, refusing to move, or may grab onto something for support; nystagmus is often noted during the attack. There is often associated anxiety, pallor, nausea, sweating, and occasionally vomiting. No pain is associated with the events, and there is no loss of consciousness. At the completion of the attack, the child usually resumes normal activity.[59] Physical examination and all imaging studies are normal. BPVC rarely occurs after age 8 years. It is reported that 43% of patients with BPVC have a positive family history of migraine. Children affected with BPVC may develop classic migraines later in life, reported at an incidence of 13%,[78] often many years after the cessation of BPVC symptoms.[79]

Paroxysmal torticollis of infancy is considered in the same spectrum as BPVC, as a component of the periodic juvenile migraine disorders.[59] Paroxysmal torticollis consists of episodic head tilt, which may have associated nausea, vomiting, pallor, and agitation. The episodes are brief and self-limited. They may alternate from side to side. The symptoms typically resolve by 2–3 years of age.[55]

Basilar migraine is a particular variant of migraine that comprises 3%–19% of childhood migraine. Vertigo may be particularly apparent in this form of migraine. Clinically, children present with an aura of vertigo, visual disturbance, or ataxia. Pain follows but may be occipital in location, unlike the frontal or bitemporal pain typical of migraine in adults.[80] The average age of onset is 7 years, and females are most often affected.

Head trauma and resultant traumatic brain injury or labyrinthine concussion can result in vestibulopathy. The reported incidence of dizziness after head trauma varies greatly in the literature, ranging from 15% to 78%. Regardless, it should be considered that even minor head trauma may result in vestibular pathology. Mechanisms for vestibular injury include direct trauma to the eighth nerve complex and root entry zone at the brainstem or labyrinthine concussion. In the latter, there are several theories as to the cause of the vestibular end-organ injury. There may be injury or disruption of the microcirculation of the vestibule with resultant hemorrhage and inflammation. The concussive pressure wave itself may cause rupture of the membranous labyrinth.[81] Typically, patients are affected immediately after the trauma. Children usually recover completely; however, rarely they may develop BPPV.[55]

CNS structural lesions are among the principle concerns in a child presenting with new-onset vertigo. In our series, CNS structural lesions accounted for 9.1% of patients with vertigo and disequilibrium. Symptomatic malformations may include Chiari malformation with syrinx formation, spinocerebellar atrophy, arachnoid cyst of the posterior fossa, and delayed myelination disorders. Tumors of the posterior fossa may also contribute to balance dysfunction. The most common posterior fossa tumors in children are astrocytoma, medulloblastoma, ependymoma, and glioma. Rarely will dizziness be the only presenting symptom.[66] Cerebellopontine angle tumors are exquisitely rare in children and if found, should prompt consideration of neurofibromatosis type II (bilateral CPA tumors). Concerns for a CNS structural lesion should be investigated with MRI with and without contrast.

Children with various behavioral and psychiatric disorders, such as sensorimotor integration disorder, conversion disorder, anxiety, tic disorder, autism, and attention deficit/hyperactivity disorder, may have associated vestibular or balance complaints. Children who present with a nonorganic cause of their balance symptoms can be identified by a mismatch of symptoms with clinical findings, evidence of secondary gain by their symptoms, and possibly by nonphysiologic responses and evidence of malingering on their objective vestibular testing. The importance of integrating the psychosocial history with the clinical picture cannot be overemphasized.[56]

Neurodegenerative disease (e.g., familial ataxia) and encephalopathy result in imbalance from dysfunction of central and sometimes peripheral vestibular pathways. We have found that up to 7% of patients referred for disequilibrium carry these diagnoses.

SUMMARY

This chapter has focused at length on the development of the human vestibular system and its associated reflexes, factors that affect the vestibular system in children, and causes of vertigo and imbalance in children.

It should be remembered that impaired vision, inability to converge or fixate with binocular vision may result in a feeling of unsteadiness or vertigo. In addition, any peripheral neuropathy that impairs proprioception may also lead to these sensations.

REFERENCES

1. Sidebotham P. Balance through the ages of man. *J Laryngol Otol.* 1988;3:203–208.
2. Brandt T, Glasauer S, Stephan T, et al. Visual-vestibular and visuovisual cortical interaction: new insights from fMRI and pet. *Ann N Y Acad Sci.* 2002;956:230–241.
3. Jeffery N, Spoor F. Prenatal growth and development of the modern human labyrinth. *J Anat.* 2004;204:71–92.
4. Richard C, Laroche N, Malaval L, et al. New insight into the bony labyrinth: a microcomputed tomography study. *Auris Nasus Larynx.* 2010;37:155–161.
5. Wright CG, Hubbard DG. SEM observations on development of human otoconia during the first trimester of gestation. *Acta Otolaryngol.* 1982;94(1–2):7–18.
6. Holt K. *Movement and Child Development. Clinics in Developmental Medicine. No. 55.* Philadelphia: Lippincott; 1975.
7. Schulte FJ, Linke I, Michaelis E, et al. Excitation, inhibition and impulse conduction in spinal motoneurones of preterm, term and small-for-dates newborn infants. In: Robinson, ed. *Brain and Early Behavior Development in the Fetus and Infants. CASDS Study Group on Brain Mechanisms or Early Behavioural Development.* New York: Academic Press; 1969.
8. Kaga K, Sakurai H, Ogawa Y, et al. Morphological changes of vestibular ganglion cells in human fetuses and in pediatric patients. *Int J Pediatr Otorhinolaryngol.* 2001;60:11–20.
9. Blayney AW. Vestibular disorders. In: Adams DA, Cinnamond MJ, eds. *Paediatric Otolaryngology.* 6th ed. Scott-Brown's Otolaryngology. Vol. 6. Oxford: Butterworth-Heinemann; 1997:1–29.
10. Swaiman KF. Neurologic examination after the newborn period until two years of age. In: *Pediatric Neurology Principles and Practice.* 3rd ed. St Louis: Mosby; 1999:31–53.
11. Eviatar L, Eviatar A, Naray L. Maturation of neurovestibular responses in infants. *Dev Med Child Neurol.* 1974;16:435–446.
12. Eviatar L, Eviatar A. The normal nystagmic response of infants to caloric and per-rotatory stimulation. *Laryngoscope.* 1979;89:1036–1044.
13. Weissman BM, Di Seenna AO, Leigh RJ. Maturation of the vestibulo-ocular reflex in normal infants during the first 2 months of life. *Neurology.* 1989;39:534–538.
14. Cohen B. Origin of quick phases of nystagmus. In: Brodal A, Pompeiano O, eds. *Basic Aspects of Central Vestibular Mechanisms.* Amsterdam: Elsevier; 1972:1–649.
15. Ornitz EM, Atwell CW, Walter DO, et al. The maturation of vestibular nystagmus in infancy and childhood. *Acta Otolaryngol.* 1979;88:244–256.

16. Ornitz EM, Kaplan AR, Westlake JR. Development of the vestibulo-ocular reflex from infancy to adulthood. *Acta Otolaryngol Stockh.* 1985;100:180–183.

17. Casselbrant ML, Mandel EM, Sparto P, et al. Longitudinal posturography and rotational testing in children three to nine years of age: normative data. *Otol Head Neck Surg.* 2010;142:708–714.

18. Donat JFG, Donat JR, Swe Lay K. Changing response to caloric stimulation with gestational age in infants. *Neurology.* 1980;30:776–778.

19. Fife TD, Tusa RJ, Furman JM, et al. Assessment: vestibular testing techniques in adults and children. *Neurology.* 2000;55:1431–1441.

20. Van der Laan FL, Oosterveld WJ. Age and vestibular function. *Clin Aviat Aerosp Med.* 1974;45:540–547.

21. Mulch G, Petermann W. Influence of age on results of vestibular function tests. Review of literature and presentation of caloric test results. *Ann Otol Rhinol Laryngol Suppl.* 1979;88:1–17.

22. Andrieu-Guitrancourt JA, Peron JM, Dehesdin D, et al. Normal vestibular responses to air caloric tests in children. *Int J Pediatr Otolaryngol.* 1981;3:245–250.

23. Staller SJ, Goin DW, Hildebrandt M. Pediatric vestibular evaluation with harmonic acceleration. *J Otolaryngol Head Neck Surg.* 1986;95:471–476.

24. Valente M. Maturational effects of the vestibular system: a study of rotary chair, computerized dynamic posturography, and vestibular evoked myogenic potentials with children. *J Am Acad Audiol.* 2007;18:461–481.

25. Rine RM. Physical therapy management of children with vestibular dysfunction. In: Herdman S, ed. *Vestibular Rehabilitation.* 4th ed. Philadelphia: F.A. Davis Co; 2014.

26. Shinjo JY, Yukiko KK. Assessment of vestibular function of infants and children with congenital and acquired deafness using ice-water caloric test, rotational chair test and vestibular-evoked myogenic potential recording. *Acta Otolaryngol.* 2007;127:736–747.

27. Kelsch TA, Schaefer LA, Esquivel CR. Vestibular evoked myogenic potentials in young children: test parameters and normative data. *Laryngoscope.* 2006;116:895–900.

28. Shumway-Cook A, Woollacott MH. The growth of stability: postural control from a development perspective. *J Mot Behav.* 1985;17:131–147.

29. Nashner LM, Stupert CL, Horak FB, et al. Organization of postural controls: an analysis of sensory and mechanical constraints. *Prog Brain Res.* 1989;80:411–418.

30. Ornitz EM. Normal and pathological maturation of vestibular function in the human child. In: Romand R, ed. *Development of Auditory and Vestibular Systems.* New York: Academic Press Inc; 1983:479–536.

31. Forssberg H, Nashner LM. Ontogenetic development of postural control in man: adaptation to altered support and visual conditions during stance. *J Neurosci.* 1982;2:545–552.

32. Wiener-Vacher SR, Toupet F, Narcy P. Canal and otolith vestibule-ocular reflexes to vertical and off vertical axis rotation in children learning to walk. *Acta Otolaryngol.* 1996;116:657–665.

33. Bucci MP, Kapoula Z, Yang Q, et al. Speed-accuracy of saccades, vergence and combined eye movements in children with vertigo. *Exp Brain Res.* 2004;157:286–295.

34. Shumway-Cook A, Woollacott M. Attentional demands and postural control: the effect of sensory context. *J Gerontol A Biol Sci Med Sci.* 2000;55:M10–M16.

35. Bradley NS. Motor control: developmental aspects of motor control in skill acquisition. In: Campbell SK, ed. *Physical Therapy for Children.* Philadelphia, PA: WB Saunders Co; 1997:39–77.

36. Burleigh AL, Horak FB, Malouin F. Modification of postural responses and step initiation: evidence for goal-directed postural interactions. *J Neurophysiol.* 1994;72:2892–2902.

37. Illingworth RS. *The Normal Child.* 8th ed. Edinburgh: Churchill Linvingstone; 1983.

38. Hatzitaki V, Zisi V, Kollias I, Kioumourtzoglou E. Perceptual-motor contributions to static and dynamic balance control in children. *J Mot Behav.* 2002;34(2):161–170.

39. Hsu YS, Kuan CC, Young YH. Assessing the development of balance function in children using stabilometry. *Int J Pediatr Otorhinolaryngol.* 2009;73:737–740.

40. Foudriat BA, Di Fabio RP, Anderson JH. Sensory organization of balance responses in children 3—6 years of age: a normative study with diagnosis implication. *Int J Pediatr Otorhinolaryngol.* 1993;27:255–271.

41. Starkes J, Riach CL. The role of vision in the postural control of children. *Clin Kinesiol.* 1990;44:72–77.

42. Woollacott MH, Debu B, Mowatt M. Neuromuscular control of posture in the infant and child: is vision dominant? *J Mot Behav.* 1987;19:167–186.

43. Hirabayashi S, Iwasaki Y. Developmental perspective of sensory organization on postural control. *Brain Dev.* 1995;17:111–113.

44. Steindl R, Kunz K, Schrott-Fischer A, et al. Effect of age and sex on maturation of sensory systems and balance control. *Dev Med Child Neurol.* 2006;48:477–482.

45. Riach CI, Hayes KC. Maturation of postural sway in young children. *Dev Med Child Neurol.* 1987;29:650–658.

46. Ionescu E, Morlet T, Froehlich P, et al. Vestibular assessment with Balance Quest: normative data for children and young adults. *Int J Pediatr Otorhinolaryngol.* 2006;70:1457–1465.

47. Ferber-Viart C, Ionescu E, Morlet T, et al. Balance in healthy individuals assessed with Equitest: maturation and normative data for children and young adults. *Int J Pediatr Otorhinolaryngol.* 2007;71:1041–1046.

48. Cherng RJ, Chen JJ, Su FC. Vestibular system in performance of standing balance of children and young adults under altering sensory conditions. *Percept Mot Skills.* 2001;92:1167–1179.

49. Charpiot A, Tringali S, Ionescu E, et al. Vestibulo-ocular reflex and balance maturation in healthy children aged from six to twelve years. *Audiol Neurotol.* 2010;15:201–210.

50. Yang Q, Bucci MP, Kapoula Z. The latency of saccades, vergence, and combined eyes movements in children and in adults. *Invest Ophthalmol Vis Sci.* 2002;43:2939–2949.

51. Peterka RJ, Black FO. Age-related changes in human posture control. Sensory organization tests. *J Vestib Res.* 1990;1:73–85.

52. Neimensivu R, Pyykko I, Wiener-Vacher S. Vertigo and balance problems in children – an epidemiologic study in Finland. *Int J Pediatr Otolaryngol.* 2006;70:259–265.

53. Vartiainen E, Karjalainen S, Kärjä J. Vestibular disorders following head injury in children. *Int J Pediatr Otorhinolaryngol.* 1985;9:135–141.

54. Halmagyi GH. History II. Patient with vertigo. In: Baloh RW, Halmagyi GH, eds. *Disorders of the Vestibular System.* Oxford University Press; 1996:171–177.

55. Casselbrant ML, Mandel EM. Balance disorders in children. *Neurol Clin.* 2005;23:807–829.

56. Wiener-Vacher SR. Vestibular disorders in children. *Int J Audiol.* 2008;47:578–583.

57. Balatsouras DG, Kaberis A, Assimakopoulos D. Etiology of vertigo in children. *Int J Pediatr Otorhinolaryngol.* 2007;71:487–494.

58. Szirmai A. Vestibular disorders in childhood and adolescents. *Eur Arch Otorhinolaryngol.* 2010 Nov;267(11):1801–4. doi: 10.1007/s00405-010-1283-2. Epub 2010 May 21.

59. Niemensivu R, Pyykko I, Erna K. Vertigo and imbalance in children. *Arch Otolaryngol Head Neck Surg.* 2005;131:996–1000.

60. Arnvig J. Vestibular function in deafness and severe hardness of hearing. *Acta Otolaryngol Head Neck Surg.* 1955;45:283–288.

61. Cushing SL, Papsin BC, Rutka JA, James AL, Gordon KA. Evidence of vestibular and balance dysfunction in children with profound sensorineural hearing loss using cochlear implants. *Laryngoscope.* 2008;118(10):1814–1823.

62. Waldron M, Matthews J, Johnson I. The effect of otitis media with effusions on balance in children. *Clin Otolaryngol Allied Sci.* 2004;29:318–320.

63. Choung YH, Park K, Moon SK, et al. Various causes and clinical characteristics in vertigo in children with normal eardrums. *Int J Pediatr Otorhinolaryngol.* 2003;67:889–894.

64. Golz A, Netzer A, Angel-Yeger B. Effects of middle ear effusion on the vestibular system in children. *Otolaryngol Head Neck Surg.* 1998;119:695–699.

65. Casselbrant ML, Redfern MS, Furman JM, Fall PA, Mandel EM. Visual induced postural sway in children with and without otitis media. *Ann Otol Rhinol Laryngol.* 1998;107:401–405.

66. Luxon L, Pagarkar W. The dizzy child. In: M Graham John, Scadding Glenis K, Bull Peter D, eds. *Pediatric ENT.* Springer; 2008:459–478.

67. Taborelli G, Melagrana A, D'Agostino R. Vestibular neuronitis in children: study of medium and long term follow-up. *Int J Pediatr Otorhinolaryngol.* 2000;54:117–121.

68. Akagi H, Yuen K, Maeda Y. Meniere's disease in childhood. *Int J Pediatr Otorhinolaryngol.* 2001;61:259–264.

69. Pryor SP, Demmler GJ, Madeo AC, et al. Investigation of the role of congenital cytomegalovirus infection in the etiology of enlarged vestibular aqueducts. *Arch Otolaryngol Head Neck Surg.* 2005;131:388–392.

70. Buchman CA, Joy J, Hodges A, et al. Vestibular effects of cochlear implantation. *Laryngoscope.* 2004;114:1–22.

71. Jacot E, Van Den Abbeele T, Wiener-Vacher S. Vestibular impairments pre- and post-cochlear implant in children. *Int J Pediatr Otorhinolaryngol.* 2009;73:209–217.

72. Migliori G, Battisti E, Pari M, et al. A shifty diagnosis: cogan's syndrome. A case report and review of the literature. *Acta Otorhinolaryngol Ital.* 2009;29:108–113.

73. Mikulec AA, McKenna MJ, Ramsey MJ, et al. Superior semicircular canal dehiscence presenting as conductive hearing loss without vertigo. *Otol Neurotol.* 2004;25(2):121–129.

74. von Brevern M, Zeise D. Acute migrainous vertigo: clinical and oculographic findings. *Brain.* 2005;128:365–374.

75. Murdin L, Premachandra P, Davies R. Sensory dysmodulation in vestibular migraine: an otoacoustic emission suppression study. *Laryngoscope.* 2010;120:1632–1636.

76. Battista RA. Audiometric findings of patients with migraine-associated dizziness. *Otol Neurol.* 2004;25:987–992.

77. Basser LS. Benign paroxysmal vertigo of childhood. (A variety of vestibular neuronitis). *Brain.* 1964;87:141–152.

78. Ralli G, Atturo F, deFilippis C. Idiopathic benign paroxysmal vertigo in children, a migraine precursor. *Int J Pediatr Otorhinolaryngol.* 2009;73:S16–S18.

79. Lempert T, Neuhauser H. Migrainous vertigo. *Neurol Clin.* 2005;23:715–730.

80. Lewis D. Pediatric migraine. *Neurol Clin.* 2009;27:481–501.

81. Fitzgerald D. Head trauma: hearing loss and dizziness. *J Trauma Inj Infect Crit Care Issue.* 1996;40(3):488–496.

CHAPTER 4

Assessment Techniques for Vestibular Evaluation in Pediatric Patients

L. MAUREEN VALENTE, PHD

INTRODUCTION

Pediatric vestibular evaluation has become more established in audiology and otolaryngology clinics over recent years. Along with early identification of hearing impairment, early identification of vestibular disorders has allowed earlier and perhaps more effective remediation strategies in children complaining of dizziness or balance disorders. Researchers and clinicians have contributed valuable information related to vestibular disorders that may be diagnosed in the pediatric population. There has been a paucity of both clinical and research work related to vestibular evaluation techniques that may be used with young children. The current chapter focuses on the adaptation of adult vestibular evaluation techniques for use with pediatric patients, beginning with the medical/physical examination and progressing through major tests of vestibular function. An important concept recurring throughout is that the use of pediatric normative data is crucial so that results obtained after testing a child are not compared with adult normative data.

TAKING THE HISTORY

Many clinicians who perform vestibular evaluation have remarked that the case history is one of the most important diagnostic tools available when evaluating a dizzy patient. Although the author firmly believes that this premise also holds true for pediatric patients, a need exists within the profession for the development of a reliable parent questionnaire. Clearly, answers to certain questions are invaluable: concerns related to the child's development and gross motor skills, description of episodes encountered, time course of symptoms, onset of symptoms, complaints that may be interpreted as peripheral signs, and complaints that may be interpreted as central signs. On searching the literature regarding vestibular evaluation in children, one may view several different bodies of work. On the one hand, physical therapy and occupational therapy studies document evaluation and remediation techniques used with disorders such as autism, motor delay, learning disability, and behavioral disorders.[1–7] Although the evaluative

tools are fascinating, they are very different from those discovered within the audiology and otolaryngology bodies of literature. Many studies within the latter group link vestibular disorders to entities such as migraine syndrome, benign paroxysmal vertigo of childhood, otitis media, sensorineural hearing loss, and a myriad of childhood syndromes.[8–16] Additional research related to vestibular consequences of such syndromes is in order, including CHARGE (coloboma, heart defects, atresia choanae, growth retardation, genital abnormalities, ear abnormalities) association, Cogan syndrome, Usher syndrome, Waardenburg syndrome, and others. Inasmuch as evaluative tools and remediation strategies are highly variable among groups of practitioners, a secondary goal would be improved opportunities for interprofessional education and practice.

Many challenges have historically existed with regard to vestibular evaluation of children. One critical challenge is that pediatric patients may not be able to thoroughly describe dizziness and other "vestibular" symptoms, giving rise to the necessity of developing appropriate checklists and parent questionnaires. Another challenge related to vestibular evaluation in general is that the cost of many pieces of technologically advanced equipment is prohibitive, regardless of patient age. Here, we start with the basics, the history and physical examination.

THE INFORMAL EVALUATION (MEDICAL-PHYSICAL EXAMINATION)

Following the history, the physical examination is undertaken to search for possible etiologies of dizziness or balance disturbance. This section highlights the adaptation of adult screening techniques for pediatric patients and describes the relative ease of performance in an office setting with little or no elaborate equipment. The clinician starts with the standard physical examination with special attention to the eye/visual examination, ear examination, and neurologic examination. Of particular interest in the eye examination is the presence of nystagmus. The clinician begins the informal evaluation by checking for spontaneous nystagmus and/or gaze-evoked nystagmus. One simple method is to have the child look straight ahead, if the child is able to follow such verbal commands. This portion of the evaluation may be referred to as the "static evaluation," in that the examiner is not eliciting nystagmus in any way. The examiner looks for horizontal or vertical nystagmus. Nystagmus in any direction should not be present under typical conditions (unless congenital), and additional testing helps determine if the disorder is peripheral or central in nature.

The "dynamic evaluation" involves a battery of testing that attempts to elicit nystagmus and observe various types of oculomotor tasks. While assessing gaze nystagmus, the examiner asks the child to follow the examiner's finger as it moves to the right and left and in upward and downward directions. Modifications for young patients may include the use of puppets or cartoon videos to encourage the child to look in cardinal positions of gaze. Presence or absence of nystagmus is observed, bearing in mind that nystagmus should not be present with a typically functioning vestibular system. Tasking (keeping the child mentally alert through informal conversation, establishing rapport, easy mental "tasks" such as counting) is important with regard to many vestibular tests, including the assessment of spontaneous nystagmus and especially gaze-evoked nystagmus, such that any nystagmic response is robust and not suppressed. Tasking must be geared toward the child's age and capabilities. It may be possible to use Frenzel lenses for eye magnification and alleviation of visual fixation suppression, depending on the child's age. At this point, the clinician may also briefly check to determine that the eyes are moving conjugately.

As the clinician continues with the dynamic evaluation, "head-shake nystagmus" (HSN) may be considered. According to Fife,[17] the vestibulo-ocular reflex (VOR) should be readily observable by the age of 9–12 months in typically developing infants. The purpose of the VOR is to stabilize gaze, particularly as the body and head are moving. The horizontal VOR is the most commonly studied and is represented by the following example. When the head moves to the right in a sustained rotation, the right vestibular system is excited while the left is inhibited. This is often referred to as a "push–pull" mechanism. The eyes move to the left (slow phase in the opposite direction) and rapidly snap back to the right. This process continues, enabling the examiner to observe a right-beating nystagmus. Nystagmus direction is named for the fast phase and is measured according to its slow phase velocity in degrees

per second. The opposite is true with leftward rotation, resulting in left-beating (fast phase) nystagmus.

The presence of nystagmus and other eye movements may be enhanced via Frenzel lenses, electrooculography (EOG), or infrared videooculography (VOG). As with adults, the child's head may be gently rotated to the left and right (as though shaking the head "no") in a rhythmic manner at approximately 1–2 Hz to check for the presence of HSN. Theoretically, symmetrically functioning vestibular systems do not induce symptoms in view of alternating the excitation and inhibition process between systems as the head moves from right to left. Some children may not be in a position developmentally to verbalize the presence of symptoms, such as dizziness or vertigo, on head rotation. Nystagmus should not be observed with symmetric peripheral vestibular systems, although it may be observed in the presence of an asymmetry. Such HSN screening may be advantageous in situations where caloric irrigations and/or rotary chair (RC) testing may not be feasible. If such measures are available, HSN screening may provide complementary information by incorporating higher frequencies of head motion. It should be noted that much of the standard vestibular test battery assesses low-frequency reactivity of peripheral vestibular organs.

Head thrust testing (HTT), also termed head impulse testing (HIT), may be performed with young children. This procedure is also based on the VOR. The examiner gently rotates the child's head approximately 30 degrees to the right or left while asking the child to focus on the examiner's nose or some other stable target. One may creatively devise placement of colorful stickers or cartoon characters for facilitation of such head movement and have the child focus on the target. The examiner incorporates a brief and rapid head thrust back to midline while making certain that visual fixation is maintained. A corrective "catch-up" saccade may be seen in the form of deviation from the target and a rapid refixation of the eyes on the target. This abnormality may indicate a disorder of the ipsilateral horizontal semicircular canal. Thus, if the refixation saccade is identified on head thrust to the right, it is the right horizontal semicircular canal that is impaired (and the converse is true for the left). Fig. 4.1 displays the successful demonstration of the HTT with a 3-year-old child. The technique for HSN would look very similar.

Children may also be evaluated via dynamic visual acuity (DVA) techniques, with modification of the typical Snellen eye chart for this population. Familiar to most, this chart is highly used during eye examinations

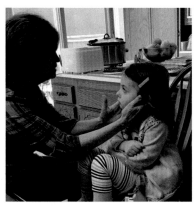

FIG. 4.1 Example of clinician preparing to perform head impulse testing/screening with a 3-year-old child.

as the patient reads smaller and smaller lines of various letter "E" configurations. Child-friendly characters may easily be substituted for the more traditional letters that become smaller with each line. With this procedure, a baseline is obtained in the form of the smallest line of characters that the child may discern from a calibrated distance. The child again attempts to read the smallest line of figures during horizontal rotation of the head, approximating 1–2 Hz. On reading, a loss of one line may be considered insignificant, whereas a loss of three lines or more may indicate VOR deficiency. Advances in computerized technology may facilitate obtaining results.

The clinician may also perform rudimentary oculomotor tasks, such as checking saccadic eye movement. This may be performed by rapidly moving a finger or some other target, ensuring that the child follows the rapidly moving stimulus and meets the target. With more formal measures, the child may follow a series of rapidly moving lights, even described as "ladybugs moving across a screen," and the examiner assesses the latencies obtained. Latency refers to time parameters and indicates whether the speed of attaining each target is within normative data parameters. Oculomotor testing may also determine the "smoothness of pursuit" by asking the child to follow a visual target (e.g., finger, puppet, or cartoon) moving rhythmically from right to left. This cycle is repeated, and the eyes are observed to note any deviation from a smooth pursuit of the target.

Although children rarely demonstrate the true benign paroxysmal positional vertigo (BPPV) that may be present in adults, they may experience positional vertigo and/or sudden vertiginous episodes. They also may experience benign paroxysmal vertigo of childhood that is not positional but occurs at random times and is episodic. Positioning and positional testing, therefore, may be successfully performed with children.

With all procedures, establishing rapport with the child is critical, and the child's comfort level may be increased by being seated on a parent lap and/or by having a parent present. The traditional Dix-Hallpike maneuver is the classic assessment tool for the determination of BPPV. This maneuver involves rapidly moving the patient from a seated position to a lying position with the head turned in one direction. The clinician observes the presence or absence of nystagmus. Subjective symptoms are also noted. A positive Dix-Hallpike maneuver occurs with the elicitation of torsional nystagmus and a report of dizziness. If positive, it is beneficial to repeat this measure to help determine if the response fatigues. The procedure is repeated as the patient lies back and turns the head in the opposite direction. As this *positioning* procedure is time-efficient and noninvasive, this procedure and more traditional *positional* testing may be performed with children. It is important for the child to be able to understand instructions and to receive continual reassurance, in view of a potentially darkened-room environment.

With *positional* testing, the examiner places the head and body in various positions to help determine if any such change in head/body position elicits nystagmus and/or dizziness. Typical head and body positions may be similar to those performed with adults: supine, head right, head left, right lateral, and left lateral. As the clinician searches for the presence of nystagmus, it is also important to supplement this information with any subjective reports of symptoms that the child may express.

Finally, the clinician may ask the child to perform various types of standing balance tasks for screening postural stability. Examples may include Romberg maneuvers where the child stands with feet together, and sway is noted with eyes both open and closed. A variation is the tandem Romberg, where such stability is evaluated with one foot in front of the other, touching heel to toe. Fig. 4.2 depicts the author teaching a 3-year-old patient the tandem Romberg test.

The examiner may ask the child to march in place with eyes closed to determine straightness versus deviation of marching or may encourage the child to walk forward in a heel-to-toe pattern. With the latter, cerebellar dysfunction may be suspected if difficulties arise.[18,19] Other cerebellar signs may include slurring of speech, upper or lower extremity dysfunction, ataxia, muscle incoordination, dysmetria, tremors, or abnormalities noted on oculomotor tasks.

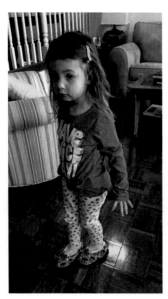

FIG. 4.2 A 3-year-old child learning tandem Romberg techniques.

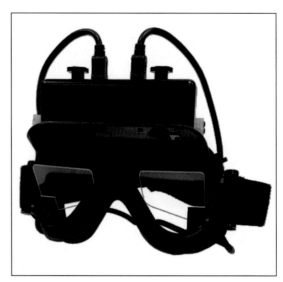

FIG. 4.3 Goggles used for videooculography and rotary chair testing. (Courtesy of and with permission from Micromedical Technologies, Inc.)

FORMAL VESTIBULAR EVALUATION MEASURES

Videonystagmography and Video-oculography

The formal vestibular evaluation is a battery of tests that assists the clinician in determining if dizziness is of central or peripheral origin. With the advent of infrared cameras mounted in eye goggles to replace electrodes for recording and measuring eye movement, VOG, or videonystagmography (VNG), has replaced EOG, also called electronystagmography (ENG), in most clinics. An example of such goggles is shown in Fig. 4.3, with the clinician making use of the smallest size possible for evaluation of the pediatric patient. Electrodes may be challenging with children, in view of discomfort in application and removal. Many children accept the eye goggles used for VNG, especially if their placement is framed by the examiner in a "gamelike" manner.

VNG has revolutionized oculomotor assessment and vestibular testing, in that there are now mechanisms to better observe, record, and measure eye movements. If VNG results suggest peripheral vestibular dysfunction, components of the test battery may help the clinician determine the affected inner ear. Components of this test battery include testing for spontaneous nystagmus and gaze nystagmus, performing various oculomotor tests, measuring positioning and positional nystagmus, and performing caloric irrigations. Several investigators have effectively described some of the adaptations of adult VNG techniques that may be used with children.[20]

As the parent makes certain that the child is optimally prepared for vestibular evaluation, it is important that certain medications (such as those for cough or cold) be withheld for 24–48 h under medical supervision. As some aspects of the test battery may induce nausea, it is important that the child eats only *lightly* before the appointment time. VNG should be performed in a darkened room so that visual fixation of nystagmus does not occur; therefore children may feel more comfortable when a parent is present in the examining room. At the beginning of the VNG, a calibration procedure is performed using a light bar, and the patient is asked to look repeatedly from left to right. Children's attention may be maximized if asked to focus on interesting cartoon characters that illuminate in place of the lights. Oculomotor tests may also be performed with a light bar or flat-screen television. These tests include measurement of saccades or rapid eye movements, optokinetic testing (reflexively following lights that induce the slow and then fast phase of nystagmic eye movements), and sinusoidal tracking to evaluate smooth pursuit.

With all of these oculomotor tests, interesting cartoon characters may replace the traditional lighting, resulting in greater ease of testing the pediatric patient. Just as with audiometry, the clinician may wish to use an assortment of cartoon characters to regain attention, should habituation or fatigue take place.

Measurement of spontaneous nystagmus, addressed in a previous section, may be more formally measured as an initial component of the VNG test battery. The child is asked to sit quietly as the clinician records and analyzes eye movement with eyes open and with vision compromised (e.g., with Frenzel lenses). Contrasting of measurements with eyes open and vision compromised may better enable the examiner to pinpoint peripheral versus central pathology. Eye movement is not elicited in any way during spontaneous nystagmus testing, and the examiner exercises care in making certain that tasking measures appropriate for the individual child are carried out. For example, the child may listen to nursery rhymes or familiar children's songs. As a more active approach, the child may be able to tell a story about a recent cartoon or movie. Gaze nystagmus may be recorded by having the child look at a light bar displaying interesting cartoons, or the clinician may ask the child to "look at the lightning bugs" if a traditional light bar is used. In this manner, it is feasible to measure gaze nystagmus in cardinal gaze positions. The Dix-Hallpike maneuver, traditionally performed with adult patients to help diagnose BPPV, may be easily performed with children. The clinician thoroughly explains to the child that a positioning procedure will take place as the clinician assists the child in progressing from the sitting to lying position with the head turned either to the right or the left. The examiner checks for the presence of nystagmus and elicits a subjective report of symptoms, if the child is capable of reporting such symptoms. Traditional positional testing may also be carried out with children, with the most common positions: supine, head right, and head left. The clinician may use judgment regarding expanding the test battery to include right and left lateral, as well as other, positions.

Such positioning and positional testing may prove challenging with young children, especially if the child has difficulty following instructions. Adaptations of positioning and positional testing with children include the establishment of excellent rapport, having a parent present, and ensuring that the child is comfortable at all times. The clinician should be conscious of allaying fears throughout the evaluation, especially if the testing is performed in a darkened room. Many children with hearing loss exhibit vestibular disorders and may be referred for vestibular testing. Such children may need specific modifications, such as making certain that hearing devices are in place and/or providing signs with written instructions when necessary. Children who communicate via sign language may be effectively tasked by asking them to sign stories or

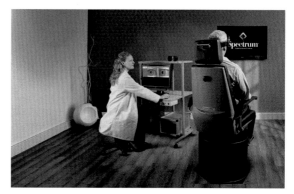

FIG. 4.4 Videooculography equipment, including flat screen television, goggles, and computerized console for test performance and data analysis. (Courtesy of and with permission from Micromedical Technologies, Inc.)

words to familiar children's songs.[11] The examiner may creatively think of additional modifications that may be implemented with children demonstrating other types of disability.

Bithermal caloric irrigation, considered "a gold standard" in evaluating the status of each ear independently, is arguably the most challenging to implement with a pediatric patient. In this author's experience, this section of the test battery may reliably be performed by the developmental age of 5–6 years (although much variability exists among children). The clinician irrigates each ear canal with warm and cool water or air, stimulating the vestibular system and recording slow-phase eye movement velocity with each of four responses. Nystagmus *should* be induced here, as the vestibular systems are being excited (warm irrigations) and inhibited (cool irrigations) with such procedures. Small children may not tolerate this stimulating irrigation or lying still for several minutes as the postirrigation nystagmic response is measured. Children may be fearful of the irrigation equipment and procedure and also of becoming dizzy or experiencing the sensation of movement following stimulation. Fig. 4.4 displays state-of-the art VNG equipment that may be easily adapted for children, including the goggles, light bar/flat-screen television, and computerized recording equipment.

Adaptations are numerous, including selection of water, closed loop (water), or air irrigation systems. With a closed loop system, a balloonlike sleeve is placed upon the irrigator tip such that the water warms or cools the system while not actually touching the tympanic membrane. Some clinicians have experienced success with closed loop or air systems, whereas others have found that children enjoy a water and "bathlike"

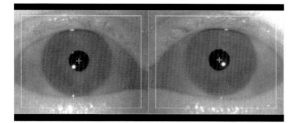

FIG. 4.5 Television monitor that allows clinician to subjectively view patient's eye movements. (Courtesy of and with permission from Micromedical Technologies, Inc.)

analogy. When using water irrigation, it is important to ensure the tympanic membranes are intact; water irrigation in the setting of a tympanic membrane perforation or ventilation (tympanostomy) tube is contraindicated.

Many pediatric evaluative techniques approach a screening, as opposed to thorough diagnostic evaluation, and this may be the case with caloric testing. The examiner, for example, may choose to perform two instead of four irrigations to achieve success in obtaining some type of reliable measure for each ear. Although there may be equipment challenges in doing so, it also may be possible to perform bilateral simultaneous irrigations to diminish test time, number of irrigations, and negative postirrigation patient response. Tasking during caloric testing is critical. It is also very important to calm fears and to view the resulting nystagmus on a video monitor, in addition to viewing computer calculations following each irrigation. In other words, one is observing the recording of eye movement as it occurs following each caloric irrigation and noting computer calculations in degrees of eye movement per second as a system of checks and balances. Fig. 4.5 demonstrates the image of the eye projected on a computer screen, so that the clinician may supplement computerized data analysis with subjective viewing of nystagmus.

Along with advances in computerized technology, additional vestibular evaluative procedures have been developed for use with adults: rotary chair, video head impulse test (vHIT), gaze stabilization test (GST), computerized dynamic posturography (CDP), and vestibular evoked myogenic potentials (VEMPs). Adaptation of these techniques has been very valuable with children, especially in view of the challenges faced in performing some aspects of the VNG test battery with very young children.

Rotary Chair

Use of computerized RC has served to complement the vestibular evaluation battery with adult patients. RC results may help substantiate questionable VNG results and also may help evaluate the VOR at additional test

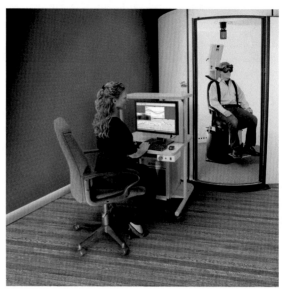

FIG. 4.6 Rotary chair equipment that may be used across the lifespan. (Courtesy of and with permission from Micromedical Technologies, Inc.)

frequencies. Fig. 4.6 shows an example of the RC equipment that is currently available and that may easily be adapted for patients of all ages.

Precursors to such advanced technology with pediatric patients included evaluation of per-rotation and post-rotation nystagmus as part of a medical evaluation.[21,22] In evaluating the VOR during and after rotational stimulation, it was common for the clinician to evaluate parameters such as frequency and amplitude of nystagmic beats, as well as duration of nystagmic activity. Cyr and colleagues[23,24] were among the first investigators to evaluate and clinically use RC techniques with pediatric patients, some of whom were premature infants and others who were full-term infants within the first year of life. Cyr and colleagues painted their darkened enclosure to resemble a spaceship, piped in familiar children's songs for tasking purposes, and seated the children on parents' laps. Techniques approached a screening in that examiners successfully evaluated the VOR at 0.08 Hz. Staller and colleagues also successfully performed RC techniques with very young children, advocating the importance of testing sinusoidal harmonic acceleration (SHA) at more than one test frequency whenever possible.[25] The SHA protocol induced the horizontal VOR through repeated rightward and leftward chair rotations. More than one frequency is recommended during testing because the vestibular system is not linear and varying responses may be noted at different test frequencies. In addition to obtaining computerized measurements following rotation, investigators have stressed the importance of also subjectively observing the VOR via infrared camera and video monitor.

As demonstrated, SHA seems to be the most popular subtest that has been performed with pediatric patients. In 2007 the author performed SHA at 0.08 and 0.50 Hz with two age groups of typically developing children: preschoolers and preadolescents.[26] These children were successfully evaluated via the previously mentioned modification of adult techniques, and it was noted that most children readily adapt to "ride-like" techniques. Appropriate tasking is implemented, and chair restraints may be either adapted or foregone for such a diminutive-sized patient. Children may sit on a parent's lap. It is important for the examiner to be in continual contact with the child via a talk-back system, and the door may be opened between subtests.

Similar to adult patients, VOR parameters of gain, phase, and symmetry may be accurately measured. Gain is a measure that refers to the reflex strength and may be defined as slow-phase eye velocity divided by chair (i.e., head) velocity. The phase measure refers to timing of the response, specifically of head movement in one direction as compared with compensatory eye movement in the other direction. When the calculated phase measure is less than zero, eye velocity "lags" head velocity, and when the phase measure is greater than zero, eye velocity "leads" head velocity.[27] Symmetry helps the examiner compare contribution of the right ear with contribution of the left ear toward the total response. This is accomplished by comparing slow component eye velocity during rightward rotation with slow component eye velocity during leftward rotation. These primary measures must be reliable, which may present challenges with small children and may also vary as a function of frequency. It is critical for the clinician and researcher to gather normative data as a function of age within their facility.

Although the author's study did not find significant gain, phase, or symmetry differences between the two previously described groups of children, she did report that children's gain measures were significantly higher at 0.08 and 0.5 Hz than adult normative data indicated. She further reported successfully performing step velocity (SV) testing with preschool- and adolescent-aged children. SV testing is an additional RC subtest whereby the patient is rotated in one direction at approximately 100 degrees per second, then abruptly stopped. The clinician observes and records nystagmic activity that diminishes as the rotation at constant velocity is sustained. This per-rotation nystagmus is measured as the vestibular time constant is calculated (in seconds) for each rotation. The vestibular time constant is defined as the time it takes for the nystagmic response to diminish to 37% of its original velocity and is compared with normative data to assist in differential diagnosis.[27] On sudden stopping of the chair, post-rotation nystagmus (beats in the opposite direction) is also noted. A post-rotation vestibular time constant may also be measured as the nystagmus begins to diminish; this too is defined as the time it takes for the nystagmus to diminish to 37% of its original velocity. Although SV testing may be performed efficiently on many young children, it is important to further explore head restraint methodologies so that the most reliable measures possible may be obtained because a basic assumption underlying performance and interpretation of RC is that the head and body are moving in accordance with the movement of the chair.

Cyr and colleagues[20,24] demonstrated the efficacy of performing optokinetic testing with children using RC enclosures. Children tend to automatically follow lights or stripes, and the enclosure allows the examiner to fill the visual field with eliciting stimuli so that visual fixation does not interfere with test findings. The clinician may also adequately assess visual fixation skills through the use of RC equipment and accompanying stimuli. If nystagmus diminishes upon visual fixation of a target, such as a light, this is a normal finding or may be more indicative of a peripheral (as opposed to central) pathology.

RC involves numerous other subtests, such as assessment of visual vestibular interactions and dynamic subjective visual vertical testing. With the former, the patient views stripes projected on the enclosure wall as the chair rotates. The patient tracks stimuli through integration of the VOR and the visual pursuit systems. With the latter, patients adjust a luminous line in darkness according to their perceptions of an upright earth-vertical position. Deviation from the straight vertical in degrees is measured, and individuals with otolith organ injury may show alteration in judgment of vertical positioning. Although RC and other vestibular evaluation measures have gained popularity with children, especially before and after cochlear implantation,[28–31] much research and clinical work are still needed regarding the performance of all subtests with pediatric populations.

With regard to various disorders, RC may also provide benefit in evaluating children who have affected/hypoactive systems such as in conjunction with a sensorineural hearing loss, vestibular system damage as a result of ototoxic medications, and vestibular loss associated with many other disorders.[32–34] In summary, RC using the adaptation of adult techniques may serve as a highly successful assessment tool to evaluate children, particularly when caloric irrigations may be unsuccessful. Main adaptations include a more "child friendly" enclosure, asking the child to be seated on a parent lap, and making certain that tasking techniques are appropriate for a pediatric patient. The test may serve as more of a screening than a diagnostic evaluation, particularly if the entire frequency range cannot be tested owing to limited attention span. If a limited frequency range is implemented, it is important to represent low-, medium-, and high-frequency stimuli whenever possible. As the clinician evaluates more objective computerized measurements, it is also critical to view actual nystagmic activity projected on the video monitor. SV testing may be successfully performed with many children, especially if appropriate head restraints are implemented. Per- and post-rotation vestibular time constants may be measured in seconds for both rightward and leftward sustained rotations, although more research is needed regarding test-retest reliability and obtaining the most accurate possible measures. It is crucial to obtain additional normative data for children, as well as additional studies regarding differential diagnosis and anticipated findings with various disorders and syndromes.

Video Head Impulse Testing and Gaze Stabilization Test

Video head impulse testing is a newer technique in the vestibular evaluation battery (See Chapter 8). vHIT involves the patient wearing specialized goggles with recording cameras such that the VOR may be measured upon head impulse movement. The advantages are that precise VOR measurements may be attained, and these techniques may be more easily tolerated than VNG and RC techniques. Although this test has primarily emerged with test batteries involving adult patients, investigators have reported successful use with children.[35-37] The advantages are evident, related to such quick, objective measures with children and such precise measures of eye velocity and any saccadic activity resulting from HIT. It has been reported that children fearing darkened testing environments may also be more amenable to tasks required for vHIT testing. Child adaptations will continue to emerge, such as describing wearing of the goggles in a positive light and framing the entire test as being "ridelike." As with all vestibular tests, pediatric normative data are needed.

The GST has also made valuable contributions toward the adult vestibular test battery over recent years. This test assesses VOR involvement in gaze stabilization

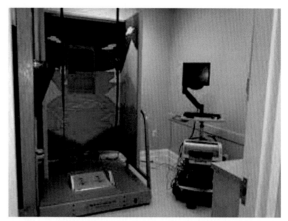

FIG. 4.7 NeuroCom/Natus Balance Manager System used for computerized dynamic posturography. (Courtesy of and with permission from NeuroCom/Natus International, Inc.)

as the head is rotated at higher frequencies and velocities. Visual targets may be randomized and unpredictable with regard to direction and timing. Performance is measured according to symmetry between right and left head movements, as well as parameters related to maximum gaze velocity (in degrees per second) that the patient achieves. As with the evolution of other newer techniques for vestibular evaluation in adults, it is expected that researchers will investigate efficacy of this test with children, particularly because this is a quick and objective test. The creative examiner will continue to adapt adult techniques toward those that are more child-friendly. Future research will focus on the development of normative data banks for children of various ages, particularly as related to velocity and symmetry measures.

Computerized Dynamic Posturography

CDP has been clinically useful over recent years in assessing functional balance and relative contributions of visual, proprioceptive, and vestibular cues. The patient is placed on a platform with safety harnesses in place and faces a visual surround. Sensors within the platform footplate measure the force exerted from the feet when the patient's center of gravity is displaced.[38] The CDP equipment is shown in Fig. 4.7.

Perhaps the most commonly implemented subtest is the sensory organization test (SOT). This test is composed of six conditions that become progressively more difficult, whereby the patient must maintain the best balance possible in the face of compromising visual and/or proprioceptive cues (Table 4.1). There are

TABLE 4.1
Compromising Visual and/or Proprioceptive Cues of Sensory Organization Test

	Platform	Visual Surround
Condition 1	Stable	Stable – Eyes Open
Condition 2	Stable	Stable – Eyes Closed
Condition 3	Stable	Sway – Referenced – Eyes Open
Condition 4	Sway – Referenced	Stable – Eyes Open
Condition 5	Sway – Referenced	Stable – Eyes Closed
Condition 6	Sway – Referenced	Sway – Referenced – Eyes Open

three trials of each condition for reliability purposes; although equipment and protocols may vary, each trial lasts approximately 20 seconds. Scores are reported out of a maximum score of 100, which would indicate perfect balance and absence of sway. In addition to scores reported for each condition, there is also a composite score noted that represents all scores, with heavier weighting on those conditions that rely more heavily on the use of vestibular cues alone. Sway referencing refers to movement of the platform and/or visual surround in response to the body's own sway, typically in an anterior-posterior direction with patients who demonstrate vestibular disorders.

In 1996, DiFabrio and Foudriat[39] reported that a child as young as 3 years old may be tested via CDP techniques, although performance increases as the child ages. Hirabayashi and Iwasaki[40] conducted a CDP study with a large number of children and reported that the proprioceptive system matures by approximately 4 years of age and the visual system by 15 years of age. These researchers believed that the vestibular system is the last to mature and that many children did not reach maturity by 15 years of age. Shimizu et al.[41] found that CDP performance varied greatly between pediatric and adult populations, when studying performance of children aged 6 through 13 years. Cyr and colleagues[20,24] believed that CDP should be performed with children when parents report a history of imbalance, "clumsiness," neurologic impairment, or suspected organic disease. More recently, Rine and colleagues[42,43] performed SOT measurements on young children 3–7 years old. They concluded that CDP testing provides useful measures of all systems involved and conveyed important information related to system maturation. In 2007 the

author compared SOT findings of preschool children with those of preadolescent children, with further comparisons of pediatric findings to adult normative data.[26] Importantly, it was reported that younger children performed significantly poorer than older children on all six conditions. Furthermore, children of both age groups performed significantly poorer on all SOT conditions compared with adult normative data. These points reiterate that pediatric results should be compared and interpreted with reference to pediatric (and not adult) normative data, that one should obtain normative data in one's own clinic for all measures, and that special adaptations should be made for testing children.

When performing CDP with pediatric patients, the smallest harness may be utilized for safety. With all subjects, height and weight should be ascertained to ensure proper platform and sensor calibration, as well as to ensure accuracy of measures. The clinician should consult with the manufacturer's equipment manual to determine minimum weight requirements for proper measurement. As with any pediatric assessment tool, the clinician should establish excellent rapport and calm fears, although many children feel that CDP is "ridelike." Parents may be present, and positive reinforcement appropriate for the individual child is always in order. As the child faces the visual surround, the clinician may consider arranging a more interesting or "child-friendly" visual stimulus. For example, this visual surround could display interesting cartoon characters, a nursery rhyme, or other familiar landscape, or even photos of the child himself. The creative clinician may also devise other means to maintain attention, such as an interesting video or video game. Three trials of the six SOT conditions may tax the attention span of a small child, even though each trial is a mere 20 seconds in duration. At the risk of compromising reliability, the examiner may forego all three trials for a smaller number of trials; future research may explore the validity of results if the clinician were to forego earlier conditions and test only the more difficult conditions when fatigue is present.

The motor control test (MCT) is a second CDP subtest whereby the platform moves in unexpected perturbations: in both forward and backward directions. Latencies in milliseconds are measured from the start of the platform translation to the initiation of force exerted by the feet as the patient attempts to maintain balance.[38] As previously stated, perturbations are proportional to the height of the patient, so perturbations are smaller with a child than with an adult. The MCT is quick and efficient to use with children, although some children may fear the unexpected platform movement. In 2007 the author found that pediatric results are comparable with those obtained with adults, although there is a need for additional pediatric normative data.[26] With both SOT and MCT, a learning curve may be seen from trial to trial.

A third subtest of CDP is the adaptation test, whereby the platform moves unexpectedly to "toes up" or "toes down" position. The regaining of balance on such disruption is measured, along with how well the patient adapts to change from trial to trial. There is a paucity of both clinical and research work related to the adaptation test of CDP with children.

It may be helpful for children to receive a sticker or other tangible reward following completion of each subtest trial. CDP provides much valuable information for the clinician in addition to the subtest scores, and much of this information is unexplored with children. For example, there are strategy scores that provide helpful information about the correct use of the ankle, hip, and step strategies for maintaining balance. Information may be gained regarding how well a patient integrates visual, vestibular, and proprioceptive cues and whether the child is overly dependent on one modality. There are measures that help determine if a patient is equally distributing weight on the right and left sides of the body. Although remediation is beyond the scope of this chapter, it is clear that this wealth of information may provide great benefit to those patients in whom remediation is in order. Directions for future research are many, including development of equipment and test procedures for younger and younger children. Recent investigations have studied CDP results with children before and after cochlear implant, as well as anticipated results with various childhood disorders and syndromes.[44-46] Further studies will serve as a welcome addition to the body of literature, as will further adaptations of techniques for use with children and further establishment of pediatric normative data for all aspects of all subtests.

Vestibular Evoked Myogenic Potentials

VEMPs have gained much popularity over the past few decades, as their usage has transitioned from animal to human studies and continues to move toward clinical vestibular evaluation. VEMPs are quick and efficient to perform and objective in interpretation. Their debut within the vestibular evaluation arena was welcome, in that most vestibular tests assessed the function of the horizontal semicircular canals and VOR. Clinicians have had few assessment tools at their disposal to measure the function of otolith structures,

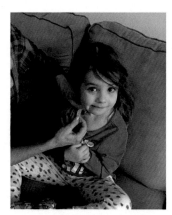

FIG. 4.8 Electrode placement for vestibular evoked myogenic potential testing being initiated with a 3-year-old child.

the utricle and the saccule. Via evidence-based principles, investigators[47,48] have demonstrated that these auditory stimulus-driven evoked potentials arise from the saccule, in that some subjects with severe to profound sensorineural hearing loss have normal VEMP responses. In contrast, some patients with normal hearing sensitivity and impaired function of the inferior branch of the vestibular nerve have exhibited abnormal or absent VEMP responses. Eliciting the cervical VEMP (cVEMP) involves placement of electrodes in the following manner: ground on the forehead, noninverting electrodes on each contracted sternocleidomastoid muscle (SCM), and inverting electrodes on the sternum or sternoclavicular juncture. Fig. 4.8 demonstrates electrode placement for cVEMP testing with a 3-year-old child.

Standard auditory brainstem response equipment may be adapted for elicitation of VEMPs via the electrode array, signal averaging equipment, and appropriate stimulus and recording parameters.[49] As the auditory stimulus is presented via air conduction or bone conduction, the afferent auditory pathway involves stimulation of the saccule, eighth nerve, and vestibular nuclei.[50] Efferent pathways travel to the motor neurons of the neck muscles, including the SCM. Current VEMP elicitation techniques were originally described by Colebatch and colleagues,[51] although VEMP tracings have been recorded from other parts of the body. Current research involves enhancing and refining the clinician's test administration techniques and interpretation of results. To keep the SCM contracted so that the evaluation may be performed, the patient may be placed in several different positions. One is to turn the head to the right or to the left to elicit

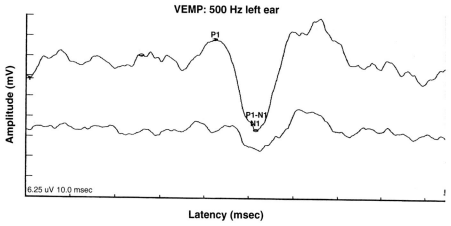

FIG. 4.9 Vestibular evoked myogenic potential tracing obtained with a 6-year-old patient.

muscle contraction while remaining in a seated position. Some examiners may have the patient gently push the head against an object to create resistance so that the neck may be optimally contracted. Other examiners may ask the patient to lie in a supine position and raise the head to contract the neck muscles in either a chin-to-chest position or a head-turned-to-right or left position. Clever adaptions for children include wall-mounted video cartoons that activate only when the child lifts the head or sufficiently contracts the SCM.

VEMP tracings typically are collected using a two-channel recording paradigm and 25 millisecond prestimulus baseline of raw electromyography (EMG) activity, followed by a tracing that highlights a positive peak (P1) and a negative peak (N1). A cVEMP tracing, obtained on a 6-year-old patient, is seen in Fig. 4.9.

To interpret the results, the audiologist may first observe wave morphology to ensure that the waveform displays the proper pattern and waves P1 and N2 are easily discernible. The audiologist obtains normative data and compares the patient's P1 and N1 latencies in milliseconds with normative clinic data for that particular age group. Research has shown that there is an indirect correlation between auditory tone burst stimulus frequency and latency of P1 and N1 waveforms,[49] at least in the cVEMP. That is, lower-frequency stimuli typically elicit waveforms with more delayed latencies, whereas higher-frequency stimuli typically elicit waveforms with earlier latencies. Another important parameter to consider in VEMP interpretation is the P1-N1 amplitude, labeled in microvolts and described as the difference from the peak of P1 to the trough of N1. This parameter has been challenging in measurement and interpretation for two major reasons. First, the P1-N1

amplitude of the cVEMP is directly related to the tonic level of neck contraction, which may vary from patient to patient. Second, this amplitude measure is also positively correlated with the intensity level of the acoustic stimulus.

Investigators have reported important ways to control for neck contraction variability, including incorporating additional electrodes and computer software so that the patient may monitor SCM contraction levels to meet specific targets displayed on a computer screen.[49] Clinicians may also calculate a normalized amplitude measure, dividing raw amplitude by the average amplitude of prestimulus EMG baseline activity. Some clinicians calculate an amplitude asymmetry ratio, defined as the difference between amplitudes of unaffected and affected sides divided by the amplitude sum of both sides. With these calculations, a smaller number indicates greater symmetry, whereas a larger number indicates greater asymmetry. Each clinic should establish normative values for asymmetry ratio, and most clinics report asymmetry ratios of 40% or greater as an abnormal finding.

Minor and colleagues have reported clinical utility of the VEMP threshold measure, especially as a diagnostic tool in the evaluation of patients with superior canal dehiscence syndrome (SCDS).[52] Such a threshold measure is generally defined as the lowest level of auditory intensity that elicits a discernible VEMP tracing. In such a case, a VEMP tracing on the affected (e.g., SCDS) side would yield a much lower threshold (lower auditory stimulus intensity) than the VEMP response on the unaffected side. Again, a large asymmetry would be noted in patients with SCDS. Congenital SCDS has been reported in children.

The efficiency and objectivity of VEMP testing facilitate its use with pediatric patients. In 2005 Sheykholeslami and colleagues studied a group of typically developing neonates and a group of neonates exhibiting "clinical findings."[53] They reported that VEMP tracings, readily obtained in this population, demonstrate morphology that is similar to that of adult populations. They noted shorter latencies of the N1 peak and greater amplitude variability with children as compared with adult patients. In 2006 Kelsch concurred that VEMP testing is easily accomplished with children 3–11 years old and found earlier initial peak latencies than those occurring in adult patients.[54] The author studied samples of preschool- and adolescent-aged children in 2007 and found shorter P1 and N1 latencies with pediatric, as contrasted with adult, participants.[26] VEMPs were readily measured with children through the use of 500 Hz tone burst and click stimuli. Recommendations toward a VEMP battery for children suggested that such testing may also screen for vestibular pathology rather than serve as a full diagnostic assessment. Furthermore, it was reported that testing with both stimuli may prove redundant if children have very limited attention span, although it is always crucial to repeat each waveform. In this study, the most robust waveforms were obtained through the use of lower-frequency tone burst stimuli.[26]

The ocular VEMP or oVEMP has also gained clinical prominence over recent years. The oVEMP is elicited via air conduction or bone conduction, and the response is recorded from the ocular muscles. Generally, surface electrodes are placed just below the eye, and the patient is asked to look in an upward direction. oVEMPs are felt to be utricular in origin, entering the central nervous system through the superior vestibular nerve.[55] oVEMP tracings also display a positive peak (P1) and a negative peak (N1), with interpretation parameters being very similar to those of the cVEMP: primarily morphology, latency, and amplitude. oVEMP amplitudes are typically very small, requiring care in acquisition and interpretation. oVEMP tracings have been recorded in children as young as 3 years old.[56] Examiner challenges may lie in coaxing the child to look in an upward direction and to hold that gaze.

As adult techniques are modified for children, the clinician may find that pediatric patients do not view VEMP testing as "fun" or "ridelike" as with other vestibular evaluation measures discussed. The clinician may refer to electrodes as "stickers," promising a "prettier and more fun" sticker on completion of the test. This author has attempted the use of EMG-monitoring software with young children and found that attempting to use multiple electrodes on a small neck was challenging and that

some electrodes are very heavy and cumbersome. Such monitoring software is being developed and perfected for children, and one may creatively devise avenues for maintaining attention and helping children maintain computer screen visual targets. The child may be seated on a parent's lap for testing and will require much positive reinforcement as with other test techniques. It may be beneficial for the child to turn the head 90 degrees to contract the SCM and focus upon a wall-mounted sticker or cartoon character. The parent may also provide hand, shoulder, and upper body resistance to steady the child and help create resistance during data collection. Pediatric insert earphones are available for presentation of acoustic stimuli, and most children readily accept these transducers. Although protocols vary, some examiners present 128 stimulus sweeps for obtaining a cVEMP tracing, whereas many examiners find that interpretable tracings are obtained following fewer (64) stimulus sweeps. In the event of limited time and attention span, the clinician may also choose to obtain binaural recordings, as opposed to testing in a monaural fashion. VEMP testing techniques continue to evolve and further develop with the pediatric patient.[57,58]

CONCLUSIONS

In summary, vestibular testing is appropriate and "doable" for pediatric patients. Testing techniques and protocols may be easily adapted for children. The audiologist may be only one member of a multidisciplinary team, with other members including an otolaryngologist, neurologist, psychologist, educators, physical therapists and occupational parents, and others. The audiologist bears in mind that the scope of practice is very broad and that other evaluative measures may be performed with a particular child: thorough audiologic evaluation, electrophysiologic testing, hearing aid evaluation, cochlear implant assessment, and various (re)habilitative strategies.

There are many preevaluation measures that the physician and the audiologist may obtain before performing a more formal assessment. Examples are gait and balance screenings, observation of spontaneous nystagmus and gaze nystagmus, oculomotor testing, and HTT. With creativity and warm interpersonal skills, these measures may easily be performed with many pediatric patients. VNG has been performed successfully with adults and older children for many years, and this equipment is readily available in most clinics. Adaptations have been described, such as substitution of cartoon characters for lights when performing oculomotor testing, having the parent present at all times (including sitting with the child on the RC), and reward/reinforcement strategies. Challenges with children include positional testing and especially the successful performance of bithermal caloric irrigations. Newer technologies, such as the RC and CDP, may be more easily adapted for vestibular evaluation with pediatric patients. Adaptation of adult techniques, such as child-friendly tasking measures with RC testing and incorporating a more child-friendly visual surround with CDP testing, have been highly successful. Finally, cVEMPs and oVEMPs may successfully be obtained with children, with adaptations such as seating the child on a parent lap, maintaining head and body position via parental support, and focusing on child-friendly cartoon characters.

Adult techniques can be adapted for use with younger and younger children, and it is important to obtain pediatric normative data. Clearly, results obtained during the evaluation of a child should not be interpreted in the context of adult normative data.

Future areas of research are many. Studies regarding anticipated findings with various RC and CDP subtests are in order, especially as related to various pathologies in children. CDP seems to provide the clinician with much useful information that may be applied toward remediation. Additional studies are in order regarding best rehabilitative practice with pediatric patients, with additional collaboration of all team members involved in diagnostic and treatment processes. Additional VEMP studies will examine the bone-conducted VEMP, types of tracings obtained via presentation of various auditory stimuli, and expected results with various disorders and syndromes.[31] More adequate targeting procedures of EMG activity and neck contraction are recommended, as well as investigations related to measuring the VEMP from alternative anatomic sites of the body.

Through the gathering of evidence from vestibular testing and clinical practice, clinicians will gain a greater understanding of who should be tested, associated diagnoses, and who should be referred for treatment, as well as optimal test strategies and techniques. As with hearing impairment, the earlier a pediatric vestibular disorder is identified, the earlier the remediation may be initiated.

REFERENCES

1. Ayers AJ. Learning disabilities and the vestibular system. *J Learn Disabil*. 1978;11(1):18–29.
2. Ottenbacher K, Watson PJ, Short MA. Association between nystagmus hyporesponsivity and behavioral problems in learning-disabled children. *Am J Occup Ther*. 1979;33(5):317–322.
3. Ottenbacher K. Excessive postrotary nystagmus duration in learning-disabled children. *Am J Occup Ther*. 1980;34(1):40–44.
4. Polatajko HJ. A critical look at vestibular dysfunction in learning-disabled children. *Dev Med Child Neurol*. 1985;27:283–292.
5. Shumway-Cook A, Horak F, Black FO. A critical examination of vestibular function in motor-impaired learning-disabled children. *Int J Pediatr Otorhinolaryngol*. 1987;14:21–30.
6. Horak FB, Shumway-Cook A, Crowe TK, Black FO. Vestibular function and motor proficiency of children with impaired hearing, or with learning disability and motor impairments. *Dev Med Child Neurol*. 1988;30:64–79.
7. Crowe TK, Horak FB. Motor proficiency associated with vestibular deficits in children with hearing impairments. *Phys Ther*. 1988;68(10):1493–1499.
8. Casslebrandt ML, Furman JM, Mandel EM, Fall PA, Kurs-Lasky M, Rockette HE. Past history of otitis media and balance in four-year-old children. *Laryngoscope*. 2000;110:773–778.
9. Mira E, Piacentino G, Lanzi G, Balottin U. Benign paroxysmal vertigo in childhood. *Acta Otolaryngol Suppl*. 1984;406:271–274.
10. Mira E, Piacentino G, Lanzi G, Balottin U. Benign paroxysmal vertigo in childhood: a migraine equivalent. *ORL*. 1984;46(20):97–104.
11. Brookhouser PE, Cyr DB, Beauchaine KA. Vestibular findings in the deaf and hard of hearing. *Otolaryngol Head Neck Surg*. 1982;90:773–777.
12. Cyr DG, Brookhouser PE, Beauchaine KA. Language and learning skills of hearing-impaired children: vestibular evaluation. *ASHA Mono*. 1986;23:21–23.
13. Huygen PLM, van Rijn PM, Cremers CWRJ, Theunissen EJJM. The vestibulo-ocular reflex in pupils at a Dutch school for the hearing-impaired: findings related to acquired causes. *Int J Pediatr Otorhinolaryngol*. 1993;25:39–47.
14. Wiener-Vacher SR, Amanou L, Denise P, Narcy P, Manach Y. Vestibular function in children with the CHARGE association. *Arch Otolaryngol Head Neck Surg*. 1999;125:342–347.
15. Ndiaye IC, Rassi SJ, Wiener-Vacher SR. Cochleovestibular impairment in pediatric cogan's syndrome. *Pediatrics*. 2002;109(2):1–7.
16. Fishman GA, Kumar A, Joseph ME, Torok N, Anderson RJ. Usher's syndrome: ophthalmic and neuro-otologic findings suggesting genetic heterogeneity. *Arch Opthalmol*. 1983;101:1367–1374.
17. Fife TD, Tusa RJ, Furman JM, et al. Assessment: vestibular testing techniques in adults and children. *Neurology*. 2000;55:1431–1441.
18. Desmond A. *Vestibular Function: Evaluation and Treatment*. New York: Thieme Medical Publishers; 2004:52–59.
19. McFeely WJ, Bojrab DI. Performing the physical exam: posture and gait tests. In: Goebel JA, ed. *Practical Management of the Dizzy Patient*. Philadelphia: Lippincott, Williams and Wilkins; 2001:107–111.

20. Cyr DG. The vestibular system: pediatric considerations. *Sem Hear.* 1983;4(1):33–45.

21. Eviatar L, Eviatar A. Neurovestibular examination of infants and children. *Adv Otorhinolaryngol.* 1978;23:169–191.

22. Eviatar L, Eviatar A. The normal nystagmic response of infants to caloric and perrotatory stimulation. *Laryngoscope.* 1979;89:1036–1045.

23. Cyr DG. Vestibular testing in children. *Ann Otorhinolaryngol.* 1980;89:63–69.

24. Cyr DG, Brookhouser PE, Valente M, Grossman A. Vestibular evaluation of infants and preschool children. *Otolaryngol Head Neck Surg.* 1985;93(4):463–468.

25. Staller SJ, Goin DW, Hildebrandt M. Pediatric vestibular evaluation with harmonic acceleration. *Otolaryngol Head Neck Surg.* 1986;95(4):471–476.

26. Valente LM. Maturational effects of the vestibular system: a study of rotary chair, computerized dynamic posturography, and vestibular evoked potentials with children. *J Am Acad Audiol.* 2007;18(6):461–481.

27. Goebel JA, Hanson JM. Vestibular physiology. In: Hughes GB, Pensak ML, eds. *Clinical Otology.* 2nd ed. New York: Thieme Medical Publishers; 1997:43–52.

28. Licamelli G, Zhou G, Kenna MA. Disturbance of vestibular function attributable to cochlear implantation in children. *Laryngoscope.* 2009;119(4):740–745.

29. Cushy SL, Papsin BC, Rutka JA, James AL, Blaser SL, Gordon KA. Vestibular end organ and balance deficits after meningitis and cochlear implantation with children. *Otol Neurotol.* 2009;30:488–495.

30. Jacot E, Van Den Abbele T, Debri HR, Wiener-Vacher SR. Vestibular impairment pre- and post-cochlear implant. *Int J Pediatr Otorhinolaryngol.* 2010;74(1):105.

31. Janky K, Givens D. Vestibular, visual acuity and balance outcomes in children with cochlear implants. A preliminary report. *Ear Hear.* 2015;36(6):e364–e372.

32. De Kegel A, Maes L, Baetens T, Dhooge I, Van Waelvelde H. The influence of a vestibular dysfunction on the motor development of hearing impaired children. *Laryngoscope.* 2012;122:2837–2843.

33. Inoue A, Iwasaki S, Ushio M, Chihara Y, Fujimoto C, et al. Effect of vestibular dysfunction on the development of gross motor function in children with profound hearing loss. *Audiol Neurootol.* 2013;18:143–151.

34. Christy JB, Payne J, Azuero A, Formby C. Reliability and diagnostic accuracy of clinical tests of vestibular function for children. *Pediatr Phys Ther.* 2014;26:180–189.

35. Hamilton S, Zhou G, Brodsky J. Video head impulse testing in the pediatric population. *Int J Pediatr Otorhinolaryngol.* 2015;79(8):1283–1287.

36. Sommerfleck P, Macchi M, Weinschelbaum R, De Bagge M, Bernaldez P, Carmona S. Balance disorders in childhood: main etiologies according to age and usefulness of the video head impulse test. *Int J Pediatr Otorhinolaryngol.* 2016;87:148–153.

37. Nassif N, Balzanelli C, DeZenis O. Preliminary results of video head impulse testing in children with cochlear implants. *Int J Pediatr Otorhinolaryngol.* 2016;88:30–33.

38. Nashner LM. Computerized dynamic posturography. In: Goebel JA, ed. *Practical Management of the Dizzy Patient.* Philadelphia: Lippincott, Williams and Wilkins; 2001:143–170.

39. DiFabio RP, Foudriat BA. Responsiveness and reliability of a pediatric strategy score for balance. *Phys Res Int.* 1996;1(3):180–194.

40. Hirabayashi S, Iwasaki Y. Developmental perspective of sensory organization on postural control. *Brain Dev.* 1995;17(2):111–113.

41. Shimuzu K, Asai M, Takata S, Watanabe Y. The development of equilibrium function in childhood. In: Taguchi K, Igarashi M, Mori S, eds. *Vestibular and Neural Front.* New York: Elsevier Science BV; 1994:183–186.

42. Rine RM, Rubish K, Feeney C. Measurement of sensory system effectiveness and maturational changes in postural control in young children. *Pediatr Phys Ther.* 1998;10:16–22.

43. Rine RM, Cornwall G, Gan K, et al. Evidence of progressive delay of motor development in children with sensorineural hearing loss and concurrent vestibular dysfunction. *Percept Mot Skills.* 2000;90:1101–1112.

44. Casselbrant M, Mandel E, Sparto J, et al. Longitudinal posturography and rotational testing in children three to nine years of age: normative data. *Otolaryngol Head Neck Surg.* 2010;142(5):708–714.

45. Yi SH, Hwang JH, Kim SJ, Kwon JY. Validity of pediatric balance scales in children with spastic cerebral palsy. *Neuropediatrics.* 2012;43(6):307–313.

46. Cushing S, Papsin B, Rutka J, James A, Gordon K. Evidence of vestibular and balance dysfunction in children with profound sensorineural hearing loss using cochlear implants. *Laryngoscope.* 2008;118:1814–1823.

47. Halmagyi GM, Colebatch JG. Vestibular evoked myogenic potentials in the sternocleidomastoid muscle are not of lateral canal origin. *Acta Otolaryngol Suppl.* 1995;520(1):1–3.

48. Murofishi T, Halmagyi GM, Yavor RA, Colebatch JG. Absent vestibular evoked myogenic potentials in vestibular neurolabyrinthitis: an indicator of vestibular nerve involvement? *Arch Otolaryngol Head Neck Surg.* 1996;122(8):845–848.

49. Akin FW, Murnane OD. Vestibular evoked myogenic potentials: preliminary report. *J Am Acad Audiol.* 2001;12(9):445–452.

50. Halmagyi GM, Curthoys LS. Otolith function tests. In: Herdman SJ, ed. *Vestibular Rehabilitation.* Philadelphia: FA David; 2000:196–214.

51. Colebatch JG, Halmagyi GM, Skuse NF. Myogenic potentials generated by click-evoked vestibulocollic reflex. *J Neurol Neurosurg Psychiatry.* 1994;57(2):190–197.

52. Manzari L, Burgess A, Curthoys I. Ocular and cervical vestibular evoked myogenic potentials in response to bone-conducted vibration in patients with probable inferior vestibular neuritis. *J Laryngol Otol.* 2012;126(7):683–691.

53. Minor LB, Cremer PD, Carey JP, Della Santina CC, Streubel SO. Symptoms and signs in superior canal dehiscence syndrome. *Ann N Y Acad Sci.* 2001;942:445–452.

54. Sheykholeslami K, Megerian CA, Arnold JE, Kaga K. Vestibular evoked myogenic potentials in infancy and early childhood. *Laryngoscope*. 2005;115(8):1440–1444.

55. Kelsch TA, Schaefer LA, Esquivel CR. Vestibular evoked myogenic potentials in young children: test parameters and normative data. *Laryngoscope*. 2006;116(6):895–900.

56. Young Y. Assessment of functional development of the otolithic system in growing children: a review. *Int J Pediatr Otorhinolaryngol*. 2015;79(4):435–442.

57. Maes L, De Kegel A, Van waelvelde H, Dhooge I. Rotatory and colic vestibular evoked myogenic potential testing in normal hearing and hearing impaired children. *Ear Hear*. 2014;35:E21–E32.

58. Xu X, Zhang X, Zhang Q, Hu J, Chen Y, et al. Ocular and cervical vestibular evoked myogenic potentials in children with cochlear implant. *Clin Neurophysiol*. 2014;126(8):1624–1631.

CHAPTER 5

An Update on the Predominant Forms of Vertigo in Children and Their Associated Findings on Balance Function Testing

DEVIN L. MCCASLIN, PHD • JAMIE M. BOGLE, PHD • GARY P. JACOBSON, PHD

INTRODUCTION

There are many disorders that can cause "dizziness" in the pediatric population.[1-5] In 1999, Russell and Abu-Arafeh[6] published an epidemiological study showing that in their sample, 15% of school-age children had experienced at least one episode of vertigo in the previous year. In a further effort to describe the prevalence and causes of dizziness in the pediatric population, O'Reilly et al.[7] searched electronic medical records (i.e., ICD-9 codes) of 561,151 inpatient and outpatient visits during a 4-year period. These investigators reported that approximately 1% of this cohort met criteria for presenting with a primary complaint related to balance. Further analysis revealed that 2283 patients (0.4%) received a diagnosis of unspecified dizziness, and of these, 6.2% were diagnosed with a peripheral cause of dizziness while 4.1% were diagnosed with a central cause. The total prevalence of diagnoses related to balance in the records reviewed was determined to be 0.45%. These data serve to highlight the relative rarity of seeking medical attention for symptoms of dizziness and imbalance in young children. Numerous investigators have described the most common disorders causing vertigo and imbalance in children in their clinics.[5,8-10] Even though these reports originate from different clinics and regions of the world, there is surprisingly good agreement regarding primary causes of dizziness in the pediatric population. Nevertheless, children experiencing vertigo and imbalance have received less attention in the literature than their adult counterparts. This is most likely due to the difficulty that young children have in describing their symptoms, coupled with challenges that exist for clinicians in working through the differential diagnostic process with children. Despite these limitations, it is now known that the most common disorders in children that cause dizziness manifest themselves as abnormalities on quantitative balance function testing (i.e., rotary chair testing, videonystagmography/electronystagmography, and vestibular evoked myogenic potential [VEMP] testing).

BACKGROUND

Assessment of vestibular system function in the pediatric population is gaining interest for several reasons. First, determining vestibular system integrity can assist physicians in diagnosing impairment and in defining the most appropriate course of treatment. Second, some children with dizziness and balance problems have serious health issues, and vestibular system assessment can help identify patients whose symptoms may stem from neurologic impairment secondary to intracranial abnormality (e.g., head trauma, brain tumor) versus developmental delay. However, unlike in adults, episodic vertigo occurs rarely in children and may manifest itself in many forms.[11] For example, a child with acute vestibular system impairment may present with many of the same symptoms as adults (e.g., vomiting, nystagmus, hearing loss, ataxia) or may have subtler symptoms such as visual disturbance, motor delay, or headache.[7] As with adults, children with vestibular disorders may also present with loss of vestibular function, which is progressive or chronic, thereby affecting development of postural control.[12] Identifying whether dizziness in a pediatric patient is of vestibular origin requires a team approach, beginning with an assessment by a physician. During this initial visit, a detailed case history should be obtained along with comprehensive neurologic and otologic examinations. Once neurologic impairments are excluded, quantitative balance function testing may help identify both peripheral and central vestibular system deficits.

Despite the fact that dizziness and vertigo occur in children, there are few dizziness clinics that have made a commitment to test this population. One explanation for this is the challenge of extracting clinical and laboratory information from children. According to Wiener-Vacher,[9] children will often not report vertiginous symptoms because of their inability to verbalize the abnormal sensations they are experiencing. Vestibular disorders in young children often are dismissed by professionals and caregivers alike, and the symptoms are consequently attributed to behavioral problems (i.e., finding ways to attract attention) or simply being "clumsy." Additionally, diseases that affect the vestibular system in adults have a different frequency of occurrence in the pediatric population. For example, benign paroxysmal positional vertigo (BPPV) is generally quoted as the most common form of vertigo in adults.[13-15] It has been estimated to have a prevalence of 2.4% in the general adult population.[16] In children, BPPV has been reported to occur in up to 6% of those presenting with dizzy concerns.[10,17,18] This means that the provider must approach the diagnosis of childhood dizziness and vertigo with a very different background of knowledge. Finally, although there continues to be interest in the development of techniques for assessing the vestibular system in adults, the same energy has not been directed toward adapting these techniques for application to children. One of the pioneers in the assessment of vestibular function in the pediatric population was Dr. David Cyr who worked at the Boys Town Institute. Much of his work in the 1980s focused on adapting existing adult protocols for use with children.[19,20] Many of these adaptations are still in use today (see Chapter 4). Although interest in the assessment of the vestibular system in children has led manufacturers to develop both age-adjusted pupil tracking algorithms and age-appropriate visual targets, the majority of manufacturers at the time of this report do not offer videonystagmography goggles that are appropriately sized for children. Having equipment that allows for accurate assessment of children is critical because many disorders causing dizziness and vertigo in children have a vestibular origin. Although the clinical utility of quantitative balance function testing is well-documented in children, continued research and development in balance assessment techniques will further our understanding of pediatric dizziness and vertigo.

ASSESSING DIZZINESS HANDICAP IN PEDIATRIC PATIENTS

It is now standard practice to evaluate the impact that balance disorders have on an individual's ability to participate in age-appropriate activities and document any restrictions that may be imposed by the impairment. This is referred to in the literature as a patient's dizziness-related quality of life (DRQoL). There are a number of important reasons to measure patients' DRQoL. First, these metrics provide the treating clinician with information that can be used to design and guide treatment of a patient's symptoms. Specifically, a clinician can administer a handicap measure to a patient, provide treatment designed to mitigate the origin of the impairment, and then reassess to determine if there has been any change. Historically, psychometric investigations have been performed describing how much change in the score is needed to be considered significant. Having outcome measures that include the patient's perception of their symptoms in addition to findings on the vestibular test battery as well as their subsequent response to intervention provides a multidimensional profile of the patient's symptom status. Secondly, it has been shown that there is often a disparity between a patient's symptoms and their findings on vestibular function studies.[21] That is, there are no semiobjective measures of vestibular impairment that are strongly predictive of dizziness handicap and/or disability. Lastly, in the current health care environment, evidence-based practice is important to all parties involved, including insurance carriers.

DRQoL has been typically assessed using validated self-report measures. These appraisals are most commonly done in a paper-pencil format, are brief to complete, and are psychometrically robust (i.e., test-retest reliability is high). There are a number of tools that assess DRQoL including the Vertigo Handicap Inventory and the Dizziness Handicap Inventory (DHI).[22] Until recently, there was no single measure of dizziness handicap and/or disability for children. In 2015, the Vanderbilt Pediatric Dizziness Handicap Inventory of Patient Caregivers (DHI-PC) was introduced and validated for use with children aged 5–12 years.[23] Questions on the DHI-PC are written in such a way that they may be answered by the child or their proxy. The DHI-PC form is shown in Fig. 5.1.

DIFFERENTIAL DIAGNOSIS

The differential diagnostic process is more complex in children reporting dizziness or balance problems than in adults for several reasons. First, symptoms of dizziness can manifest differently in children than in adults. Moreover, young children have limited verbal skills and often the clinician must rely on the caregiver's observations for the case history. Accordingly, determining which pediatric patients should receive vestibular

NAME: _____   DATE: _____

VANDERBILT PEDIATRIC DIZZINESS HANDICAP INVENTORY- PATIENT CAREGIVER (DHI-PC) (AGES 5-12 YEARS)

Instructions: The purpose of this questionnaire is to identify difficulties that your child may be experiencing because of his or her dizziness or unsteadiness. Please answer "yes", "no", or "sometimes" to each question. **Answer each question as it pertains to your child's dizziness problem only**.

	Yes (4)	Sometimes (2)	No (0)
1. Does your child's problem make him/her feel tired?			
2. Is your child's life ruled by his/her problem?			
3. Does your child's problem make it difficult for him/her to play?			
4. Because of his/her problem, does your child feel frustrated?			
5. Because of his/her problem, has your child been embarrassed in front of others?			
6. Because of his/her problem, is it difficult for your child to concentrate?			
7. Because of his/her problem, is your child tense?			
8. Do other people seem irritated with your child's problem?			
9. Because of his/her problem, does your child worry?			
10. Because of his/her problem, does your child feel angry?			
11. Because of his/her problem, does your child feel "down"?			
12. Because of his/her problem, does your child feel unhappy?			
13. Because of his/her problem, does your child feel different from other children?			
14. Does your child's problem significantly restrict his/her participation in social or educational activities, such as going to dinner, meeting with friends, field trips, or to parties?			
15. Because of your child's problem, is it difficult for him/her to walk around the house in the dark?			
16. Because of his/her problem, does your child have difficulty walking up stairs?			
17. Because of his/her problem, does your child have difficulty walking one or two blocks?			
18. Because of his/her problem, does your child have difficulty riding a bike or scooter?			
19. Because of his/her problem, does your child have difficulty reading or doing schoolwork?			
20. Does your child's problem make it difficult to successfully do activities that others his/her age can do?			
21. Because of his/her problem, does your child have trouble concentrating at school?			
	TOTAL SCORE		

FIG. 5.1 The Vanderbilt Pediatric Dizziness Handicap Inventory for Patient Caregivers (DHI-PC). (From McCaslin DL, Jacobson GP, Lambert W, English LN, Kemph AJ. The development of the Vanderbilt pediatric dizziness handicap inventory for patient caregivers (DHI-PC). *Int J Pediatr Otorhinolaryngol.* 2015;79(10):1662–1666; with permission.)

testing can be difficult. In this regard, several investigators have designed structured case histories to be used for the evaluation of vertiginous children.[8,24–26] One example set forth by Ravid et al.[25] consists of a set of structured questions coupled with a computer algorithm designed to aid in the differential diagnosis of the dizzy child.

To validate the effectiveness of the questionnaire, the authors performed a retrospective analysis of data collected from all children presenting with dizziness to their clinic over a 2-year period. Responses to the structured questionnaire were compared with the computer algorithm, and both were compared against the final diagnoses in the medical record. The questionnaire-derived diagnoses matched the medical record diagnoses in 92% of the patients, and results of the computer-assisted algorithm were identical to the final diagnoses in the medical record in 84% of patients. Similarly, Niemensivu et al.[26] evaluated a structured case history for the diagnosis of dizziness in children and, following thorough clinical examination and vestibular laboratory testing, found that the most common disorders identified using this approach were otitis media–related vertigo, migraine-associated dizziness, and benign paroxysmal vertigo of childhood (BPVC).

In our experience, using a structured case history coupled with a decision tree has worked well to identify patients who will benefit from vestibular testing. For instance, if the algorithm suggests that the patient may have labyrinthitis, then quantitative testing can be performed to determine whether the child has a peripheral impairment, whether it is unilateral or bilateral, if unilateral how severe, and whether the child is compensating centrally for the impairment. Conversely, if a child presents with chronic dizziness, no hearing loss, and a documented neurologic deficit(s), balance function testing would most likely not be indicated, and other issues would need to be ruled out (e.g., degenerative disease or posterior fossa tumor) using different techniques. This information is useful to both the physician and the pediatric physical therapist when considering management options. This approach also streamlines the differential diagnostic process and affords the physician the ability to be selective in determining which tests will be beneficial in deriving the diagnosis and which will not.

Recently, Pavlou, Whitney, and associates[27] developed and validated the Pediatric Vestibular Symptom Questionnaire (PVSQ). This instrument is designed to identify and quantify subjective vestibular symptoms (e.g., dizziness, imbalance) in children aged 6–17 years. The study also had a secondary

component, which described relationships among symptoms in children with vestibular impairment versus dizziness or imbalance secondary to concussion. This instrument can be used not only as an indicator for whether a child requires further assessment to investigate a potential balance impairment, but also as a metric that can be used to evaluate the effectiveness of treatment (Fig. 5.2).

THE MOST COMMON DISORDERS

After otitis media, the two most common conditions reported in the literature causing dizziness/vertigo in children are migraine headache and BPVC. The next most common disorders are trauma and vestibular neuritis. Interestingly, all of these disorders can result in patients who have abnormal findings on balance function testing. This reinforces the importance of having vestibular testing available in the pediatric dizzy clinic. Two recent studies illustrate this argument well. First, a recent report by Szirmai[5] evaluated vestibular function in children (<14 years of age, $n = 66$) and adolescents (14–18 years of age, $n = 79$). The author reported that migrainous vertigo (MV) was the most common disorder causing dizziness in this cohort, followed by extravestibular disease (e.g., anxiety, panic disorder) and then labyrinthitis. Only 36% of the patients in this study demonstrated normal vestibular system function. In the group of adolescents, extravestibular disease was the most common cause of vertigo followed by migraine. Only 39% of the adolescents demonstrated normal vestibular results.

A report by Wiener-Vacher[9] reviewed the most common vestibular disorders in over 2000 children over a 14-year period. Patient records were examined retrospectively to determine the most common diagnoses in children presenting with dizziness and vertigo. Consistent with many earlier reports, the most commonly diagnosed vestibular disturbance was MV, which was responsible for nearly 25% of patients. BPVC represented 20% of the diagnoses, and cranial trauma and ophthalmologic disorders each accounted for 10% of the diagnoses. In this cohort, vestibular neuritis (5%) and posterior fossa tumors (<1%) were less often encountered.

Table 5.1 provides a summary of findings from a series of studies each describing the most frequent causes of pediatric dizziness/vertigo that are encountered clinically. Characteristics of these conditions (i.e., pathophysiology and balance function test findings) are described.

> The following questions ask about how often you feel dizziness and unsteadiness. Please circle the best answer for you.
> How often in the past month have you felt the following?
> 1. A feeling that things are spinning or moving around
>
> | 3 | 2 | 3 | 4 | ? |
> |---|---|---|---|---|
> | Most of the time | Sometimes | Almost never | Never | Don't know |
>
> 2. Unsteadiness so bad that you actually fall
>
> | 3 | 2 | 3 | 4 | ? |
> |---|---|---|---|---|
> | Most of the time | Sometimes | Almost never | Never | Don't know |
>
> 3. Feeling sick
>
> | 3 | 2 | 3 | 4 | ? |
> |---|---|---|---|---|
> | Most of the time | Sometimes | Almost never | Never | Don't know |
>
> 4. A light-headed or swimmy feeling in the head
>
> | 3 | 2 | 3 | 4 | ? |
> |---|---|---|---|---|
> | Most of the time | Sometimes | Almost never | Never | Don't know |
>
> 5. Feeling of pressure in the ear(s)
>
> | 3 | 2 | 3 | 4 | ? |
> |---|---|---|---|---|
> | Most of the time | Sometimes | Almost never | Never | Don't know |
>
> 6. Blurry vision, difficulty seeing things clearly, and/or spots before the eyes
>
> | 3 | 2 | 3 | 4 | ? |
> |---|---|---|---|---|
> | Most of the time | Sometimes | Almost never | Never | Don't know |
>
> 7. Headache or feeling of pressure in the head
>
> | 3 | 2 | 3 | 4 | ? |
> |---|---|---|---|---|
> | Most of the time | Sometimes | Almost never | Never | Don't know |
>
> 8. Unable to stand or walk without holding on to something or someone
>
> | 3 | 2 | 3 | 4 | ? |
> |---|---|---|---|---|
> | Most of the time | Sometimes | Almost never | Never | Don't know |
>
> 9. Feeling unsteady, about to lose balance
>
> | 3 | 2 | 3 | 4 | ? |
> |---|---|---|---|---|
> | Most of the time | Sometimes | Almost never | Never | Don't know |
>
> 10. A fuzzy or cotton wool feeling in the head
>
> | 3 | 2 | 3 | 4 | ? |
> |---|---|---|---|---|
> | Most of the time | Sometimes | Almost never | Never | Don't know |
>
> 11. Do any of these symptoms stop you doing what you want to do?
> If yes, which ones? ....

Questionnaire copy not to scale.

FIG. 5.2 The pediatric vestibular symptom questionnaire. (From Pavlou M, Whitney S, Alkathiry AA, et al. The pediatric vestibular symptom questionnaire: a validation study. *J Pediatr.* 2016;168:171–177e1. https://doi.org/10.1016/j.jpeds.2015.09.075; with permission.)

MIGRAINE-ASSOCIATED VERTIGO IN CHILDREN

A number of epidemiologic investigations of dizziness in childhood have been published recently. Pacheva and Ivanov[28] reported their observations from a sample of 2509 pediatric migraine patients who were evaluated in a pediatric neurologic clinic. These investigators reported that migraine variants were responsible for symptoms in 24% of the patients, basilar migraine (BM) was diagnosed in 6% of patients, and BPVC and hemiplegic migraine were responsible for 5% and 4% of diagnoses, respectively.

Teixeira et al.[29] reported findings of patients with migraine equivalents who were evaluated in an outpatient pediatric neurology clinic. Of the 674 pediatric headache patients, 38 (5.6%) had migraine equivalents, and the majority were males. Further review revealed that 15 patients had abdominal migraine, 12 had BPVC, 5 had confusional migraine, 3 had aura without migraine, 2 had paroxysmal torticollis, and 1 patient had cyclic vomiting. A family history of migraine was common.

Marcelli et al.[30] conducted an investigation focusing on BPVC, which is one of the most common pediatric

TABLE 5.1
Literature Reports of the Most Common Causes of Vertigo/Dizziness in Children

			Balatsouras et al.[10]	Bower and Cotton[11]	Choung et al.[17]	D'Agostino et al.[109]	Erbek et al.[18]	Ravid et al.[25]	Riina et al.[3]	Weisleder and Fife[36]	Szirmai[5]	Wiener-Vacher[9]
Total subjects	832	%	54	34	55	282	50	62	119	31	145	More than 2k
Migraine	n (%)	17.19	11 (20.4)	4 (11.8)	17 (30.9)	15 (5.4)	17 (34)	24 (39)	17 (14.3)	11 (35.5)	27 (18.6)	25%
	143											
BPVC	n (%)	15.99	9 (16.7)	5 (14.7)	14 (25.5)	60 (21)	6 (12)	10 (16)	23 (19.3)	6 (19.4)		20%
	133											
Otitis media	n (%)	2.64	5 (9.2)	5 (14.7)	d		d		12 (10.1)			
	22											
Viral infection	n (%)	15.63	15 (27.7)	4 (11.8)	1 (1.8)	53 (18.8)	2 (4)	9 (14)	14 (11.8)		32 (22.1)	5%
	132											
Trauma	n (%)	13.1	3 (5.5)	3 (8.8)	4 (7.3)	85 (30.3)		2 (3)	6 (5)		6 (4.1)	10%
	109											

Some studies excluded children with otitis media (denoted with d); BPVC, benign paroxysmal vertigo of childhood.

migraine equivalents. It was the authors' objective to characterize the progression of BPVC by conducting a 10-year longitudinal investigation with a sample of 15 children. These investigators reported that 67% of the patients reported either the onset or worsening of migraine over this interval. Furthermore, the neurootologic assessment was abnormal for 20% of patients during the symptom-free period and was abnormal for 67% of patients during the episode.

Another epidemiologic investigation by Raucci et al.[31] reported their experience assessing vertigo and dizziness in a pediatric emergency department over a 5-year period. They found that dizziness and/or vertigo was the presenting complaint in 616 out of a total of 248,834 visits (or 2.5 dizzy patients per 1000 visits). The most common dizziness disorders were migraine, which accounted for 25% of visits, and BPVC, which accounted for 6% of the diagnoses.

Sommerfleck et al.[32] reported the primary dizziness diagnoses of 206 patients aged 1–18 years (median age: 10 years). These investigators commented that 39% of the sample met criteria for definite vestibular migraine and another 13% satisfied criteria for probable MV. Interestingly, before puberty more boys than girls had migraine diagnoses. Following puberty the sex ratio favored girls. The most common disorder affecting children aged 1–5 years was BPVC. For the group between 6–11 and 12–18 years of age, the most common disorder was vestibular migraine.

The general view is that vestibular migraine coupled with BPVC account for approximately 37% of dizzy/vertiginous diagnoses in pediatric patients. The dizziness is described as moderate to severe in intensity and should be present for at least 5 minutes and no more than 72 hours. In fact, one-third of patients experience dizziness lasting minutes, one-third experience dizziness lasting hours, and one-third experience dizziness lasting days. Approximately 10% of patients experience short-lasting dizziness (seconds). Dizziness may precede or follow the headache, and the dizziness perception may be either spinning or a rocking sensation.

There are a number of "episodic syndromes" that may be migraine variants that can affect pediatric dizzy patients. These syndromes include infantile colic, benign paroxysmal torticollis, benign paroxysmal vertigo, cyclical vomiting syndrome, and abdominal migraine. These are referred to as episodic syndromes because head pain may be completely absent. These variants may occur in isolation or may coexist with other migrainous diagnoses. Furthermore, the prevalence of these syndromes has been reported to range from 2% to 4% of the pediatric dizzy population.[33]

Treatments for vestibular migraine range from sleep hygiene and diet control to prophylactic treatment with medications that include flunarizine, propranolol, metoprolol, topiramate, clonazepam, lamotrigine, nortriptyline, amitriptyline, verapamil, and lomerizine.[34]

As mentioned previously, the most common diagnosis in children with vertigo and dizziness is migraine headache or migraine equivalent, although the temporal relationship of headache and dizziness has been reported to be variable. That is, vertigo may precede, follow, or occur simultaneously with dizziness/vertigo, and often there are accompanying symptoms such as nausea and/or sensory distortions (i.e., sensitivity to light, sound, taste, smell, and motion). The clinical features of migraine in children can be different from those seen in adults.[35] In childhood, migraines often are localized to the frontal or periorbital region, last less than 2 hours and may not manifest themselves as the typical throbbing pain often described by adults.[36] Approximately 20% of children with migraine have associated dizziness. There are three commonly reported migraine variants that can produce abnormal findings on quantitative vestibular system testing[37]: BM, MV, and BPVC.[38,39] Reports estimate that BM occurs in 3%–19% of children with migraine and usually occurs around age 7 years.[35] Many migraines present with an aura consisting of different sensory sensations (e.g., olfactory, visual, or vestibular). BM has been described in the literature as presenting with an aura consisting of audiovestibular manifestations, such as tinnitus, loss of hearing, acute imbalance, and vertigo.[40] Usually, the neurologic examination in pediatric patients with BM is normal. According to Eggers,[41] only a very small proportion of patients with MV meet criteria for BM.

Etiology and Pathophysiology of Migraine

The pathophysiology of vestibular migraine is currently unresolved. In BM, the root cause has been suggested to be asymmetrical activation of brainstem vestibular nuclei or defective Ca^{2+} channels, which are shared by the brain and the inner ear.[38,42] MV is considered by most to be a distinct entity, and as with BM the pathophysiology of MV is still not completely understood. Investigators have set forth hypotheses, which include cortical spreading depression affecting the parietoinsular vestibular cortex, and changes in activity between the parietal cortex and vestibular nuclei.[43–45]

Balance Function Findings in Children With Migraine

Laboratory findings in patients with MV can consist of both central and peripheral impairment and have been well-documented in adults. Olsson[46] evaluated 50 patients with BM and 49 of the participants demonstrated abnormal ocular motor testing. When caloric test findings are combined across studies, the frequency with which unilateral impairment was observed ranged from 8% to 60% of patients.[43,44,46,47] Marcelli et al.[48] reported vestibular findings in 22 children diagnosed with migraine. In this sample, 73% of participants with MV demonstrated either peripheral or central vestibular abnormalities. The vestibular manifestations varied and included spontaneous-positional nystagmus, post head-shaking nystagmus, benign paroxysmal positional vertigo, vibration-induced nystagmus, the absence of VEMPs, and reduced responses to caloric stimuli—unilaterally or bilaterally. Vestibular system testing may be a useful tool in the differential diagnosis of children with migraine, especially in those children whose headaches are associated with vertigo or dizziness.

BENIGN PAROXYSMAL VERTIGO OF CHILDHOOD

BPVC was initially reported by Basser in 1964, who described the clinical presentation of BPVC in 17 children ≤ 4 years of age.[49] Primary symptoms include episodic attacks of vertigo lasting from seconds to minutes resulting in the child being unable to stand without support. Additional symptoms include nystagmus, tinnitus, pallor, diaphoresis, and vomiting. BPVC is a pediatric migraine equivalent recognized by the International Headache Society classification system.[50] During attacks of BPVC, there is no loss of consciousness, and there is a complete recovery following an attack. A child who is capable will describe a sensation of spinning. The age of onset of BPVC has been reported to occur before 4 years of age and is rarely seen after 8 years of age.[49] In an epidemiologic study by Russell and Abu Arafeh,[6] it was determined that 2% of school-age children met criteria for BPVC, defined as at least three transient episodes of the sensation of rotation, either of the child or of the surrounding environment severe enough to interfere with normal activity and not associated with loss of consciousness or any neurologic auditory abnormality.

Etiology and Pathophysiology of Benign Paroxysmal Vertigo of Childhood

While the pathophysiology of BPVC is currently unknown, there is strong supporting evidence that BPVC is a migraine headache variant. Many children with BPVC will go on to develop migraine later in life.[6,51–55] There is mounting evidence suggesting that in many patients, BPVC is vascular in origin.[42,49,56,57] For example, an episodic vasospasm could result in ischemia to the inner ear culminating in end-organ impairment and consequently vertigo. A central mechanism postulated is an interruption in blood flow to the vestibular nuclei and associated pathways.[49,56] Regardless of etiology, the variable nature of laboratory findings makes diagnosing this disorder difficult. Currently, the diagnosis of BPVC is primarily dependent on a reliable and characteristic history.

Balance Function Findings in Children With Benign Paroxysmal Vertigo of Childhood

There is great variability in quantitative vestibular test results obtained from patients with BPVC. Several studies have reported that children with BPVC commonly present with significant bithermal caloric asymmetry.[49,58,59] However, other investigators have found no such relationship.[60,61] Mierzwinski et al.[62] evaluated 124 children with vertigo, 13 of whom presented with characteristics commonly associated with BPVC. Results showed that of this subset of 13 patients, 5 had normal electronystagmography (ENG) test results. In addition, one patient was found to have significant unilateral caloric weakness, and the other seven patients had either central vestibular impairments or a mixture of peripheral and central vestibular system deficits.

TRAUMA

Traumatic brain injury (TBI) in young children is common, and significant attention has been given to these conditions recently because of increased public awareness of concussion in sports. A TBI is disruption of typical brain function following a sudden blow to the head or body. This can occur because of direct trauma to the head (i.e., blunt force, penetrating injury) or indirectly through whiplash mechanisms. The Centers for Disease Control and Prevention have stated that children under 14 years of age comprise approximately 500,000 emergency department visits for TBI each year.[63] Most TBIs are classified as "mild" or "concussions" with a large proportion occurring because of sports- or recreation-related injuries. An estimated 3.8 million sports-related concussions occur in the United States annually[64] with fewer than 10% seeking evaluation in emergency departments.[65] Unfortunately, these numbers may not represent the scope of concussion-related injuries, as up to half of concussions may go unrecognized or unreported.[64,66]

Postinjury, children may present with a wide range of symptoms such as headache, dizziness, imbalance, cognitive impairment, changes in personality, and sleep disturbance. Vestibular-related abnormalities noted at initial presentation have been associated with delayed return to academics and sports or recreational activities.[67,68]

Etiology and Pathophysiology of Trauma

Children with TBIs may demonstrate peripheral, central, or mixed vestibulopathy. The majority of reports in the literature regarding objective measurement of vestibular dysfunction following trauma have been collected in adults. In adults, peripheral vestibulopathy has been associated with direct end-organ damage, especially to otolith organs.[69] Labyrinthine concussion is thought to be due to microscopic hemorrhages or damage to the sensory epithelium.[70] Perilymph fistula,[71] posttraumatic endolymphatic hydrops,[72] superior semicircular canal dehiscence,[73] and BPPV have also been reported following trauma.[74-76] Peripheral vestibulopathy has been associated with penetrating or blunt head trauma, especially when temporal bone fracture occurs.[77,78] If the vestibular labyrinth and/or vestibular nerve are affected following head injury, children can experience severe vertigo with nystagmus and nausea consistent with acute unilateral peripheral vestibular impairment. Posttraumatic BPPV has a reported incidence of 11% in adults,[74] and while pediatric vestibular clinics report the prevalence of BPPV between 5% and 12%,[18,79] the rate of postinjury BPPV is not yet known. Case studies have demonstrated this possibility[75,76] and BPPV should be considered for children with posttraumatic vertigo.

Central vestibulopathy associated with dizziness and imbalance is common following head injury and may be related to various causes. These include diffuse axonal injury, migraine-associated dizziness, and/or psychologic considerations. These are not exclusive categories, and a child's dizziness may be related to multiple underlying causes. Furthermore, it may be that a child presents to the clinic with both peripheral and central involvement, which can lead to complicated management. In general, concussions are minimally associated with peripheral vestibulopathy[80,81]; however, up to 81% of adolescent and collegiate athletes report difficulty with dizziness and imbalance postinjury, thought to be related to atypical central vestibular functioning.[82,83] Alhilali et al.[84] hypothesized that patients with mild TBI likely present with dizziness symptoms because of diffuse axonal injury. This study evaluated 30 children and adults with reported dizziness and/or imbalance following mild TBI. All patients were evaluated using tract-based spatial statistics of diffusion-tensor imaging on magnetic resonance imaging

(MRI). These data provided radiologic evidence of atypical cerebellar and fusiform gyri function, which are regions associated with sensorimotor processing, balance, and visually guided movement. Furthermore, these authors noted that injury to the cerebellum in those patients with mild TBI and vestibular symptoms was associated with prolonged symptom recovery, which has previously been noted only using clinical signs and symptoms.[82,83]

Balance Function Findings in Children With Trauma

Objective vestibular diagnostic testing is rarely documented in children following head injury, and currently available studies often provide mixed results because of the small number of participants as well as the wide range of likely injuries included in the sample. Peripheral end-organ damage should especially be suspected if the child also presents with hearing loss. Several cases of posttraumatic perilymph fistula have been reported. For example, Neuenschwander et al.[85] and Kim et al.[86] described cases of ataxia and/or vertigo following penetrating and blunt head injuries in children. Three of the five case studies resulted in diagnoses of perilymphatic fistula, one with dehiscence of the oval window, and one with ossicular chain damage without surgical evidence for fistula. All of the children in these case studies demonstrated hearing impairment; four were sensorineural and one was conductive. Spontaneous nystagmus was observed in three of the five patients. Although not commonly reported, these studies demonstrate the possibility of perilymph fistula presenting in pediatric head trauma patients and should be considered, especially in the presence of concurrent hearing loss.

In one of the most comprehensive studies describing effects of blunt head injury in children, Vartiainen et al.[87] described findings in 199 children. These investigators compared 61 children treated for acute blunt head injury with 59 age-matched controls. An additional 138 children with previous diagnosis of blunt head trauma were invited for examination to determine posttraumatic findings in the long term. Thirty-nine patients (19.6%) had sustained skull fracture. The results of this study are summarized in Table 5.2.

Spontaneous nystagmus and/or positional nystagmus was defined by a maximum slow-phase eye velocity that was ≥7 degrees/second. Abnormal smooth pursuit and failure of fixation suppression for a minimum of two caloric irrigations was considered a central ENG finding. These authors also studied subjective vestibular disturbances

TABLE 5.2
Summary of Large-Scale Study by Vartiainen et al.[87] Describing Findings in 199 Children With Blunt Head Trauma at Different Intervals Postinjury

	Blunt Trauma (n = 61, Caloric Testing Performed on 41)		Blunt Trauma (n = 138, Caloric Testing Performed on 113)
	Immediately Following Trauma	6–12 months Posttrauma	2–8 years Posttrauma
Spontaneous nystagmus and/or positional nystagmus	21 (46%)	8 (17%)	22 (18%)
Central ENG finding	20 (43%)	10 (24%)	14 (12%)
Caloric testing (*performed in 154 of 190 total patients*)	40 (21%)	13 (7%)	11 (6%)

Results are presented in *n* (%) format.

in their patients. Of the 61 patients with acute head injury, only 1 (2%) complained of vertigo. The severity of abnormal vestibular diagnostic results was associated with the severity of injury, noting that children with positive imaging findings or loss of consciousness greater than 15 minutes had two to four times the likelihood of abnormal ENG findings than children with less severe injuries. Of 138 patients who were evaluated 12 months or more post–head injury, 2 patients (1%) described vertigo. Authors of this study hypothesize that while objective vestibular lesions are common in children with head injuries, children rarely express subjective symptoms. This may indicate that children are able to compensate quickly for unilateral vestibular system disturbance.[87]

Surprisingly, reports describing findings on quantitative vestibular and balance function testing in children following significant head trauma are rare with the exception of the large-scale study by Vartiainen et al.[87] It may be more likely that children who have sustained head trauma are referred for hearing evaluation. When it is determined that the child has hearing loss, quantitative vestibular testing may be indicated as well. In particular, sensorineural hearing loss is often a sentinel symptom of temporal bone fracture or perilymphatic fistula. Children presenting with audiovestibular signs (e.g., ataxia, vertigo, hearing loss, tinnitus) should be receive both auditory and vestibular assessment to reduce possible sequelae from unmanaged symptoms.

With the increase in attention provided to concussion in recent years, more data are available concerning mild TBI or concussion. These injuries can be sustained with direct or indirect injury to the head and are quite commonly associated with dizziness and imbalance in children. Traditional vestibulo-ocular reflex (VOR) testing (i.e., caloric, video head impulse testing) has not been contributory to the diagnosis for these patients.[80,81] For example, Alshehri et al.[80] evaluated 56 children and adults postconcussion using video head impulse testing (vHIT) to describe the presence of VOR pathway dysfunction. No patient demonstrated abnormal vHIT responses; however, significant increases in headache, dizziness, and nausea were noted posttest.

While peripheral vestibulopathy has not been well studied in children following concussion, up to 81% demonstrate abnormalities of functional VOR (i.e., gaze stability) as well as dynamic balance.[67,68] These reports suggest that evaluation of the vestibular and balance systems, especially in a dynamic or functional manner, is particularly important for appropriate management of children following concussion to facilitate academic success and return to sport/recreational activities. Zhou and Brodsky[81] provide one of the most comprehensive pediatric postconcussion datasets including objective vestibular evaluations, finding that dynamic or integrative evaluations, such as dynamic visual acuity testing and computerized dynamic posturography, were most often abnormal in children with dizziness and balance complaints following concussion. In this sample, significant abnormalities in dynamic visual acuity were noted in 57% of the children, while compromised balance was found in 40%. Diagnostic impairments noted on caloric testing were found in 21%, while rotary chair abnormalities were noted in up to 27% depending on the metric used. Otolith reflex abnormalities, as measured by cervical VEMPs, were found in 18%. These data suggest that including evaluations of dynamic function improves the ability to identify atypical vestibular function in children postconcussion. This has been replicated in adult studies, finding that abnormalities in dynamic sensory integration are common after injury.[88]

COCHLEAR IMPLANTATION

Cochlear implantation has provided access to auditory information in children with significant hearing loss. This technology utilizes an electrode array inserted into the cochlea to stimulate the auditory nerve. Depending on the etiology of inner ear pathology, vestibular dysfunction may be present in up to half of these children.[89,90] Additionally, the cochlear implant procedure itself may cause dizziness and imbalance postoperatively.

Dizziness and imbalance are the most commonly reported complications for children post–cochlear implantation. Sivan et al.[91] provide a retrospective chart review of 579 pediatric cochlear implant recipients. Both unilaterally and bilaterally implanted users across all ages (1–17 years) reported dizziness and imbalance complaints. Thirty-two percent of children experienced dizziness or imbalance postoperatively; however, those with anatomical anomalies (e.g., enlarged vestibular aqueduct) were up to four times more likely to experience these complications. In addition, the percentage of dizziness and balance complaints was significantly increased for those undergoing revision surgery, likely related to increased trauma associated with removal and reinsertion of the electrode array.

The long-term effects of cochlear implantation on the developing balance system are not well known. De Kegel et al.[92] noted that children receiving cochlear implants between 6 and 18 months of age have significantly different gross motor skill development when compared with the developmental trajectory of children with normal hearing or deaf children without cochlear implantation. Initial data suggest that these trajectories can be corrected, but that longitudinal studies are needed to better understand the impact of early cochlear implantation on vestibular and balance development of young children.

Etiology and Pathophysiology of Cochlear Implant–Related Dizziness

Risk factors associated with dizziness and imbalance after cochlear implant surgery are related to structural anomalies of the inner ear that can be identified on imaging studies before surgery and intraoperative factors related to trauma to the inner ear. Children with significant sensorineural hearing loss may also demonstrate atypical inner ear structures or etiologies associated with concomitant vestibulopathy. In some patients, these underlying structural abnormalities may result in vestibular dysfunction. Cushing et al.[89] evaluated 153 children and found that the rate of vestibular dysfunction was higher for those with cochleovestibular abnormalities that included common cavity and enlarged vestibular aqueduct. Horizontal semicircular canal function, as measured by caloric irrigations, was abnormal in 39% (11 of 28 children), with abnormalities in rotary chair tests noted in approximately half of those evaluated. Furthermore, saccular reflex testing was abnormal in 46% of patients. These authors also found that as the complexity of anatomical abnormality increased, so did the likelihood of vestibular dysfunction.

As the cochlea is proximal to vestibular end organs, vestibular trauma may occur because of electrode array insertion. As the electrode array is inserted into the cochlea, significant pressure can be exerted, especially along the 180 degrees mark of the cochlea. As the saccule is positioned opposite the basal turn of the cochlea, pressure from electrode insertion is exerted on the saccule. Tien and Linthicum[93] evaluated a sample of 11 pairs of temporal bones from patients with unilateral cochlear implants. They noted significant damage to vestibular end organs in 55%, with the majority of damage occurring in the saccule. In addition, Handzel et al.[94] found collapse of the saccule in 53% (9 of 17 temporal bones). Postoperatively, endolymphatic hydrops due to electrode insertion trauma or postoperative inflammatory processes has been demonstrated in up to 57% in small samples of cochlear implant users.[94–96] The prevalence of altered labyrinthine structures postoperatively is obviously limited but seems likely to some extent as demonstrated by histopathologic studies as well as functional findings described below.

Balance Function Findings in Children Post–Cochlear Implantation

Vestibular diagnostic information has been documented for children and adults post–cochlear implantation with the overall consensus showing some level of vestibular impairment in up to half of patients.[97] In a systematic review of 439 cochlear implant recipients, Kuang et al.[98] noted that approximately one-third of cochlear implant recipients demonstrated reduced vestibular function as measured by caloric testing. Furthermore, Jacot et al.[99] evaluated 89 children between 7 months and 16.5 years of age both before and after cochlear implantation, with half demonstrating atypical vestibular function prior to surgery. Of those with appropriate VOR function (i.e., caloric testing) prior to implantation, 60.5% demonstrated symmetrical responses at their postoperative evaluation. The majority of change noted on testing demonstrated a significant decrease in function; however, a small subset of patients actually demonstrated hyperactive caloric response of the operated ear, perhaps consistent with irritation within the labyrinth. Abnormalities in VOR pathways are not universally reported. Ajalloueyan et al.[100] did not find any change in VOR test results as measured with caloric and vHIT in children between 1 and 4 years of age. Unfortunately, because of the tolerance limits of these young children, only 13 children were evaluated with caloric irrigations and 8 with vHIT. However, these data are in agreement with Nassif et al.[101] who evaluated 16 older children (5–17 years) with unilateral or bilateral cochlear implants and found no difference in VOR gain as measured by vHIT. Further evaluation of the postoperative effects on VOR is needed to systematically evaluate the effects of surgery on the inner ear.

As the otolith organs may be at increased risk for damage during cochlear implantation due to their proximity to the cochlea, changes in saccular and utricular function have been studied. Several studies have reported reduced cervical VEMP responses in up to half of recipients post–cochlear implantation.[97,102-104] Krause et al.[105] reported on 25 adolescent and adult cochlear implant recipients; only 8 patients demonstrated appropriate cervical VEMPs preoperatively and half lost function after implantation. These authors hypothesize that this may be related to the higher risk of saccular injury during surgery. Interestingly, fewer than 40% of those with reduced otolith responses reported concerns with balance or dizziness following surgery. Similarly, Devroede et al.[104] evaluated 26 children between 1 and 13 years of age who were under evaluation for their second cochlear implant. The majority of children (79%) demonstrated appropriate cervical VEMP responses prior to implantation; however, 21% had abnormal VEMPs after surgery. The otolith organs are important in developing appropriate balance function,[92,106] and the saccule may be particularly vulnerable to injury during the implantation process.[93,94] These findings suggest that further investigation of the vestibular system before and possibly after cochlear implantation may provide important information to

achieve optimal management for a child who may be at risk for gross motor delay.

Gross motor skills, including balance function, have been evaluated in children following cochlear implantation. Ebrahimi et al.[107] evaluated 85 children between 7 and 12 years of age with congenital or early onset bilateral profound hearing loss and compared these children with age-matched controls. Forty-one percent of the children with hearing loss also had a unilateral cochlear implant at a mean age of 4.5 years. Balance testing was completed, finding that children with hearing loss, especially those with a cochlear implant, demonstrated reduced balance function as compared with controls. An additional study by Huang et al.[108] evaluated the standing balance of 24 adolescents with at least 5 years of cochlear implant use, finding that they demonstrated significantly poorer balance than their peers. An effect of etiology was possible in this study; however, results highlight the potential for long-term balance dysfunction that may occur in these patients. It is unclear if there is sufficient compensation over time.

While there is considerable variability in vestibular system outcomes for children post–cochlear implantation, the overall consensus in the literature is that there is some level of risk, at least for a subset of children. As such, discussing this with caregivers (and patients when possible) preoperatively is essential for managing expectations for the postoperative period.

VESTIBULAR NEURITIS

Vestibular neuritis in adults presents as a sudden onset of rotary vertigo and vomiting lasting for several days to weeks (see Chapter 10). Children experiencing an attack of vestibular neuritis often present with the same symptoms as their adult counterparts.[10,11,17,18,109-113]

Etiology and Pathophysiology of Vestibular Neuritis

While the cause of vestibular neuritis is somewhat controversial, many investigators have suggested that vestibular neuritis is viral in origin, although bacterial and other types of infections have also been suggested.[114-116] It has also been suggested that unknown factors may contribute to reactivation of a latent virus (e.g., herpes zoster oticus), resulting in inflammation of the nerve and potentially causing cell damage.[116,117]

Balance Function Findings in Children With Vestibular Neuritis

Vestibular neuritis is uncommon in children. However, there have been a few published accounts of quantitative vestibular assessment of children after vestibular neuritis. The caloric examination is the gold standard for documenting the side and degree of peripheral vestibular impairment and can provide information regarding integrity of lateral semicircular canals and/or superior vestibular nerves. The clinical utility of the caloric examination for measuring peripheral vestibular function in children was demonstrated by Balatsouras et al.[10] who evaluated 54 children with dizziness, 15 of whom received a final diagnosis of viral infection. Abnormal peripheral ENG findings were documented in 13 of these children and were defined as the presence of spontaneous nystagmus, directional preponderance, and/or caloric weakness. The remaining two children had a combination of peripheral findings as well as a central finding, defined as one or more of the following: saccadic pursuit, gaze-evoked nystagmus, spontaneous central nystagmus, positional central nystagmus, or impaired fixation suppression during caloric testing. In three separate studies, caloric responses in five children diagnosed with vestibular neuritis demonstrated a significant deficit.[17,18,113] Other studies have supported the role of caloric testing for quantifying vestibular impairment in children with vestibular neuritis. Bower and Cotton[11] reported their findings for three children with vestibular neuritis, one of whom demonstrated significant caloric weakness. Melagrana et al.[112] reported findings from 72 children with unilateral sensorineural hearing loss of possible viral origin. In their sample, 20 children (28%) displayed significant unilateral vestibular weakness during caloric examination. Additionally, they noted either spontaneous nystagmus or positional nystagmus in 53% of the children.

Rotary chair testing can also be a useful tool in assessing children with suspected vestibular neuritis. Choung et al.[17] reported results of positional, rotary chair, and caloric testing in 55 children with the chief complaint of vertigo or dizziness, one of whom was diagnosed with vestibular neuritis. This lone patient demonstrated unilateral caloric weakness and no significant positional nystagmus. In addition, abnormal VOR gain, phase, or symmetry (not specified by authors) during rotary chair testing was observed, and normal VOR fixation further suggested a peripheral origin of the dizziness.

Other investigators have described characteristics of children with vestibular neuritis during the physical examination and bedside testing. In a review of 282 children with vertigo by D'Agostino et al.,[109] 50 children were diagnosed with labyrinthitis, 2 with vestibular neuritis, and 1 with cochleovestibular neuritis. The

two patients with diagnosed vestibular neuritis demonstrated spontaneous nystagmus and positive Romberg's sign, and one demonstrated "moderate" positional nystagmus. In separate case studies of children with vestibular neuritis, Ergul et al.[110] and Zannolli et al.[113] also described findings from bedside testing. Both patients presented with vestibular spontaneous nystagmus, a positive head thrust test in the direction of suspected impairment, and a positive Romberg's sign.

One must be careful not to rely on vestibular testing alone to diagnose vestibular neuritis but rather consider it a part of the entire evaluation (including history, physical, and neurologic examinations). In a recent study, Goudakos et al.,[118] evaluated adult patients with vestibular neuritis. When caloric responses were analyzed, 90% of patients maintained a significant vestibular weakness after 1 month. When patients were evaluated 6 months post–symptom onset, 80% of patients continued to have abnormal caloric findings. In this regard, Eviatar and Eviatar[111] identified 5 of 50 children in their cohort with vestibular neuronitis. Each of these children had an acute onset of vertigo and nausea without impairment of hearing following an upper respiratory infection and mild earache. Vestibular testing was completed 2 weeks postonset, and two of the five children demonstrated directional preponderance on caloric stimulation with no caloric weakness. The remaining three children demonstrated normal vestibular examinations implying spontaneous recovery (or no acute loss).

The majority of studies to date have utilized caloric testing and bedside testing to describe impairments in the vestibular system believed to be due to viral origin. Further investigations centered on the clinical utility of tests such as cVEMP and oVEMP for assessing pediatric dizziness will certainly be done in the coming years. There remains a paucity of data describing effects of central nervous system compensation in children and how this can affect quantitative vestibular testing. While these data are available in adults, it is currently unclear how the rate of recovery may differ in children with vestibular neuritis.[119]

In a recent investigation, Brodsky et al.[120] described both the clinical features of, and recovery from vestibular neuritis in children. Their sample included 11 children between the ages of 5 and 19 years, with an average vertigo duration of 10 days. These investigators reported that both caloric and rotary chair testing were abnormal in 100% of the patients, vHIT was abnormal in 62% of patients, subjective visual vertical testing was abnormal in 50% of the sample, and none of the children had abnormal cVEMPs (most likely because the superior division of the vestibular nerve was affected in each case). Interestingly, 36% of the patients failed to recover completely, and these children were older (≥15 years of age) at the time of symptom onset. Furthermore, those who failed to recover completely also were found to have initiated vestibular rehabilitation later from the onset of symptoms (i.e., >90 days) compared with those patients who recovered completely (i.e., initiated vestibular rehabilitation therapy ≤14 days from the onset of the symptoms). This information highlights importance of early intervention during the post–acute period.

OTITIS MEDIA

Otitis media and middle ear effusion are frequently quoted as a common cause of vestibular complaints in children.[2,8,11,121,122] The reported symptoms are typically "unsteadiness" and "clumsiness" rather than true vertigo. A longitudinal, population-based investigation of 21,962 adults examining the relationship between presence of otitis media during childhood and occurrence of dizziness during adulthood has been reported.[123] Patients were evaluated at ages 7, 10, and 13 years and underwent a hearing screening in a longitudinal school hearing evaluation. Children identified with hearing loss were referred to otolaryngologists for assessment and treatment. The same individuals, as adults, completed a health questionnaire that contained questions focused on dizziness. These investigators reported that adults who, as children, had a history of either chronic suppurative otitis media or recurrent acute otitis media were 2.1 and 1.3 times, respectively, more likely to experience dizziness as adults.

Etiology and Pathophysiology of Otitis Media

Different theories have been proposed as to how middle ear pathologies can affect the vestibular labyrinth. Golz et al.[124] postulated that toxins present in middle ear fluid could enter the inner ear fluid via the round window, blood vessels, or the lymphatic system and cause serous labyrinthitis. Other researchers have proposed that pressure changes in the middle ear may result in displacements of the round and oval windows, leading to secondary movement of labyrinthine fluids.[125,126] While the etiology remains unclear, several research studies have focused on how otitis media with effusion (OME) affects vestibular test results in pediatric patients.[122,124,127–130]

Balance Function Findings in Children With Otitis Media

The traditional vestibular test battery can be difficult to perform in the pediatric OME population. Conductive hearing loss frequently accompanies OME, which makes

testing VEMPs with air-conducted stimuli impractical. In addition, OME is prevalent in very young children who may not tolerate caloric or rotary chair testing. A study by Golz et al.[124] used ENG to compare 136 children with OME history and 74 children without history of middle ear pathology. Neither study group showed abnormalities during optokinetic or pursuit testing; however, 42 children with OME (31%) demonstrated spontaneous nystagmus, and 24 (17.5%) showed positional nystagmus consistent with BPPV. Thirteen children showed both spontaneous nystagmus and positional nystagmus. Therefore, 79 children with OME (58%) had abnormal ENG findings compared with 3 children (4%) in the control group. In line with this study, Koyuncu et al.[129] evaluated spontaneous nystagmus and positional nystagmus in 30 children with OME and 15 matched controls. Spontaneous nystagmus of greater than 7 degrees/second was observed in 1 child with OME; positional nystagmus was observed in 10 children with OME. The control group demonstrated no abnormalities on ENG testing. The study group was then reevaluated 1 month following myringotomy and tube insertion. Neither spontaneous nystagmus nor positional nystagmus was observed postoperatively.

Rotary chair testing was performed on 40 children with a history of OME and compared with 31 children with no significant history.[131] Three stimuli were used: 0.02 Hz rotation at 50 degrees/second, 0.1 Hz rotation at 50 degrees/second, and 0.1 Hz at 150 degrees/second. The study group showed significantly poorer VOR gain than controls during the latter test, with comparable VOR phase and symmetry. These same 71 children were also evaluated using computerized dynamic posturography with no significant differences observed between groups. Posturography results of this study are contradicted by findings in other research articles. Casselbrandt et al.[122] showed higher velocity of sway in a group of children with OME. Jones et al.[128] showed that body sway was more common in children with secretory otitis media compared with a control group. Finally, a study by Waldron et al.[130] of 20 children with OME before and after pressure equalization (PE) tube insertion showed poorer results on sway posturography preoperatively versus postoperatively. Although the origin of balance dysfunction relative to middle ear pathology may be debated, it is certain that more research is needed to evaluate vestibular function in children with OME.

SUMMARY

In children with vertigo and imbalance, a thorough physical and neurotologic examination is required. Tools such as the structured case history approach presented in this chapter can assist the clinician in the determination of who may benefit from quantitative vestibular testing. The five most common disorders affecting pediatric balance all may result in abnormal performance on quantitative vestibular testing. Vestibular tests assess function and are inexpensive compared with neuroimaging tests, which often are ordered as part of the assessment of the dizzy child (e.g., MRI and CT). However, as this review illustrates, there are currently no clear patterns in the results from vestibular testing that can be expected from any of the five most common disorders causing dizziness/vertigo in children. There are several reasons for this. First, balance function test results that have been reported in various impairments causing dizziness in children all have different criteria for what is determined to be normal as well as different methodology (e.g., air vs. water caloric stimulation). This highlights the urgent need to establish pediatric normative data for all vestibular function tests. Second, there is most certainly variability in the criteria for diagnosis between dizziness centers. What is abnormal for one laboratory may not be for another. Finally, children are difficult to assess, as discussed earlier in this chapter. Often it will not be possible to sustain a child's cooperation and complete the entire vestibular test battery; therefore, the clinician will need to be highly selective and flexible with regard to which tests to perform. Regardless, what is critical is documenting whether a vestibular impairment exists in a child. Vestibular system impairments in children can lead to motor incoordination and visual disturbances that can slow normal locomotion development. For appropriate rehabilitative therapy to be suggested, the presence or absence of vestibular system impairment should be documented to guide management and treatment. It is undisputed that large-scale studies using comparable test methods and criteria need to be completed in children with dizziness. The resurgence of interest in pediatric balance function testing will surely lead to new techniques and research studies that will advance our understanding of how to incorporate evidence-based practice in this population.

ON THE HORIZON

"Auditory neuropathy (AN) or auditory neuropathy spectrum disorder (ANSD)" is a term that describes a condition consisting of a distinct collection of auditory abnormalities. The ANSD pattern is commonly composed of abnormal results from tests assessing the function of the vestibulocochlear nerve and normal findings from tests, which evaluate the function of the outer hair cells. However, it is not only hearing loss that distinguishes AN patients from their normal counterparts. Recently, evidence has been emerging that this group of patients with "AN" may also demonstrate "vestibular neuropathy." Currently, there are very few studies examining vestibular function in patients with confirmed AN. However, there is mounting evidence that these patients demonstrate abnormal findings on balance function testing as well, which suggests that the vestibular branch of the vestibulocochlear nerve is also impaired in children with AN.[132-135]

REFERENCES

1. Fried MP. The evaluation of dizziness in children. *Laryngoscope*. 1980;90(9):1548–1560.
2. Busis SN. Dizziness in children. *Pediatr Ann*. 1988;17:648.
3. Riina N, Ilmari P, Kentala E. Vertigo and imbalance in children. *Arch Otolaryngol Head Neck Surg*. 2005;131:996–1000.
4. Tusa RJ, Saada AA, Niparko JR. Dizziness in childhood. *J Neurol*. 1994;9(3):261–274.
5. Szirmai A. Vestibular disorders in childhood and adolescents. *Eur Arch Otorhinolaryngol*. 2010;267(11):1801–1804.
6. Russell G, Abu-Arafeh I. Paroxysmal vertigo in children-an epidemiological study. *Int J Pediatr Otorhinolaryngol*. 1999;49(suppl 1):S105–S107.
7. O'Reilly RC, Morlet T, Nicholas BD, et al. Prevalence of vestibular and balance disorders in children. *Otol Neurotol*. 2010;31(9):1441–1444. http://dx.doi.org/10.1097/MAO.0b013e3181f20673.
8. Blayney AW, Colman BH. Dizziness in children. *Clin Otolaryngol*. 1984;9(2):77–85.
9. Wiener-Vacher SR. Vestibular disorders in children. *Int J Audiol*. 2008;47:578–583.
10. Balatsouras DG, Kaberos A, Assimakopoulos D, Katotomichelakis M, Economou NC, Korres SG. Etiology of vertigo in children. *Int J Pediatr Otorhinolaryngol*. 2007;71(3):487–494.
11. Bower CM, Cotton RT. The spectrum of vertigo in children. *Arch Otolaryngol Head Neck Surg*. 1995;121:911–915.
12. Eviatar L, Miranda S, Eviatar A, Freeman K, Borkowski M. Development of nystagmus in response to vestibular stimulation in infants. *Ann Neurol*. 1979;5(6):508–514.
13. von Brevern M, Radtke A, Lezius F, et al. Epidemiology of benign paroxysmal positional vertigo: a population based study. *J Neurol Neurosurg Psychiatry*. 2007;78(7):710–715.
14. Furman JM, Cass SP. Benign paroxysmal positional vertigo. *N Engl J Med*. 1999;341(21):1590–1596.
15. Johkura K, Momoo T, Kuroiwa Y. Positional nystagmus in patients with chronic dizziness. *J Neurol Neurosurg Psychiatry*. 2008;79(12):1324–1326.

16. Fife TD. Benign paroxysmal positional vertigo. *Semin Neurol.* 2009;29(5):500–508.
17. Choung YH, Park K, Moon SK, Kim CH, Ryu SJ. Various causes and clinical characteristics in vertigo in children with normal eardrums. *Int J Pediatr Otorhinolaryngol.* 2003;67(8):889–894.
18. Erbek SH, Erbek SS, Yilmaz I, et al. Vertigo in childhood: a clinical experience. *Int J Pediatr Otorhinolaryngol.* 2006;70(9):1547–1554.
19. Cyr DG. Vestibular testing in children. *Ann Otol Rhinol Laryngol.* 1980;89:63–69.
20. Cyr DG. The vestibular system: pediatric considerations. *Semin Hear.* 1983;4(1):33–45.
21. Jacobson GP, Calder JH. Self-perceived balance disability/handicap in the presence of bilateral peripheral vestibular system impairment. *J Am Acad Audiol.* 2000;11(2):76–83.
22. Jacobson GP, Newman CW. The development of the dizziness handicap inventory. *Arch Otolaryngol Head Neck Surg.* 1990;116(4):424–427.
23. McCaslin DL, Jacobson GP, Lambert W, English LN, Kemph AJ. The development of the Vanderbilt pediatric dizziness handicap inventory for patient caregivers (DHI-PC). *Int J Pediatr Otorhinolaryngol.* 2015;79(10):1662–1666.
24. Eviatar L. Dizziness in children. *Otolaryngol Clin North Am.* 1994;27(3):557–571.
25. Ravid S, Bienkowski R, Eviatar L. A simplified diagnostic approach to dizziness in children. *Pediatr Neurol.* 2003;29(4):317–320.
26. Niememsivu R, Kentala E, Wiener-Vacher S, Pyykkö I. Evaluation of vertiginous children. *Eur Arch Otorhinolaryngol.* 2007;264(10):1129–1135.
27. Pavlou M, Whitney S, Alkathiry AA, et al. The pediatric vestibular symptom questionnaire: a validation study. *J Pediatr.* 2016;168:171–177e1. http://dx.doi.org/10.1016/j.jpeds.2015.09.075.
28. Pacheva IH, Ivanov IS. Migraine variants – occurrence in pediatric neurology practice. *Clin Neurol Neurosurg.* 2013;115(9):1775–1783. http://dx.doi.org/10.1016/j.clineuro.2013.04.012.
29. Teixeira KCS, Montenegro MA, Guerreiro MM. Migraine equivalents in childhood. *J Child Neurol.* 2013;29(10):1366–1369. http://dx.doi.org/10.1177/0883073813504459.
30. Marcelli V, Russo A, Cristiano E, Tessitore A. Benign paroxysmal vertigo of childhood: a long-term follow-up. *Cephalalgia.* 2015;35(6):538–544. http://dx.doi.org/10.1046/j.1468-2982.1994.1406458.x.
31. Raucci U, Vanacore N, Paolino MC, et al. Vertigo/dizziness in pediatric emergency department: five years' experience. *Cephalalgia.* 2016;36(6):593–598. http://dx.doi.org/10.1177/0333102415606078.
32. Sommerfleck PA, González Macchi ME, Weinschelbaum R, De Bagge MD, Bernáldez P, Carmona S. Balance disorders in childhood: main etiologies according to age. Usefulness of the video head impulse test. *Int J Pediatr Otorhinolaryngol.* 2016;87:148–153. http://dx.doi.org/10.1016/j.ijporl.2016.06.020.

33. Lebron D, Vasconcellos E. The episodic syndromes that maybe associated with migraines. *Semin Pediatr Neurol.* 2016;23(1):6–10. http://dx.doi.org/10.1016/j.spen.2016.01.003.
34. Lagman-Bartolome AM, Lay C. Pediatric migraine variants: a review of epidemiology, diagnosis, treatment, and outcome. *Curr Neurol Neurosci Rep.* 2015;15(6). http://dx.doi.org/10.1007/s11910-015-0551-3.
35. Lewis DW. Pediatric migraine. *Neurol Clin.* 2009;27(2):481–501.
36. Weisleder P, Fife T. Dizziness and headache: a common association in children and adolescents. *J Child Neurol.* 2001;16:727–730.
37. Prensky AR, Sommer D. Diagnosis and treatment of migraine in children. *Neurology.* 1979;29(4):506–510.
38. Cass SP, Furman JM, Ankerstjerne K, Balaban C, Yetiser S, Aydogan B. Migraine-related vestibulopathy. *Ann Otol Rhinol Laryngol.* 1997;106(3):182–189.
39. Lewis DW, Middlebrook MT, Mehallick L, Rauch TM, Deline C, Thomas EF. Pediatric headaches: what do the children want? *Headache.* 1996;36(4):224–230.
40. Johnson GD. Medical management of migraine-related dizziness and vertigo. *Laryngoscope.* 1998;108:1–28.
41. Eggers SD. Migraine-related vertigo: diagnosis and treatment. *Curr Neurol Neurosci Rep.* 2006;6(2):106–115.
42. Baloh RH, Honrubia V. Childhood onset of benign positional vertigo. *Neurology.* 1998;50(5):1494–1496.
43. Dieterich M, Brandt T. Episodic vertigo related to migraine (90 cases): vestibular migraine? *J Neurol.* 1999;246(10):883–892.
44. Cutrer FM, Baloh RW. Migraine-associated dizziness. *Headache.* 1992;32(6):300–304.
45. Furman JM, Sparto PJ, Soso M, Marcus D. Vestibular function in migraine-related dizziness: a pilot study. *J Vestib Res.* 2005;15(5–6):327–332.
46. Olsson JF. Neurotologic findings in basilar migraine. *Laryngoscope.* 1991;101(1 Pt 2 suppl 52):1–41.
47. Kayan A, Hood JD. Neuro-otological manifestations of migraine. *Brain.* 1984;107(4):1123–1142.
48. Marcelli V, Furia T, Marciano E. Vestibular pathways involvement in children with migraine: a neuro-otological study. *Headache.* 2010;50(1):71–76.
49. Basser LS. Benign paroxysmal vertigo of childhood. (A variety of vestibular neuronitis). *Brain.* 1964;87:141–152.
50. Olesen J. The classification and diagnosis of headache disorders. *Neurol Clin.* 1990;8(4):793–799.
51. Fenichel GM. Migraine as a cause of benign paroxysmal vertigo of childhood. *J Pediatr.* 1967;71(1):114–115.
52. Herraiz C, Calvin FJ, Tapia MC, de Lucas P, Arroyo R. The migraine: benign paroxysmal vertigo of childhood complex. *Int Tinnitus J.* 1999;5(1):50–52.
53. Mira E, Piacentino G, Lanzi G, Balottin U. Benign paroxymal vertigo in childhood. Diagnostic significance of vestibular examination and headache provocation tests. *Acta Otolaryngol Suppl.* 1984;406:271–274.

54. Lanzi G, Balottin U, Borgatti R. A prospective study of juvenile migraine with aura. *Headache*. 1994;34(5): 275–278.

55. Moretti G, Manzoni GC, Caffarra P, Parma M. "Benign recurrent vertigo" and its connection with migraine. *Headache*. 1980;20(6):344–346.

56. Finkelhor BK, Harker LA. Benign paroxysmal vertigo of childhood. *Laryngoscope*. 1987;97(10):1161–1163.

57. Slater R. Benign recurrent vertigo. *J Neurol Neurosurg Psychiatry*. 1979;42(4):363–367.

58. Dunn DW, Snyder CH. Benign paroxysmal vertigo of childhood. *Am J Dis Child*. 1976;130(10):1099–1100.

59. Koenigsberger MR, Chutorian AM, Gold AP, Schvey MS. Benign paroxysmal vertigo of childhood. *Neurology*. 1968;18(3):301–302.

60. Eeg-Olofsson O, Odkvist L, Lindskog U, Andersson B. Benign paroxysmal vertigo in childhood. *Acta Otolaryngol*. 1982;93(1–6):283–289.

61. Lanzi G, Balottin U, Fazzi E, Mira E, Piacentino G. Benign paroxysmal vertigo in childhood: a longitudinal study. *Headache*. 1986;26(10):494–497.

62. Mierzwinski J, Polak M, Dalke K, Burduk P, Kazmierczak H, Modrzynski M. Benign paroxysmal vertigo of childhood. *Otolaryngol Pol*. 2007;61(3):307–310.

63. Faul M, Xu L, Wald MM, Coronado VG. *Traumatic Brain Injury in the United States: Emergency Department Visits, Hospitalizations, and Deaths*. Atlanta, GA; 2010.

64. Harmon KG, Drezner JA, Gammons M, et al. American medical society for sports medicine position statement: concussion in sport. *Br J Sports Med*. 2013;47(1):15–26.

65. Coronado VG, Haileyesus T, Cheng TA, et al. Trends in sports- and recreation-related traumatic brain injuries treated in US emergency departments: the national electronic injury surveillance system – all injury program (NEISS-AIP) 2001-2012. *J Head Trauma Rehabil*. 2015;30(3):185–197.

66. McCrea M, Hammeke T, Olsen G, Leo P, Guskiewicz K. Unreported concussion in high school football players: implications for prevention. *Clin J Sport Med*. 2004;14(1): 13–17.

67. Corwin DJ, Wiebe DJ, Zonfrillo MR, et al. Vestibular deficits following youth concussion. *J Pediatr*. 2015;166(5): 1221–1225.

68. Ellis MJ, Cordingley DM, Vis S, Reimer KM, Leiter J, Russell K. Clinical predictors of vestibulo-ocular dysfunction in pediatric sports-related concussion. *J Neurosurg Pediatr*. 2017;19(1):38–45.

69. Akin FW, Murnane OD. Head injury and blast exposure: vestibular consequences. *Otolaryngol Clin North Am*. 2011;44(2):323–334.

70. Penner M, Rumney P. Balance problems in children and youth with acquired brain injuries. In: O'Reilly RC, Morlet T, Cushing SL, eds. *Manual of Pediatric Balance Disorders*. San Diego: Plural; 2013:199–209.

71. Whitelaw AS, Young I. A case of perilymphatic fistula in blunt head injury. *Emerg Med J*. 2005;22(12):921. http://dx.doi.org/10.1136/emj.2004.020495.

72. Ferster APO, Cureoglu S, Keskin N, Paparella MM, Isildak H. Secondary endolymphatic hydrops. *Otol Neurotol*. 2017:1. http://dx.doi.org/10.1097/MAO.0000000000001377.

73. Peng KA, Ahmed S, Yang I, Gopen Q. Temporal bone fracture causing superior semicircular canal dehiscence. *Case Rep Otolaryngol*. 2014;2014:817291. http://dx.doi.org/10.1155/2014/817291.

74. Ahn S-K, Jeon S-Y, Kim J-P, et al. Clinical characteristics and treatment of benign paroxysmal positional vertigo after traumatic brain injury. *J Trauma Inj Infect Crit Care*. 2011;70(2):442–446. http://dx.doi.org/10.1097/TA.0b013e3181d0c3d9.

75. Norgaard MS, Rokkjaer MS, Berg J, Luscher M. Benign paroxysmal positional vertigo in children after head trauma. *Ugeskr Laeger*. 2015;177(25):V12140706.

76. Shetye A. Benign paroxysmal positional vertigo in a child: an infrequent complication following a fairground ride and post-cochlear implant surgery. *Cochlear Implants Int*. 2012;13(3):177–180.

77. Eviatar L, Berstraum M, Randel RM. Post-traumatic vertigo in children: a diagnostic approach. *Pediatr Neurol*. 1986;2(2):61–66.

78. Moller C. Balance disorders in children. In: Luxon L, Furman JM, Martini A, Stephens D, eds. *Textbook of Audiological Medicine: Clinical Aspects of Hearing and Balance*. London: Martin Dunitz; 2003:861–868.

79. Lee JD, Kim C-H, Hong SM, et al. Prevalence of vestibular and balance disorders in children and adolescents according to age: a multi-center study. *Int J Pediatr Otorhinolaryngol*. 2017;94:36–39.

80. Alshehri MM, Sparto PJ, Furman JM, et al. The usefulness of the video head impulse test in children and adults post-concussion. *J Vestib Res*. 2016;26(5–6):439–446.

81. Zhou G, Brodsky JR. Objective vestibular testing of children with dizziness and balance complaints following sports-related concussions. *Otolaryngol Head Neck Surg*. 2015;152(6):1133–1139. http://dx.doi.org/10.1177/0194599815576720.

82. Lau BC, Kontos AP, Collins MW, Mucha A, Lovell MR. Which on-field signs/symptoms predict protracted recovery from sport-related concussion among high school football players? *Am J Sports Med*. 2011;39(11):2311–2318. http://dx.doi.org/10.1177/0363546511410655.

83. Merritt VC, Rabinowitz AR, Arnett PA, et al. Injury-related predictors of symptom severity following sports-related concussion Injury-related predictors of symptom severity following sports-related concussion. *J Clin Exp Neuropsychol*. 2015(October);3395:265–275. http://dx.doi.org/10.1080/13803395.2015.1004303.

84. Alhilali LM, Yaeger K, Collins M, Fakhran S. Detection of central white matter injury underlying vestibulopathy after mild traumatic brain injury. *Radiology*. 2014;272(1):224–232. http://dx.doi.org/10.1148/radiol.14132670.

85. Neuenschwander MC, Deutsch ES, Cornetta A, Willcox TO. Penetrating middle ear trauma: a report of 2 cases. *Ear Nose Throat J*. 2005;84(1):32–35.

86. Kim SH, Kazahaya K, Handler SD. Traumatic perilymphatic fistulas in children: etiology, diagnosis and management. *Int J Pediatr Otorhinolaryngol.* 2001;60:147–153.

87. Vartiainen E, Karjalainen S, Karja J. Vestibular disorders following head injury in children. *Int J Pediatr Otorhinolaryngol.* 1985;9:135–141.

88. Gottshall K, Drake A, Gray N, McDonald E, Hoffer ME. Objective vestibular tests as outcome measures in head injury patients. *Laryngoscope.* 2003;113(10):1746–1750. http://www.ncbi.nlm.nih.gov/pubmed/14520100.

89. Cushing SL, Gordon KA, Rutka JA, James AL, Papsin BC. Vestibular end-organ dysfunction in children with sensorineural hearing loss and cochlear implants: an expanded cohort and etiologic assessment. *Otol Neurotol.* 2013; 34(3):422–428.

90. Cushing SL, Papsin BC, Rutka JA, James AL, Gordon KA. Evidence of vestibular and balance dysfunction in children with profound sensorineural hearing loss using cochlear implants. *Laryngoscope.* 2008;118:1814–1823.

91. Sivam SK, Syms CA, King SM, Perry BP. Consideration for routine outpatient pediatric cochlear implantation: a retrospective chart review of immediate post-operative complications. *Int J Pediatr Otorhinolaryngol.* 2017;94:95–99. http://dx.doi.org/10.1016/j.ijporl.2016.12.018.

92. De Kegel A, Maes L, Van Waelvelde H, Dhooge I. Examining the impact of cochlear implantation on the early gross motor development of children with a hearing loss. *Ear Hear.* 2015;36(3):e113–e121.

93. Tien HC, Linthicum FH. Histopathologic changes in the vestibule after cochlear implantation. *Otolaryngol Head Neck Surg.* 2002;127(4):260–264. http://dx.doi.org/10.1067/mhn.2002.128555.

94. Handzel O, Burgess BJ, Nadol Jr J. Hispathology of the peripheral vestibular system after cochlear implantation in the human. *Otol Neurotol.* 2006:57–64.

95. Smeds H, Eastwood HT, Hampson AJ, et al. Endolymphatic hydrops is prevalent in the first weeks following cochlear implantation. *Hear Res.* 2015;327:48–57. http://dx.doi.org/10.1016/j.heares.2015.04.017.

96. Richard C, Fayad JN, Doherty J, Linthicum Jr FH. Round window versus cochleostomy technique in cochlear implantation: histologic findings. *Otol Neurotol.* 2012;33(7):1181–1187. http://dx.doi.org/10.1097/MAO.0b013e318263d56d.

97. Chen X, Chen X, Zhang F, Quin Z. Influence of cochlear implantation on vestibular function. *Acta Otolaryngol.* 2016;136(7):655–659.

98. Kuang H, Haversat HH, Michaelides EM. Impairment of caloric function after cochlear implantation. *J Speech Lang Hear Res.* 2015;58:1387–1395. http://dx.doi.org/10.1044/2015.

99. Jacot E, Van Den Abbeele T, Debre HR, Wiener-Vacher SR. Vestibular impairments pre- and post-cochlear implant in children. *Int J Pediatr Otorhinolaryngol.* 2009;73(2):209–217. http://dx.doi.org/10.1016/j.ijporl.2008.10.024.

100. Ajalloueyan M, Saeedi M, Sadeghi M, Abdollahi FZ. The effects of cochlear implantation on vestibular function in 1–4 years old children. *Otol Neurotol.* 2017;94:100–103. http://dx.doi.org/10.1097/MAO.0b013e31818d1cba.

101. Nassif N, Balzanelli C, Redaelli de Zinis LO. Preliminary results of video head impulse testing (vHIT) in children with cochlear implants. *Int J Pediatr Otorhinolaryngol.* 2016;88:30–33. http://dx.doi.org/10.1016/j.ijporl.2016.06.034.

102. Katsiari E, Balatsouras DG, Sengas J, Riga M, Korres GS, Xenelis J. Influence of cochlear implantation on the vestibular function. *Eur Arch Otorhinolaryngol.* 2013; 270(2):489–495.

103. Janky K, Givens D. Vestibular, visual acuity and balance outcomes in children with cochlear implants: a preliminary report. *Ear Hear.* 2015;36(6):e364–e372. http://dx.doi.org/10.1002/aur.1474.Replication.

104. Devroede B, Pauwels I, Le Bon SD, Monstrey J, Mansbach AL. Interest of vestibular evaluation in sequentially implanted children: preliminary results. *Eur Ann Otorhinolaryngol Head Neck Dis.* 2016;133:S7–S11. http://dx.doi.org/10.1016/j.anorl.2016.04.012.

105. Krause E, Wechtenbruch J, Rader T, Gürkov R. Influence of cochlear implantation on sacculus function. *Otolaryngol Head Neck Surg.* 2009;140(1):108–113e1. http://dx.doi.org/10.1016/j.otohns.2008.10.008.

106. Inoue A, Iwasaki S, Ushio M, et al. Effect of vestibular dysfunction on the development of gross motor function in children with profound hearing loss. *Audiol Neurotol.* 2013;18:143–151.

107. Ebrahimi A, Movallali G, Jamshidi A, Haghgoo HA, Rahgozar M. Balance performance of deaf children with and without cochlear implants. *Acta Med Iran.* 2016;54(11):738–742.

108. Huang M-W, Hsu C-J, Kuan C-C, Chang W-H. Static balance function in children with cochlear implants. *Int J Pediatr Otorhinolaryngol.* 2011;75(5):700–703. http://dx.doi.org/10.1016/j.ijporl.2011.02.019.

109. D'Agostino R, Tarantino V, Melagrana A, Taborelli G. Otoneurologic evaluation of child vertigo. *Int J Pediatr Otorhinolaryngol.* 1997;40(2–3):133–139.

110. Ergul Y, Ekici B, Tastan Y, Sezer T, Uysal S. Vestibular neuritis caused by enteroviral infection. *Pediatr Neurol.* 2006;34(1):45–46.

111. Eviatar L, Eviatar A. Vertigo in children: differential diagnosis and treatment. *Pediatrics.* 1977;59:833–838.

112. Melagrana A, Tarantino V, D'Agostino R, Taborelli G. Electronystagmography findings in child unilateral sensorineural hearing loss of probable viral origin. *Int J Pediatr Otorhinolaryngol.* 1998;42(3):239–246.

113. Zannolli R, Zazzi M, Muraca MC, Macucci F, Buoni S, Nuti D. A child with vestibular neuritis. Is adenovirus implicated? *Brain Dev.* 2006;28(6):410–412.

114. Bartual-Pastor J. Vestibular neuritis: etiopathogenesis. *Rev Laryngol Otol Rhinol.* 2005;126(4):279–281.

115. Davis LE. Viruses and vestibular neuritis: review of human and animal studies. *Acta Otolaryngol Suppl.* 1993;503: 70–73.

116. Strupp M, Brandt T. Vestibular neuritis. *Semin Neurol.* 2009;29(5):509–519.

117. Baloh RW. Clinical practice. Vestibular neuritis. *N Engl J Med.* 2003;348(11):1027–1032.

118. Goudakos JK, Markou KD, Franco-Vidal V, Vital V, Tsaligopoulos M, Darrouzet V. Corticosteroids in the treatment of vestibular neuritis: a systemic review and meta-analysis. *Otol Neurotol.* 2010;31(2):183–189.

119. Choi KD, Oh SY, Kim HJ, Koo JW, Cho BM, Kim JS. Recovery of vestibular imbalances after vestibular neuritis. *Laryngoscope.* 2007;117(7):1307–1312.

120. Brodsky JR, Cusick BA, Zhou G. Vestibular neuritis in children and adolescents: clinical features and recovery. *Int J Pediatr Otorhinolaryngol.* 2016;83:104–108. http://dx.doi.org/10.1016/j.ijporl.2016.01.027.

121. Balkany TJ, Finkel RS. The dizzy child. *Ear Hear.* 1986;7(3): 138–142.

122. Casselbrant ML, Furman JM, Rubenstein E, Mandel EM. Effect of otitis media on the vestibular system in children. *Ann Otol Rhinol Laryngol.* 1995;104(8):620–624.

123. Aarhus L, Tambs K, Hoffman H, Engdahl B. Childhood otitis media is associated with dizziness in adulthood: the HUNT cohort study. *Eur Arch Otorhinolaryngol.* 2016;273:2047–2054.

124. Golz A, Netzer A, Angel-Yeger B, Westerman ST, Gilbert LM, Joachims HZ. Effects of middle ear effusion on the vestibular system in children. *Otolaryngol Head Neck Surg.* 1998;119(6):695–699.

125. Suzuki M, Kitano H, Yazawa Y, Kitajima K. Involvement of round and oval windows in the vestibular response to pressure changes in the middle ear of Guinea pigs. *Acta Otolaryngol.* 1998;118(5):712–716.

126. Carlborg BI, Konradsson KS, Carlborg AH, Farmer JC, Densert O. Pressure transfer between the perilymph and cerebrospinal fluid compartments in cats. *Am J Otol.* 1992; 13(1):41–48.

127. Golz A, Angel-Yeger B, Parush S. Evaluation of balance disturbances in children with middle ear effusion. *Int J Pediatr Otorhinolaryngol.* 1998;43:21–26.

128. Jones NS, Radomskij P, Prichard AJ, Snashall SE. Imbalance and chronic secretory otitis media in children: effect of myringotomy and insertion of ventilation tubes on body sway. *Ann Otol Rhinol Laryngol.* 1990;99(6 Pt 1):477–481.

129. Koyuncu M, Saka MM, Tanyeri Y, et al. Effects of otitis media with effusion on the vestibular system in children. *Otolaryngol Head Neck Surg.* 1999;120(1):117–121.

130. Waldron MN, Matthews JN, Johnson IJ. The effect of otitis media with effusions on balance in children. *Clin Otolarnygol Allied Sci.* 2004;29(4):318–320.

131. Casselbrant ML, Furman JM, Mandel EM, Fall PA, Kurs-Lasky M, Rockette HE. Past history of otitis media and balance in four-year-old children. *Laryngoscope.* 2000;110(5 Pt 1):773–778.

132. Fujikawa S, Starr A. Vestibular neuropathy accompanying auditory and peripheral neuropathies. *Arch Otolaryngol Head Neck Surg.* 2000;126(12):1453–1456.

133. Akdogan O, Selcuk A, Ozcan I, Dere H. Vestibular nerve functions in children with auditory neuropathy. *Int J Pediatr Otorhinolaryngol.* 2008;72(3):415–419.

134. Sheykholeslami K, Megerian CA, Arnold JE, Kaga K. Vestibular-evoked myogenic potentials in infants and early childhood. *Laryngoscope.* 2005;115(8):1440–1444.

135. Sazgar AA, Yazdani N, Rezazadeh N, Yazdi AK. Vestibular evoked myogenic potential (VEMP) in patients with auditory neuropathy: auditory neuropathy or audiovestibular neuropathy? *Acta Otolaryngol.* 2010;130(10):1130–1134.

CHAPTER 6

Dizziness and Vertigo in the Adolescent

HOWARD P. GOODKIN, MD, PHD • JENNIE TAYLOR, MD, MPH • DENIA RAMIREZ-MONTEALEGRE, MD, MPH, PHD

THE ADOLESCENT BRAIN

Adolescence, the developmental transition between the dependency of childhood and the independency of adulthood, encompasses the approximate period between 12 and 18 years of age. Behavior during this developmental stage is frequently characterized by risk taking, impulsivity, and poor choices. The indestructible attitude of the adolescent, which can be met by negative consequences, promotes experimentation of adult practices, development of self-esteem, and eventually social acceptance.[1]

Although the brain reaches 90% of its adult size by 6 years of age, pruning (resulting in decreasing synaptic density) and cortical thinning occur throughout childhood and adolescence. The volume of white matter continues to increase until approximately 20 years of age and is the result of ongoing myelination of white matter tracts. One of the last regions to undergo maturational processes is the prefrontal cortex, the region of the brain that participates in executive, attentional, and regulatory functions.[2]

Adolescence represents a unique period of brain development marked by changes in neuroconnectivity and functional activation. Casey and colleagues[1] suggested that the differential developmental trajectories of the limbic system and subcortical structures (e.g., basal ganglia) as compared with the prefrontal cortex could, in part, explain the impulsivity and risk-taking behavior that occur during adolescence. In their model, earlier maturation of the limbic system and subcortical structures during adolescence drives the adolescent behavior. As connections of the prefrontal cortex mature, influence of the limbic system and subcortical structures is reduced and the prefrontal cortex dominates, resulting in improved ability to suppress impulses and greater emphasis on goal-driven choices. Their model is supported by recent demonstrations of an exaggerated response of the nucleus accumbens in the adolescent as compared with the adult and child in a task that manipulated reward values,[1,3] and correlation of the development of fiber tracts between the prefrontal cortex and basal ganglia with performance on a go/no-go task, a measure of inhibitory control.[4]

Vertigo represents the sensation of inappropriate or abnormal motion and can be related to dysfunction of the vestibular system. Although morphologic development of the vestibular system is complete by term gestation,[5] studies of the development of postural balance suggest that functional maturation of the vestibular system is ongoing during childhood and adolescence (see Chapter 3). For example, Steindl and colleagues[6] used the sensory organization subtest of computerized dynamic posturography to measure postural stability in 140 children aged 3.5–16 years without known peripheral or central vestibular, proprioceptive, or visual disorders or medications that could affect balance. They observed increasing maturation of the vestibular afferent system up to 16 years of age. Their findings were in contrast to those of a prior study[7] suggesting that vestibular development was not complete by 16 years of age. However, Steindl and colleagues[6] observed reduced vestibular influence on postural control in adults as compared with the 15- to 16-year-old age groups. Cumberworth and colleagues[8] suggested that the late functional development of the vestibular system as compared with the somatosensory and visual control of balance may explain differential rates of motion sickness in children and adolescents as compared with adults.

VERTIGO AND DIZZINESS IN THE ADOLESCENT

Vertigo and dizziness are not synonymous terms, although they are often used interchangeably. Individuals with vertigo will often describe a rotational or room-spinning sensation. They may feel as though they are on a carousel or bobbing in a boat. Nausea and vomiting are often associated complaints. True vertigo implies an equilibrium disturbance associated with dysfunction of either the central or peripheral vestibular system. In contrast, dizziness is a term that may be used by patients to describe a distorted perception of the environment[9] associated with etiologies that range from true vertigo to imbalance to presyncope to somatoform disorders. The majority of adults who presented to emergency departments (EDs) in the United States between 1993 and 2005 with a chief complaint of dizziness did not have a vestibular disorder and ultimately were diagnosed with cardiovascular, neurologic, or metabolic/toxic illnesses.[10]

Complaints of dizziness and vertigo are common in the general population, occurring more frequently in women and those older than 60 years.[11] In a review of National Hospital Ambulatory Medical Care Survey data of persons who presented to the ED with a chief complaint of vertigo/dizziness or the final diagnosis of a vestibular disorder, 16- to 19-year-old patients represented the smallest fraction.[10] More recently, Li and colleagues used data from the 2012 National Health Interview Survey, which included a total of 10,954 children to study the prevalence of dizziness and balance problems in children aged 3–17 years (mean = 10.2 years) and found that the overall prevalence for the year analyzed was 5.3%, with a higher incidence in children aged 12–17 years (6.8%).[12] When further classified, vertigo prevalence was 2.8% for adolescents (twice that of younger children), whereas the prevalence of lightheadedness was 3.7%. These authors noted a consistent age-related increase in the prevalence of dizziness and balance problems.

In contrast, population-based studies suggest that episodic vertigo and dizziness may be more common during adolescence than initially proposed. Russell and Abu-Arafeh[13] provided a screening questionnaire to 2165 children ranging in age from 5 to 15 years who attended school in the city of Aberdeen, Scotland. Of the children surveyed, 314 (14%) reported at least one episode of dizziness in the previous year and 92 children (4%) reported three or more episodes of dizziness. Although complaints of dizziness occurred at all ages in this study, it was more common in adolescents, with a peak onset at 12 years of age. In contrast, Niemensivu and colleagues,[14] based on prospective polling of children and adolescents ranging in age from 1 to 15 years, found that 8% (75 of 938) experienced an episode of vertigo or dizziness at some point during their life, predominantly between 11 and 15 years of age. These studies and future studies that attempt to define the true prevalence of vertigo and dizziness during childhood

and adolescence have many potentially confounding variables: young children and adolescents may have difficulty accurately describing their symptoms; dizziness often resolves quickly in children and thus may be disregarded by the child or their family; and vertigo or dizziness may be reported by the adolescent or family as clumsiness.[15] Furthermore, extrapolating findings in different populations may be difficult as prevalence may be influenced by environmental and genetic factors.

Vertigo and dizziness during adolescence can be the presenting symptom or, more typically, can be part of a complex of symptoms in a wide range of disorders that includes viral illnesses and intracranial tumors (see Box 6.1). In a hospital-based study, Fried[16] reviewed medical records of all admissions to the Boston City Hospital for the 12-month period that spanned July 1976 to June 1977. The majority of adolescents admitted for dizziness during this period had experienced a concussion (4 of 9). This was also a common cause for dizziness and balance problems as reported by Li and colleagues.[12]

In contrast, retrospective reviews of *outpatient* medical records of adolescents evaluated in either neurology or otolaryngology clinics[14,15,17–19] consistently report vestibular migraine and benign paroxysmal vertigo of childhood (BPVC) as the most common causes of vertigo and dizziness in adolescents and children. For example, Weisleder and Fife[20] reviewed charts of 31 children and adolescents ranging in age from 6 to 17 years who were referred for

---

BOX 6.1
Common Etiologies for Vertigo and Dizziness in Adolescents

MOST COMMON
Migraine
Migraine equivalent with benign paroxysmal vertigo of childhood being much more common in children than adolescents
Psychogenic
Viral infections or otitis media

COMMON
Chronic daily headache
Trauma
Postural orthostatic tachycardia syndrome

LESS COMMON
Intracranial tumor
Epilepsy
Benign paroxysmal positional vertigo
Vestibular neuritis
Demyelinating disease

vestibular testing at a tertiary care center over a 6-year period. The majority of patients ($n=11$; 35%) were diagnosed with vestibular migraine. Other diagnoses included BPVC ($n=6$; 20%), anxiety attacks ($n=3$; 10%), Meniere's disease ($n=2$), idiopathic sudden-onset sensorineural hearing loss ($n=1$), familial vertigo/ataxia syndrome (episodic ataxia type II, $n=1$), and malingering ($n=1$).

In addition to vestibular migraine, these clinic-based studies have consistently observed a high incidence of depression and somatoform disorders among children and adolescents evaluated in these specialty clinics for complaints of vertigo or dizziness. For example, Ketola and colleagues[21] reported that psychogenic vertigo accounted for 8% (9 of 119) of children and adolescents with the chief complaint of vertigo who were evaluated at the Otolaryngologic Clinic of Helsinki University Central Hospital between the years 2000 and 2004. Following psychiatric consultation, three children (aged 10 to almost 13 years) were diagnosed with depression; one adolescent (age 13.5 years) was diagnosed with a combination of conversion disorder, hyperventilation, and depression; one adolescent (age 15.6 years) was diagnosed with psychotic episode and depression; and the other four children (aged 9–11 years) were diagnosed with psychogenic headache, obsessive-compulsive disorder, panic disorder, or conversion disorder. Compared with children and adolescents who were identified as having an organic cause for vertigo, this group of children and adolescents had more frequent attacks or a complaint of constant vertigo, were more likely to suffer from school absenteeism, and were more likely to have dysfunctional relationships at school or at home. In addition, Emiroglu and colleagues[22] found that 29 of 31 patients (93.5%) who presented to a pediatric neurology clinic for complaints of dizziness, headache, or fainting met criteria of the *Diagnostic and Statistical Manual of Mental Disorders (DSM-IV)* for a psychiatric comorbidity, even when the primary diagnosis was some type of migraine headache.

Not all adolescents complaining of vertigo and dizziness will be referred for specialty clinic evaluation; therefore, many causes of dizziness in the adolescent are likely to be underreported in neurology and otolaryngology clinic-based studies. For example, complaints of vertigo or dizziness in the setting of concussion are likely to be principally managed by the pediatrician[23]; the child with dizziness in the setting of syncope or presyncope may be managed by the pediatrician or is more likely to be referred to a cardiologist than to a neurologist or to an otolaryngologist for further management; and the child with a brain tumor is most likely to be diagnosed in the ED and be managed by the oncologist, neuro-oncologist, and/or the neurosurgeon.

DIAGNOSIS AND TREATMENT OF SPECIFIC CAUSES OF VERTIGO IN THE ADOLESCENT
Migraine
Approximately 30% of adolescent girls experience migraine headaches,[24-26] and along with variants, migraines are the most common episodic disorder of childhood with an estimated incidence of 5%–15%.[26,27] Migraine and BPVC, considered by many to be a migraine variant in younger children,[28] account for 50%–75% of children who present to specialty clinics with vertigo and a normal otologic examination. Migraine frequency increases and BPVC frequency decreases with age.[17,18]

The vertigo associated with migraine may precede the headache (aura), may be part of the headache itself, or may not be temporally related to the headache in up to 60% of individuals.[18] Lee et al. conducted a multicenter study of all pediatric patients (aged 0–18 years; average age 12.9 years) admitted for dizziness in 11 hospitals in Korea.[29] They found a total of 411 children aged 13–17 years who reported symptoms of vertigo and/or balance problems. Sixty percent of these patients were adolescents ($n=247$), and approximately thirty percent of the children in this age group met criteria for vestibular migraine ($n=75$) according to the International Classification of Headache Disorders third edition, beta version (ICHD-3 beta; see Box 6.2). Similarly, in a 5-year retrospective study specifically looking at vestibular migraine in patients 3–18 years of age referred to the German Center for Vertigo and Balance Disorders ($n=118$), Langhagen et al. found that 30% of these patients met ICHD-3 beta diagnostic criteria, with 28% of patients classified as probable vestibular migraine, and 6% classified as suspected vestibular migraine.[30] The incidence of definite vestibular migraine was higher in girls (31%) as compared with boys (29%), and up to 73% of patients reported headaches in all or some of their vertigo attacks. In this study, 51% of patients reported motion sickness and 65% had a positive family history of migraine headaches. Interestingly, somatoform vertigo co-occurred in 27% of patients, similar to what was reported by Batu and colleagues in a Turkish study.[31]

Furthermore, vertigo is a well-established manifestation of basilar migraine, which also has associated symptoms of ataxia, dysarthria, tinnitus, and visual changes. The vertigo associated with these headaches is often brief and frequently accompanied by nausea and vomiting.[20]

The pathophysiology of vertigo in migraines is poorly understood. Unilateral neuronal instability of the peripheral vestibular nerve, idiopathic asymmetric activation of brainstem vestibular nuclei, and

DIAGNOSTIC CRITERIA FOR VESTIBULAR MIGRAINE

1. At least five episodes fulfilling criteria (3) and (4)
2. Current or past history of migraine (without or with aura)
3. Vestibular symptoms of moderate or severe intensity for 5–72 hours
4. At least 50% of episodes associated with at least one of the following
   a. Headache with at least two of the following: unilateral headache, pulsating quality, moderate-severe intensity, aggravation by routine physical activity
   b. Photophobia and phonophobia
   c. Visual aura
5. Not better accounted for by any other ICHD-3 diagnosis or any other vestibular disorder

CRITERIA FOR PROBABLE VESTIBULAR MIGRAINE

1. At least five episodes with vestibular symptoms of moderate or severe intensity for 5–72 hours
2. Only one criteria for (2) and (4) as above
3. Not better accounted for by any other ICHD-3 diagnosis or any other vestibular disorder

vasospasm causing transient ischemia of the labyrinth or central vestibular pathways have all been suggested.[20] Vestibular laboratory testing is often abnormal and demonstrates central findings in adults and children with basilar migraines, even between attacks.[15,32]

Before making the diagnosis of migraine headache in the adolescent being evaluated for complaints of headache and vertigo, episodic ataxia type 2 (EA-2; previously known as familial cerebellar ataxia without myokymia, hereditary paroxysmal cerebellar ataxia, periodic vestibulocerebellar ataxia, and acetazolamide-responsive episodic ataxia) should be considered. This rare autosomal dominant disorder is the result of a spectrum of mutations that affect *CACNA1A*,[33] the gene that encodes the α-1A subunit of P/Q type calcium channels (Cav2.1) located on chromosome 19p. Missense mutations of this same gene are linked to familial hemiplegic migraine,[34] and a CAG expansion of exon 47 has been linked to spinocerebellar ataxia type 6.[35] EA-2 is characterized by episodic attacks that last from hours to days and can be precipitated by stress or exercise as well as caffeine and alcohol. Many features of

the attack can overlap those of migraine: headache, which is typically occipital in location,[36] vertigo, nausea, and vomiting. Indeed, most people with EA-2 also meet ICHD-3 diagnostic criteria for migraine.[37] Distinguishing features during the attack are the presence of concurrent ataxia and nystagmus as well as the strong family history consistent with autosomal dominant inheritance. During the attack, dysarthria, diplopia, tinnitus, dystonia, and hemiplegia may also be present. Onset is typically before 20 years of age with a range from 2 to 61 years.[36,38,39] Of interest, a large percentage of individuals with EA-2 develop ataxia and nystagmus in the interictal periods, and atrophy of the cerebellar vermis has been observed on MRI.[40] An important reason to recognize this syndrome early is that acetazolamide has been shown to be effective in reducing the frequency of attacks that are typically rare but have been reported as often as four times per week.[41,42]

Treatment of migraine headache is divided into abortive and prophylactic therapies. For those with vertigo as the manifestation of their migraine without significant headache, management with antimotion sickness medications, such as scopolamine, has been proposed to provide symptomatic relief.[43] Unfortunately, randomized controlled studies looking at therapeutic interventions specifically focusing on vestibular migraines are limited in the adult population and nonexistent in the pediatric population. Most specialists will focus on treating these as migraine headache variants, and triptans and nonsteroidals are generally used as first-line treatment. The American Academy of Neurology (AAN) guidelines for acute treatment of migraines in children and adolescents report level A evidence for nasal sumatriptan.[44] In patients who do not respond to nasal sumatriptan, consideration for other triptans (zolmitriptan) has been reported to be useful in small study groups in a handful of patients[45]; nonsteroidals and indomethacin should be used in place of medications with caffeine, barbiturates, or opiates, as the former are less likely to cause dependency and medication overuse headache.[46-48] Dihydroergotamine, intravenous valproate, or steroids have also been used for abortive treatment of severe migraine headaches that have not responded to other outpatient treatments.[49-51]

If the migraines are frequent or disabling (i.e., affecting school performance and/or school attendance) a prophylactic agent should be considered.[26] Nevertheless, it is important to recognize that in pediatric patients, the rate of placebo response can be as high as 25%.[26] Cognitive behavioral therapy (CBT) has been shown to be of extreme value with the added benefit of having no side effects.[26,52,53] Calcium channel blockers, β-blockers, antiepileptics, such as topiramate and valproate, or tricyclic antidepressants (e.g., amitriptyline) have shown some level of prophylactic efficacy in small studies,[15,26] although AAN guidelines report insufficient evidence to make formal recommendations for the adolescent.[44] This is further supported by a recent study of amitriptyline versus topiramate versus placebo in adolescents with episodic migraine, which was terminated early because of futility.[54] In their multicenter double-blind study, Powers and colleagues found no difference in primary outcomes, while patients in either arm of pharmacologic treatment experienced increased risk for side effects. When prophylactic treatment is considered, 1 month at a therapeutic dose, if tolerated, should be attempted before altering therapy. Lifestyle changes, including sleep hygiene, regular exercise, a balanced diet, and adequate hydration are crucial, as is early CBT.[26,47]

Chronic Daily Headaches

In contrast to people with migraine headaches who will often describe true vertigo, a more general sense of dizziness is a common complaint of adolescents with chronic daily headache. Chronic daily headaches are defined as headaches lasting longer than 4 hours per day, for more than 15 days per month, for 3 months or more, without underlying pathology.[37] Prevalence studies estimate that 2%–4% of adolescent girls and 0.8%–2.0% of adolescent boys suffer from chronic daily headaches.[55,56] A study by Mack reports that 75% of these patients have a history of episodic migraines, and the other 25% have had a recent viral illness or minor head trauma.[46] Diffuse weakness, unsteadiness, and visual changes, frequently characterized as blurry vision in both eyes, are common associated symptoms. The dizziness often worsens with changes in position, especially when getting out of bed in the morning, and syncope or near syncope can occur. Mood disorders are almost universally present in adolescents who have chronic daily headaches, and treating one may not always alleviate the other (i.e., treatments for chronic daily headaches likely will not work while the mood disorder remains untreated).[46]

Indeed, chronic daily headaches are often more difficult to treat than episodic migraine headaches and may take weeks to months to improve. Comorbidities, such as sleep disturbances, mood disorders, and medication overuse, make them even more challenging. Patient (and parent) frustrations are common and can be confounding.

As with migraine headache, treatment of chronic daily headache is also divided between abortive and prophylactic medications,[26,46] with less evidence of efficacy in the adolescent population. Amitriptyline has demonstrated safety and efficacy as a prophylactic agent in the treatment of chronic daily headache in children, although higher doses may be needed than those for migraine prevention.[46,57] Amitriptyline is also helpful in improving sleep onset, which is a common comorbidity. Cardiac side effects (e.g., prolongation of the QT interval), weight gain, and sedation should be closely monitored.[46] Fluoxetine is the only selective serotonin reuptake inhibitor approved for the treatment of mood disorders in children and may be an effective prophylactic treatment for chronic daily headache.[58] However, there is an increased risk of suicidal thoughts and suicide attempts in adolescents who take this medication. Caution should be used when fluoxetine is combined with tricyclics, as these medications are metabolized through the same pathways, which leads to higher drug levels and more serious side effects, including the risk of serotonin syndrome.[46]

Nonpharmacologic methods should be included in treatment of migraine headache and chronic daily headache. Headache diaries are invaluable to help track patterns, foods, or activities that may cause or be associated with headache. Psychological consultation for CBT and treatment of underlying mood disorders[26] and physical therapy evaluation for reintroduction of physical activity are helpful adjunctive treatments. Awareness of seasonal variations and effects on school performance also need to be addressed.[46]

Postural Orthostatic Tachycardia Syndrome

Although postural orthostatic tachycardia syndrome (POTS) was not identified as a common cause of vertigo or dizziness in the specialty clinic-based studies previously cited, the majority of persons with POTS do complain of dizziness.[59-61] Patients with POTS have orthostatic intolerance defined by an increase in heart rate (HR) of more than 40 bpm (30 bpm in adults) within 10 minutes of standing from supine position without orthostatic fall in blood pressure.[61] Young women and women of childbearing age are mainly affected (5:1 ratio). The syndrome is rarely seen in young children.

POTS is characterized by a constellation of symptoms, including dizziness, headache, and fatigue, as well as nausea, "mental fog," palpitations, diaphoresis, tachypnea, and diffuse weakness that occur on standing and are relieved by sitting or lying down. Most patients will report that their symptoms are debilitating and incapacitating.[61] Patients with POTS also complain of difficulty with sleep, depression, and anxiety, but these symptoms are usually not directly related to POTS. Precipitating factors include standing, physical activity, and heat.

Onset is often in the early teen years, can be preceded by viral illness, and may have a monophasic or relapsing-remitting course.[62] Adolescents within 1–3 years of their growth spurt, who are unable to return to normal activity after suffering a minor illness or injury that may be prolonged and lead to a period of immobility, seem susceptible to POTS. When they attempt to return to normal activity, they become symptomatic when trying to stand upright.[59]

Diagnosis is based on a thorough history and a normal neurologic examination and can be confirmed while triggering an event in the clinic. HR and blood pressure should be recorded at rest while lying down for 10 minutes, and vital signs be reassessed on standing at 1, 3, 5, and 10 minutes. An increase in the HR fulfilling criteria at any time point during the 10-minute evaluation in the absence of any other causes for vertigo is diagnostic of the syndrome.[61] A small number of patients can have significant flushing as part of the syndrome, making the diagnosis of mast cell activation disorder a consideration.[63]

POTS is seen more frequently in patients with hyperextensible joints and cellular matrix protein disorders (e.g., Ehlers-Danlos), suggesting an abnormality in smooth muscle response to the autonomic nervous system.[64,65] The coincidence with puberty in adolescent girls suggests a hormonal influence, and at least one gene mutation in norepinephrine transport protein deficiency also implicates a genetic component.[59,66] Approximately 50% of patients with POTS experience a viral infection weeks to a few months before the onset of symptoms, with as many as 30% experiencing syncopal episodes. Fatigue is a frequent comorbidity in patients with POTS, with more than 90% of patients reporting the symptom and approximately 64% of patients meeting criteria for chronic fatigue syndrome.[61,67] In a handful of studies, chronic infections with viruses such as Epstein-Barr virus and enterovirus have been proposed as triggering events,[68] and antibodies to ganglionic acetylcholine receptors and α-1 adrenergic receptors suggest an autoimmune cause.[69,70] However, the direct mechanism by which these patients develop symptoms is still not fully understood. As mentioned previously, many patients complain of mental fog. It is unclear whether this lack of focus is a result of chronic fatigue or is part of the syndrome, as the underlying mechanisms to explain the cognitive symptoms are still not well understood.[67,71,72]

Different mechanisms for POTS have been proposed, and most likely a combination of these is responsible for development of the syndrome (see Table 6.1). Proposed mechanisms are related to improper interactions between carotid baroreceptors and chemoreceptors leading to reduced blood flow to the brain and the brain's ability to cope with physiologic changes needed to sustain adequate perfusion (see Chapter 15). In general, when changing from a supine or sitting position to standing, there is an immediate decrease in venous return to the heart from the downward shift of blood in the legs. Under normal physiology, this is compensated for by an increase in HR and blood pressure. Blood is then redistributed to the vital organs by splanchnic and peripheral vasoconstriction, leading to normalization of blood distribution and therefore HR and blood pressure. Patients who suffer from POTS, however, are not able to achieve adequate venous return despite physiologic increases in HR. Therefore, their HR continues to increase without the appropriate elevation in blood pressure.[59,73]

The differential diagnosis of patients who present with autonomic dysfunction suggestive of POTS includes undiagnosed diabetes, autoimmune disorders (systemic lupus erythematosus or Sjögren syndrome), eating disorders with volume depletion, anemia, paraneoplastic syndromes, and medication effects.[74] Evaluation should include basic laboratory testing, a neurology consultation with electroencephalography to rule out seizures, and a cardiology consultation to evaluate for arrhythmias.[59,61] In patients suspected with specific pathophysiology, further testing may include electromyography (neuropathic), vitamin B12 (neuropathic), renin-aldosterone levels (hypovolemic), 24-hour urine-sodium excretion, or the

TABLE 6.1
Postural Orthostatic Tachycardia Syndrome (POTS) Classification

POTS Classification	Proposed Pathophysiology
Neuropathic	Sympathetic denervation with venous pooling and reduction in stroke volume (small fiber neuropathy)
Hypovolemic	Low serum aldosterone and low renin activity
Hyperadrenergic	Usually in combination with neuropathic and/or hypovolemic
Autoimmune	Usually after a viral infection. Some patients have antibodies to α-1 adrenergic receptors. More controversial

presence of antinuclear antibodies and/or specific anti-bodies (autoimmune). In some patients, an indication for celiac disease screening is recommended.[75] In patients suspected of having a mast cell activation disorder, a 4- to 6-hour urine collection following an episode is indicated to assess for urinary methylhistamine levels, which will be elevated.[63]

Lifestyle changes seem to be useful as initial therapeutic intervention for all patients. These changes include drinking 2–3 L of water daily.[59] Studies have shown that 24-hour urine sodium excretion of less than 100 mEq is indicative of dehydration,[69] whereas greater than 170 mEq should be satisfactory to adequately compensate for the hypovolemic state.[76] Aside from drinking more water, these patients also benefit from increased salt intake, which helps to replete their intravascular volume. Recommended intake is greater than 200 mEq of sodium daily or 8–10 g/day, which, if unable to be accomplished by salting foods, can be supplemented with salt tablets or high-salt drinks.[59,61,76] Patients should avoid high-heat environments and should be encouraged to improve physical activity.[77,78] Although exercise may seem counterintuitive to some patients, studies have shown that low-paced physical activity, usually done in a recumbent position (e.g., recumbent bicycle), significantly improves symptoms and disability in these patients.[61] Of note, most patients present with noticeable deconditioning and will experience worsening of symptoms before any improvement. It is crucial that patients are educated and warned as they may feel unmotivated and are more likely to suspend the reconditioning program.

Pharmacologic treatment is mainly aimed at treating some of the symptoms, and response to treatment is highly variable. The lack of a large population to study effects of different medications imposes a significant limitation in the interpretation and replication of findings. Among medications most commonly used, β-blockers are considered first-line and can be used to minimize the increase in HR with the change in position and inappropriate relaxation of blood vessels. One study reported that more than 90% of patients felt better after starting a low-dose β-blocker,[79] although they should be closely monitored after starting treatment because overdosing can lead to fatigue.[74] α-1-Agonists, such as midodrine, increase peripheral vascular resistance and may be beneficial. However, frequent dosing is needed and compliance may be an issue when treating adolescent patients.[74] Supine hypertension is a significant side effect, and doses should be avoided before prolonged recumbency such as sleep.[59]

Synthetic mineralocorticoids, such as fludrocortisone, act on distal renal tubules to enhance sodium reuptake and expand intravascular volume and have been used as adjuvant treatment in POTS at a starting dosage of 0.05 mg/day. Little evidence, however, is present to support its efficacy in adolescents, and care should be taken because of the risk of hypokalemia and hirsutism.[59,61,73,80] In a small group of adult women, the use of pyridostigmine decreased HR and reduced the symptoms, but no reports of its efficacy in adolescent patients are available.[61]

LESS COMMON CAUSES OF VERTIGO OR DIZZINESS IN THE ADOLESCENT

Viral labyrinthitis may be the cause of vertigo in up to 20% of children younger than 16 years.[15] Epilepsy is a rare cause of vertigo in children and adolescents and is often associated with altered awareness. Meniere's disease, with classic symptoms of episodic vertigo, unilateral hearing loss, and tinnitus, is an extremely rare cause of vertigo in this age group.[15] See Chapter 5 for additional information regarding causes of vertigo in young children.

CAUSES OF VERTIGO OR DIZZINESS IN THE ADOLESCENT REQUIRING HEAD IMAGING

Adolescents who report dizziness or vertigo should undergo extensive neurologic and neurotologic evaluation to assure the absence of intracranial masses or other treatable causes.[18] Despite extensive evaluation, a proportion of individuals are not diagnosed with a specific etiologic cause for their symptoms.[15,17,18,20]

With their propensity for risk-taking behavior, adolescents commonly suffer head trauma and concussion. Adolescents with a recent history of head trauma and new-onset vertigo (with or without headache) should be imaged to assess for the presence of skull fracture. Although CT is superior to MRI in detecting fractures, MRI should be considered in this patient population to assess for intracranial abnormalities that may not be apparent on CT, such as diffuse axonal injury that can occur after high-speed collisions.[81] Magnetic resonance angiography may also be helpful in the setting of trauma to evaluate for the presence of cervical artery dissection. Even in the absence of a visualized fracture on CT, microscopic hemorrhages in the labyrinth or labyrinthine concussion (not seen on imaging studies) may be implicated as a cause of vertigo.[82]

Intracranial abnormalities (e.g., demyelinating plaques, structural anomalies, and neoplasms) are uncommon causes of vertigo and dizziness in the adolescent. In one series of 87 patients aged 0–16 years, a new neuroimaging abnormality accounted for vertigo in only 25% of cases; 38% had old abnormalities that were not attributed to the cause of vertigo; and 57% had normal neuroimaging. For those patients who complained of vertigo alone without a history of trauma, neuroimaging did not contribute to the diagnosis.[81] For those with an abnormality, the neurologic examination was abnormal (usually a cranial nerve deficit) in more than 80%, and the other 20% of patients had new-onset intense headache. Abnormalities seen in patients older than 12 years included skull fractures, benign brain tumors, demyelinating disease, and shunt malfunctions.[81] Although uncommon, cerebellar or brainstem tumors (medulloblastoma being the most common, but also astrocytoma, ependymoma, and hemangioblastoma) are in the differential diagnosis for adolescents who present with vertigo. These patients usually complain of progressively worsening headaches and have signs of increased intracranial pressure (e.g., papilledema), cranial nerve deficits, and/or gait ataxia. These neurologic signs should prompt further evaluation with neuroimaging. Patients of all ages with vestibular schwannomas (acoustic neuromas) rarely report true vertigo, but the combination of imbalance and unilateral sensorineural hearing loss and tinnitus warrants further investigation.[15] Any adolescent diagnosed with a vestibular schwannoma should raise suspicion for neurofibromatosis Type 2 (NF-2). This patient should undergo MR imaging of the entire neuraxis.

While Chiari I malformation is present at birth, symptoms may be absent or subtle until adolescence or early adulthood. Headache, neck pain, and vertigo are the most common symptoms reported by adolescents with Chiari I malformation. Neuroimaging of these patients often reveals pointed cerebellar tonsils and compression of the retrocerebellar space.[83] Neuroimaging should be seriously considered in all adolescents with a history of trauma, an abnormal neurologic examination, and persistent headaches (see Box 6.3),[81] and in those whose vestibular testing is concerning for a central nervous system lesion.[15]

In those adolescents who have normal examinations and the clinical suspicion for a mass lesion is low, a fast MRI may be useful in providing families with significant reassurance. Imaging will not assess for structural abnormalities but will aid in determining the presence of hydrocephalus and/or a brain tumor while decreasing the risk of radiation from a CT scan. A normal MRI relays to

---

> **BOX 6.3**
> **What Not to Miss: Red Flags to Consider Brain Imaging in the Adolescent With a Complaint of Vertigo or Dizziness**
>
> **HISTORY**
> Head trauma with new-onset vertigo without or with headache
> Associated complaints of double vision, difficulty swallowing, slurred speech, changes in vision, facial numbness: all concerning for cranial nerve deficits
> Difficulty with coordination
> New-onset progressively severe headache
> Progressive symptoms of vertigo
> Episodes of loss of consciousness
> Altered mental status
> History of intracranial abnormality
>
> **EXAMINATION**
> Papilledema
> Cranial nerve deficits
> Weakness or ataxia
> Sensory deficits

---

the parents that their child's complaints are being taken seriously and may go far in strengthening the doctor-patient relationship. As discussed, the cause of dizziness in adolescents is often entwined with an underlying psychological disorder, and parents may be more receptive to pursuing these diagnoses if other causes, especially intracranial mass lesions, have been evaluated and excluded.

SUMMARY

Dizziness is an uncommon complaint in adolescent patients. Migraine headache and vestibular migraine are the most common causes of dizziness in adolescents but must be differentiated from episodic ataxia type II, chronic daily headaches, and POTS. Much less common causes include head trauma or traumatic brain injury, vestibular neuritis, and intracranial abnormalities. In the absence of other diagnoses, psychogenic causes should always be considered. Evaluation is primarily geared toward careful history and physical, neurologic, and vestibular examination. Primary vestibular disorders are rare in adolescents, and treatment of the more common causes of dizziness in the adolescent may involve some trial and error. Imaging is indicated for new-onset neurologic deficit, change in mental status, or severe progressive headache.

REFERENCES

1. Casey BJ, Jones RM, Hare TA. The adolescent brain. *Ann N Y Acad Sci.* 2008;1124:111–126.
2. Toga AW, Thompson PM, Sowell ER. Mapping brain maturation. *Trends Neurosci.* 2006;29(3):148–159.
3. Galvan A, et al. Earlier development of the accumbens relative to orbitofrontal cortex might underlie risk-taking behavior in adolescents. *J Neurosci.* 2006;26(25):6885–6892.
4. Liston C, et al. Frontostriatal microstructure modulates efficient recruitment of cognitive control. *Cereb Cortex.* 2006;16(4):553–560.
5. Blayney AW, Colman BH. Dizziness in childhood. *Clin Otolaryngol Allied Sci.* 1984;9(2):77–85.
6. Steindl R, et al. Effect of age and sex on maturation of sensory systems and balance control. *Dev Med Child Neurol.* 2006;48(6):477–482.
7. Hirabayashi S, Iwasaki Y. Developmental perspective of sensory organization on postural control. *Brain Dev.* 1995;17(2):111–113.
8. Cumberworth VL, et al. The maturation of balance in children. *J Laryngol Otol.* 2007;121(5):449–454.
9. Eviatar L. Dizziness in children. *Otolaryngol Clin North Am.* 1994;27(3):557–571.
10. Newman-Toker DE, et al. Spectrum of dizziness visits to US emergency departments: cross-sectional analysis from a nationally representative sample. *Mayo Clin Proc.* 2008;83(7):765–775.
11. Neuhauser HK, et al. Epidemiology of vestibular vertigo: a neurotologic survey of the general population. *Neurology.* 2005;65(6):898–904.
12. Li CM, et al. Epidemiology of dizziness and balance problems in children in the United States: a population-based study. *J Pediatr.* 2016;171:240–247.e1–3.
13. Russell G, Abu-Arafeh I. Paroxysmal vertigo in children—an epidemiological study. *Int J Pediatr Otorhinolaryngol.* 1999;49(suppl 1):S105–S107.
14. Niemensivu R, et al. Vertigo and balance problems in children—an epidemiologic study in Finland. *Int J Pediatr Otorhinolaryngol.* 2006;70(2):259–265.
15. Balatsouras DG, et al. Etiology of vertigo in children. *Int J Pediatr Otorhinolaryngol.* 2007;71(3):487–494.
16. Fried MP. The evaluation of dizziness in children. *Laryngoscope.* 1980;90(9):1548–1560.
17. Choung YH, et al. Various causes and clinical characteristics in vertigo in children with normal eardrums. *Int J Pediatr Otorhinolaryngol.* 2003;67(8):889–894.
18. Erbek SH, et al. Vertigo in childhood: a clinical experience. *Int J Pediatr Otorhinolaryngol.* 2006;70(9):1547–1554.
19. Szirmai A. Vestibular disorders in childhood and adolescents. *Eur Arch Otorhinolaryngol.* 2010;267(11):1801–1804.
20. Weisleder P, Fife TD. Dizziness and headache: a common association in children and adolescents. *J Child Neurol.* 2001;16(10):727–730.
21. Ketola S, et al. Somatoform disorders in vertiginous children and adolescents. *Int J Pediatr Otorhinolaryngol.* 2009;73(7):933–936.
22. Emiroğlu FN, et al. Assessment of child neurology outpatients with headache, dizziness, and fainting. *J Child Neurol.* 2004;19(5):332–336.
23. Kaye AJ, et al. Mild traumatic brain injury in the pediatric population: the role of the pediatrician in routine follow-up. *J Trauma.* 2010;68(6):1396–1400.
24. Aromaa M, et al. Childhood headache at school entry: a controlled clinical study. *Neurology.* 1998;50(6):1729–1736.
25. Abu-Arafeh I, et al. Prevalence of headache and migraine in children and adolescents: a systematic review of population-based studies. *Dev Med Child Neurol.* 2010;52(12):1088–1097.
26. Hershey AD. Pediatric headache. *Continuum (Minneap Minn).* 2015;21(4 Headache):1132–1145.
27. Parker C. Complicated migraine syndromes and migraine variants. *Pediatr Ann.* 1997;26(7):417–421.
28. Mira E, et al. Benign paroxysmal vertigo in childhood. Diagnostic significance of vestibular examination and headache provocation tests. *Acta Otolaryngol Suppl.* 1984;406:271–274.
29. Lee JD, et al. Prevalence of vestibular and balance disorders in children and adolescents according to age: a multi-center study. *Int J Pediatr Otorhinolaryngol.* 2017;94:36–39.
30. Langhagen T, Lehrer N, Borggraefe I, Heinen F, Jahn K. Vestibular migraine in children and adolescents: clinical findings and laboratory tests. *Front Neurol.* 2014;5:292.
31. Batu ED, et al. Vertigo in childhood: a retrospective series of 100 children. *Eur J Paediatr Neurol.* 2015;19(2):226–232.
32. Dieterich M, Brandt T. Episodic vertigo related to migraine (90 cases): vestibular migraine? *J Neurol.* 1999;246(10):883–892.
33. Jen J, Kim GW, Baloh RW. Clinical spectrum of episodic ataxia type 2. *Neurology.* 2004;62(1):17–22.
34. Ducros A, Denier C, Joutel A, et al. The clinical spectrum of familial hemiplegic migraine associated with mutations in a neuronal calcium channel. *N Engl J Med.* 2001;345:17–24.
35. Zhuchenko O, et al. Autosomal dominant cerebellar ataxia (SCA6) associated with small polyglutamine expansions in the alpha 1A-voltage-dependent calcium channel. *Nat Genet.* 1997;15(1):62–69.
36. Baloh RW, et al. Familial episodic ataxia: clinical heterogeneity in four families linked to chromosome 19p. *Ann Neurol.* 1997;41(1):8–16.
37. Headache Classification Committee of the International Headache Society (IHS). The international classification of headache disorders, 3rd edition (beta version). *Cephalalgia.* 2013;33(9):629–808.
38. Farmer TW, Mustain VM. Vestibulocerebellar ataxia. A newly defined hereditary syndrome with periodic manifestations. *Arch Neurol.* 1963;8:471–480.
39. Imbrici P, et al. Late-onset episodic ataxia type 2 due to an in-frame insertion in CACNA1A. *Neurology.* 2005;65(6):944–946.

40. Vighetto A, et al. Magnetic resonance imaging in familial paroxysmal ataxia. *Arch Neurol.* 1988;45(5):547–549.

41. Griggs RC, et al. Hereditary paroxysmal ataxia: response to acetazolamide. *Neurology.* 1978;28(12):1259–1264.

42. von Brederlow B, et al. Mapping the gene for acetazolamide responsive hereditary paryoxysmal cerebellar ataxia to chromosome 19p. *Hum Mol Genet.* 1995;4(2):279–284.

43. Cass SP, et al. Migraine-related vestibulopathy. *Ann Otol Rhinol Laryngol.* 1997;106(3):182–189.

44. Lewis D, et al. Practice parameter: pharmacological treatment of migraine headache in children and adolescents: report of the American Academy of Neurology Quality Standards Subcommittee and the Practice Committee of the Child Neurology Society. *Neurology.* 2004;63(12): 2215–2224.

45. Richer L, et al. Drugs for the acute treatment of migraine in children and adolescents. *Cochrane Database Syst Rev.* 2016;4:CD005220.

46. Mack KJ. Episodic and chronic migraine in children. *Semin Neurol.* 2006;26(2):223–231.

47. Langhagen T, et al. Vestibular migraine in children and adolescents. *Curr Pain Headache Rep.* 2016;20(12):67.

48. Patniyot IR, Gelfand AA. Acute treatment therapies for pediatric migraine: a qualitative systematic review. *Headache.* 2016;56(1):49–70.

49. Raskin NH. Repetitive intravenous dihydroergotamine as therapy for intractable migraine. *Neurology.* 1986;36(7): 995–997.

50. Schwartz TH, Karpitskiy VV, Sohn RS. Intravenous valproate sodium in the treatment of daily headache. *Headache.* 2002;42(6):519–522.

51. Kabbouche MA, et al. Inpatient treatment of status migraine with dihydroergotamine in children and adolescents. *Headache.* 2009;49(1):106–109.

52. Powers SW, et al. Cognitive behavioral therapy plus amitriptyline for chronic migraine in children and adolescents: a randomized clinical trial. *JAMA.* 2013;310(24):2622–2630.

53. Kroner JW, et al. Cognitive behavioral therapy plus amitriptyline for children and adolescents with chronic migraine reduces headache days to ≤4 per month. *Headache.* 2016;56(4):711–716.

54. Powers SW, et al. Trial of amitriptyline, topiramate, and placebo for pediatric migraine. *N Engl J Med.* 2017;376(2):115–124.

55. Kavuk I, et al. Epidemiology of chronic daily headache. *Eur J Med Res.* 2003;8(6):236–240.

56. Wang SJ, et al. Chronic daily headache in adolescents: prevalence, impact, and medication overuse. *Neurology.* 2006;66(2):193–197.

57. Hershey AD, et al. Effectiveness of amitriptyline in the prophylactic management of childhood headaches. *Headache.* 2000;40(7):539–549.

58. Saper JR, et al. Double-blind trial of fluoxetine: chronic daily headache and migraine. *Headache.* 1994;34(9):497–502.

59. Johnson JN, et al. Postural orthostatic tachycardia syndrome: a clinical review. *Pediatr Neurol.* 2010;42(2):77–85.

60. Fischer PR, Brands CK, Porter CJ, et al. High prevalence of orthostatic intolerance in adolescents in a general pediatric referral clinic. *Clin Autonom Res.* 2005;15:340.

61. Jones PK, Shaw BH, Raj SR. Clinical challenges in the diagnosis and management of postural tachycardia syndrome. *Pract Neurol.* 2016;16(6):431–438.

62. Stewart JM. Chronic orthostatic intolerance and the postural tachycardia syndrome (POTS). *J Pediatr.* 2004;145(6): 725–730.

63. Shibao C, et al. Hyperadrenergic postural tachycardia syndrome in mast cell activation disorders. *Hypertension.* 2005;45(3):385–390.

64. Rowe PC, et al. Orthostatic intolerance and chronic fatigue syndrome associated with Ehlers-Danlos syndrome. *J Pediatr.* 1999;135(4):494–499.

65. Gazit Y, et al. Dysautonomia in the joint hypermobility syndrome. *Am J Med.* 2003;115(1):33–40.

66. Shannon JR, et al. Orthostatic intolerance and tachycardia associated with norepinephrine-transporter deficiency. *N Engl J Med.* 2000;342(8):541–549.

67. Raj V, et al. Psychiatric profile and attention deficits in postural tachycardia syndrome. *J Neurol Neurosurg Psychiatry.* 2009;80(3):339–344.

68. Chia JK, Chia AY. Chronic fatigue syndrome is associated with chronic enterovirus infection of the stomach. *J Clin Pathol.* 2008;61(1):43–48.

69. Thieben MJ, et al. Postural orthostatic tachycardia syndrome: the Mayo clinic experience. *Mayo Clin Proc.* 2007;82(3):308–313.

70. Li H, et al. Autoimmune basis for postural tachycardia syndrome. *J Am Heart Assoc.* 2014;3(1):e000755.

71. Ocon AJ, et al. Increasing orthostatic stress impairs neurocognitive functioning in chronic fatigue syndrome with postural tachycardia syndrome. *Clin Sci (Lond).* 2012;122(5):227–238.

72. Arnold AC, et al. Cognitive dysfunction in postural tachycardia syndrome. *Clin Sci (Lond).* 2015;128(1):39–45.

73. Medow MS, Stewart JM. The postural tachycardia syndrome. *Cardiol Rev.* 2007;15(2):67–75.

74. Kanjwal MY, Kosinski DJ, Grubb BP. Treatment of postural orthostatic tachycardia syndrome and inappropriate sinus tachycardia. *Curr Cardiol Rep.* 2003;5(5):402–406.

75. Gibbons CH. Small fiber neuropathies. *Continuum (Minneap Minn).* 2014;20(5 Peripheral Nervous System Disorders):1398–1412.

76. El-Sayed H, Hainsworth R. Salt supplement increases plasma volume and orthostatic tolerance in patients with unexplained syncope. *Heart.* 1996;75(2):134–140.

77. Winker R, et al. Endurance exercise training in orthostatic intolerance: a randomized, controlled trial. *Hypertension.* 2005;45(3):391–398.

78. Fu Q, Levine BD. Exercise in the postural orthostatic tachycardia syndrome. *Auton Neurosci.* 2015;188:86–89.

79. Lai CC, et al. Outcomes in adolescents with postural orthostatic tachycardia syndrome treated with midodrine and beta-blockers. *Pacing Clin Electrophysiol.* 2009;32(2):234–238.

80. Jacob G, et al. Effects of volume loading and pressor agents in idiopathic orthostatic tachycardia. *Circulation.* 1997;96(2):575–580.
81. Niemensivu R, et al. Value of imaging studies in vertiginous children. *Int J Pediatr Otorhinolaryngol.* 2006;70(9):1639–1644.
82. Davies RA, Luxon LM. Dizziness following head injury: a neuro-otological study. *J Neurol.* 1995;242(4):222–230.
83. Aitken L, Lindan C, Sidney S, et al. Chiari type I malformation in a pediatric population. *Pediatr Neurol.* 2009;40(6):449–454.

Evaluation of Dizziness in the Litigating Patient

GERARD J. GIANOLI, MD, FACS • JAMES S. SOILEAU, MD

INTRODUCTION

Dizziness is one of the most frequent chief complaints that brings a patient to a physician's office.[1] Dizziness is also a frequent complaint among litigants who have suffered accidental or job-related injuries. Worker's compensation, disability claims, and lawsuits are filed for financial compensation because of this complaint. As health care providers, we inevitably become embroiled as either expert witnesses in our patients' lawsuits or as experts sought out by those entities being sued by individuals for the alleged injury related to the complaint of dizziness. A competent evaluation of the dizzy patient is frequently sought from otolaryngologists in the position as an expert witness. The goal of this review is to put forth some guidelines in interacting with this type of patient and the legal system. Although this article is entitled "Evaluation of Dizziness in the Litigating Patient," the principles set forth here are applicable for patients who are seeking disability status, worker's compensation claims, and any other situation where there is a significant potential for secondary gain (Table 7.1).

BASIC PRINCIPLES

Physician Role: Patient Advocate Versus Advocate/Agent of Court

As health care providers, we find ourselves in the role of patient advocate for several different causes, and we are taught that this is our role as clinicians. We advocate for their best interests in relieving their suffering and preventing further harm to their health. We advocate for our patients to get insurance approval for appropriate health care, and we advocate for their disability application when appropriate. These are all ethical and, indeed, laudable positions in which to find ourselves. However, when we are in the role of expert witness, we are no longer in the role of patient advocate. When we take on the position of medical expert, we are, in essence, enjoined as agents of the court, and it is our duty to provide a truthful and objective assessment of

an individual's physical condition.[2] To advocate for our patients in this situation would be unethical. This is important to keep in mind as the patient's best interests may not be aligned with the best interests of the court and society as a whole.

Payment

Although many physicians are uncomfortable discussing fees, it is important to be transparent regarding fees when dealing with any case involving litigation. You should have a signed contract with the attorney who has hired you before seeing the patient. This contract should detail all of your fees, including office visits, testing, record review, reports, phone conferences, depositions, and trial appearances (Fig. 7.1). Because the time, effort, and intellectual energy expended in these cases are considerably more than in routine patients, you should not accept discounted Medicare or insurance rates for the clinical components in the evaluation of these patients. You should also be paid in advance for all of your services and never accept a case with a contingency fee. Accepting a contingency fee for a case compromises your impartiality and your credibility and is unethical. Although depositions can be scheduled at your convenience, trial appearances cannot. These appearances typically will absorb most, if not all, of your working day and if there is

---

TABLE 7.1
Principles of Expert Witness Evaluation

- Physician as agent of the court
- Signed contract between physician and attorney
- Extensive documentation of H&P
- Extensive objective verification of complaints
- Extensive objective testing to exclude other pathologies
- Corroboration of objective and subjective findings
- Assessment of disability, causation, prognosis, and future needs
- Evaluation of possible malingering or exaggeration

HEADER

Date: 08/12/2014
To:

Patient: _____ Account: _____
Address:_____
_____

Attn: DOB: _____ Age/Sex: _____ - _____
Via:

Physician:_____

FINANCIAL POLICY

Thank you for your interest in our clinic. **ALL** charges for attorney represented cases, accident and/or injury cases, and Workers Compensation cases **must be paid in full, in advance, no exceptions**. We do not accept the Workers Compensation fee schedule and will not refund any services we perform.

Attached you will find an estimate with itemization of tests and fees for the initial evaluation. Prepayment for these services indicates you have accepted the policies of our office. Please do not send payment if this is not acceptable to your organization. As soon as we receive payment, we will call the patient to schedule their appointment.

The physician will require radiology and laboratory studies (i.e. Bloodwork, CT and/or MRI, etc.). A recommended facility will be provided at the time of scheduling. Payment and/or payment options should be arranged by your office and the facility prior to the date of service.

Treatment fees are not included in this estimate.

Please be informed that our fees for time spent giving medical testimony are as follows:

Review of Records:	$XXX.00 per hour
Narrative Report:	$XXX.00 per report
In-Office Conference:	$XXX.00 per hour (1/4 hour minimum)
Deposition:	$XXX.00 per hour (1 hour minimum – 2 hour deposit required)
Video Deposition:	$XXX.00 per hour (1 hour minimum – 2 hour deposit required)
Court Appearance:	$XXX.00 per day (1 day minimum)
Court Preparation time:	$XXX.00 per hour (3 hour minimum per case)
Travel Time	$XXX.00 per hour

Fees for all services listed above are due IN FULL, 14 DAYS BEFORE scheduled court date/deposition date/ date of service.

There will be a cancellation fee of 50% for all services, including any services not listed on this form, CANCELLED WITHIN 14 DAYS BEFORE scheduled date of service. There will be a cancellation fee of 100% for all services CANCELLED WITHIN 7 DAYS BEFORE scheduled date and time of service. A "No Show" without cancellation in advance will result in a cancellation fee equal to 100% of the fees for all services not cancelled in advance.

Should you have any questions concerning this invoice, please contact our office. If you have any pretrial questions, please contact my office to arrange a pretrial conference in my office.

I have read, understand and agree to all of the terms of the Financial Policy listed above.

_____   _____   _____
Signature of Attorney/Caseworker   Date   Print Name of Attorney/Caseworker

FIG. 7.1 Sample financial policy contract.

any significant travel involved, more than a day. There will be more trial appearances scheduled than actually occur, because so many cases settle at the last minute. Because it is hard to reschedule a clinical day at the last minute, payment in advance and a cancellation fee are reasonable approaches for such occurrences.

Extensive Documentation of History and Physical Examination

Extensive documentation of the history and physical examination is an important first step in the evaluation of patients who are involved in litigation. We use a comprehensive previsit questionnaire to document the patient's responses in their own handwriting. This questionnaire is filled out in our office waiting room, and then signed by the patient, dated, and witnessed by one of our staff members. This is important to document because so much of our medical opinions and diagnoses are based on information garnered from the history. This may seem elaborate, but there will be times when the patient will later deny statements made in the office. Without documentation to the contrary, the expert will either be forced to change their opinion on this "new" historical information or be caught in a "my word against his word" confrontation. Of course, if the above documentation occurs, any future changes in the history are problematic for the patient and compromise his/her reliability. Any historical information provided by the patient (or the attorney) must be corroborated by medical records, physical findings, objective testing, and the like. Memory is often swayed by potential million dollar settlements. At the same time our intake questionnaire is completed, we have the patient sign a consent form for evaluation and a complete test battery (including audiometric tests, calorics, rotary chair tests, posturography, etc.), which also includes consent for photo or video documentation. In addition, we have the attorney sign an agreement itemizing our fees for office visits, testing, record review, depositions, and court appearances. If these are not signed, we do not see the patient. Furthermore, the agreement stipulates how a no-show or last minute cancellation will be handled—for both office visits and deposition/trial appearances. Likewise, we request all existing medical records.

Extensive Objective Testing to Verify Complaints

Do not be cost-conscious. In this day of escalating health care costs, many physicians have been made ever so aware of ordering unnecessary tests. However, in the context of litigation, the concern of being cost-conscious is misplaced. A complete and thorough evaluation including history, physical examination, audiologic tests, vestibular tests, imaging, and any other ancillary tests you may need is unlikely to exceed $10,000. Any (nonnuisance) litigation concerning dizziness is almost certainly seeking redress exceeding several hundred thousand dollars, and frequently exceeding a million dollars. Consequently, the costs of the evaluation by the medical expert in these cases are almost always negligible in comparison. If an attorney is reticent to proceed with a full evaluation because of the costs, this is a good clue that they do not have a case and are hoping to settle for a nuisance fee.

Corroboration of Objective and Subjective Findings

Because litigation involving the complaint of dizziness often involves the possibility of very large monetary awards, there is significant incentive for plaintiffs to malinger, or to significantly exaggerate their symptoms. Lawyers, judges, and juries are also aware of these factors—sometimes more so than physicians. Consequently, it is imperative that any subjective complaints are objectively verified and quantified as best as possible. This process will often either bolster the plaintiff's case or destroy it. However, sometimes the result is a mixture of these outcomes—helping some aspects of the case while harming other aspects. To the expert witness, whatever the result, it should not matter.

Make Sure All Pieces Fit: Do Symptoms and Severity Correlate With Objective Findings?

Among dizzy patients who are undergoing litigation, approximately 25% will have symptoms that are corroborated by objective testing and 25% will have nonphysiologic test results with no objective findings to corroborate their subjective complaints (Fig. 7.2). These two groups would appear to be fairly straightforward—one group that appears to be honest and legitimate and the other group highly suspicious for malingering. However, there is another, larger group of patients representing approximately 50% of this population who have characteristics of both—some verification of subjective symptoms by objective testing and some nonphysiologic results suggestive of exaggeration or malingering. Putting all three groups together, you could reasonably say that 75% of all patients complaining of dizziness and involved in litigation were either malingering or exaggerating their problems. Or, you could also reasonably state that 75% of these patients had legitimate pathology. In both statements, you would be correct. Separating the true pathology from the exaggeration is the main role of the expert witness.[3]

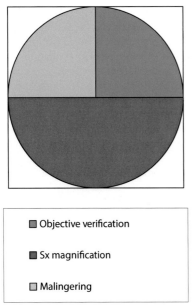

- ■ Objective verification
- ■ Sx magnification
- ☐ Malingering

FIG. 7.2 Among dizzy patients involved in litigation, objective verification of symptoms is found in approximately 25%, nonphysiologic results suggestive of frank malingering in roughly 25%, and exaggeration of symptoms in about 50%.

Assessment of Causation

Once the evaluation of objective pathology has been performed, causation must be considered. The legal hurdle for most expert witness testimony is the determination of probability. Probability is defined as more than a 50% likelihood. Consequently, when determining causation, you do not need to be absolutely certain that you are correct, but you should be more sure than not. Remember, anything is "possible," but the court wants to know what is "probable."

Two factors that need to be considered are timing and mode of injury. Timing refers to the time sequence of the event in question relative to the pathology causing the plaintiff's dizziness. Mode of injury refers to the mechanism, such as blunt head trauma, noise trauma, and explosion. Obviously, in a patient with immediate onset of vertigo after a sledge hammer impacted their occiput, both the timing and mode of injury would seem reasonable to be accepted as more probable than not that the head trauma caused the vertigo. However, if you later find out that the patient did not have any vertigo or dizziness until 1 year after the sledge hammer incident, then you would likely conclude that the vestibular problem was more probable than not to be unrelated to the head trauma. Similarly, a situation in

which a plaintiff complains of dizziness immediately after a tap on the shoulder, you might reasonably conclude that although the timing might be appropriate for causation, the mode of injury is inconsistent with the pathology observed. In this case, you would find it is more probable than not that the shoulder tap did not cause the dizziness. The two main questions to be answered are: (1) is the mechanism of trauma appropriate for the injury; and (2) is the timing appropriate to link the pathology to the alleged incident? A word of caution: it is inappropriate to take the patient's (or the attorney's) word for the mechanism of injury. You are the expert and it is your job to make this determination. Both the patient and the attorneys (defense and plaintiff) have a significant stake in the outcome of your determination. Remain objective and verify anything you are told with objective findings, such as the medical record or test findings.

Prognosis

After determination of objective pathology, causation, and probability, the next step is determination of prognosis. In this regard you need to consider the average, the best, and the worst-case scenarios. You also need to consider sequelae that may be many years in the future. For the patient who has been seriously damaged, this may be their only chance for monetary recompense. The basis for the plaintiff award is entangled in the prognosis. Any future medical and nonmedical needs should be considered. A recent conversation with a plaintiff attorney was enlightening. I had seen his patient and treated her benign paroxysmal positional vertigo (BPPV). I informed him that he had a good case and that his client was already cured. He took this as a good news/bad news moment. He had a good case, but because the client was cured, there would be little monetary award for future medical or other needs.

Interacting With Lawyers

Many physicians mistakenly believe that an attorney who hires an expert wants that expert to simply support their case. Although this may be true for a small minority of attorneys, our experience has been quite the opposite. Some of the most thankful attorneys were ones we had to give the "bad news" that their client had findings consistent with symptom amplification, nonphysiologic results, or outright malingering. Plaintiff attorneys sink a lot of their own money into their cases, and the amount of money "invested" is often substantial. The last thing a plaintiff attorney wants to do is to get all the way to a trial (read: large outlay of their own money on an expensive court trial) and then finally find out that their client is malingering. Similarly, a defense attorney who finds out that the plaintiff is legitimate and will likely win at trial is much more willing to offer a generous settlement in pretrial negotiations than risk losing at trial. Therefore, defense attorneys also generally want an objective, truthful evaluation, rather than an expert who simply supports their case.

HISTORY AND PHYSICAL EXAMINATION

Our evaluation of litigating patients starts with an extensive questionnaire as mentioned earlier. This is reviewed during the history to clarify any points that may have caused some confusion. Among important points to identify during the history are the following:

Details of the alleged trauma or inciting event
Time course for onset of symptoms
Important associated events
Progression of symptoms
Evaluation and therapeutic interventions employed
Prior history of dizziness, vertigo, tinnitus, hearing loss, or other otologic disease
Extensive medical history including:
    Surgical history
    Significant medical illnesses
    Hospitalizations
    Medication use
    Prior trauma
    Alcohol, tobacco, and drug use
    Occupational history
        Including military history, criminal convictions, and prison stay
    Family history

Physical examination should include a complete head and neck examination as well as an extensive neurootologic examination. Specifically, this should include microscopic otoscopy, documentation of facial nerve function, global neurologic examination, and eye examination using infrared videography. The eye examination should include examination of ocular movements, examination for spontaneous nystagmus (with and without visual fixation), and noting down left, right, and center gaze positions. Head-shake and head-thrust maneuvers should also be accomplished. Some will perform Dix-Hallpike testing at this time, or this can be done later as part of the formal electronystagmography/videonystagmography (ENG/VNG). The neurologic examination should include tests of the cranial nerves, cerebellar function, Romberg testing, Fukuda testing, and gait analysis.

TESTING

As mentioned, objective testing is mandatory in cases involving litigation or other situations with a potential for secondary gain such as worker's compensation and disability claims. Before objective testing is performed, there are two requirements: equipment calibration and properly trained ancillary personnel. If either of these is not present, you cannot rely on the test results. Many physicians rely on their audiologist for completion of the vestibular testing. Although there are many audiologists who are quite good at vestibular testing, many have had limited educational exposure and insufficient experience performing vestibular tests. If this is the case, appropriate additional training should be completed.

Audiologic Testing

Audiometric testing should include a basic comprehensive audiogram, with air and bone conduction thresholds (regardless of how good the hearing appears), speech audiometry, tympanometry, and acoustic reflexes. Bone conduction thresholds should be sought to −10 dB levels (supranormal levels) and not just the "cut-off" normal values of +25 dB. Appropriate validation tests should be performed when appropriate, such as the Stenger test when there is a significant asymmetric hearing pattern. One should take note of the pure tone average (PTA) in comparison with the speech reception threshold (SRT; difference between SRT and PTA should be ≤6 dB) and the sound level of conversation at which the patient is instructed in the audiometry booth (should not be at a level lower than PTA or SRT). Other factors that should be noted include whether the patient reported hearing unmasked bone stimulation appropriately, responding with "half spondees" (such as when the patient is requested to repeat the word "baseball" and he replies "base… something"), whether there are bone conduction thresholds at higher sensation levels than air conduction thresholds, and whether acoustic reflexes are present in an ear that was reported as having profound hearing loss or a conductive hearing loss. The physician should ask for a general impression of patient performance as well as the level of cooperation. Finally, the pure tone pattern should be assessed for physiologic character suggestive of organic pathology or a nonphysiologic pattern. In addition to the above audiometric testing, we feel strongly that any abnormalities should be corroborated by otoacoustic emissions and auditory evoked potential testing for threshold. We also find that adjunct testing such as electrocochleography is helpful in objectively identifying pathology. However, the decision to include such testing should be facility-specific and is dependent on the reliability of that particular facility's experience with the testing.

Vestibular Testing

Vestibular testing should include a comprehensive analysis of all aspects of the balance system that you are able to objectively evaluate. Current technology allows assessment of the vestibular system with a variety of different protocols. Among these, a bare minimum would include ENG/VNG, rotary chair testing, and computerized dynamic posturography (CDP). Additional studies that may prove helpful include vestibular evoked myogenic potentials and high-frequency vestibuloocular reflex testing (e.g., video head impulse test). Throughout these tests, the clinician should look for patterns consistent with known pathology and should be suspicious of poor results, unusual results, or failure to obtain any results at all. Poor cooperation should be noted. The clinician should also keep in mind that all of these tests can be separated into two categories determined by whether the response is voluntary or involuntary. A common mistake for inexperienced clinicians is to interpret abnormalities on the oculomotor tests as being evidence of central vestibular dysfunction. While this may be the case, keep in mind that these tests require the patient's cooperation and abnormal results could also occur with poor cooperation or malingering on the part of the patient. The clinician should be especially suspicious in cases where the patient gives nonphysiologic results in any of the test procedures (e.g., positive Stenger, aphysiologic sway on CDP). These contextual observations by the individual conducting the vestibular evaluation can be very helpful in cases where results vary significantly from the norm. The examiner should be instructed to report any erratic behavior or deviation from test protocol. These patients should never be left alone in the examination or testing rooms, and ideally, a clinic chaperone should be present as a witness to all events that take place. We have also employed video recording in various locations in our office. This helps eliminate contrary claims of their experience in our office by the plaintiffs/patients.

Video head impulse testing (vHIT) has been introduced to several laboratories recently (see Chapter 8). However, because clinical experience with this testing technology has not yet been widespread and has only been available for a limited time, we recommend caution when using this as a means to determine "normal" semicircular canal function in the context of litigation. Recent studies have shown poor correlation of vHIT with caloric irrigation studies[4]; therefore we cannot recommend using this in place of caloric irrigation. Although vHIT may eventually add to our vestibular evaluations significantly, time and clinical experience should precede its use in the evaluation of the medicolegal patient. Similarly, caution should be employed with any new testing technology as it becomes available.

Imaging

We feel that imaging (both high resolution CT scan and MRI scan) should be performed in all cases involving litigation. Because the history may not be as straightforward as we would like, a detailed analysis of the inner ear and skull base anatomy is often elucidating. Consider a patient who falls in a "Big Box" store claiming hearing loss and balance dysfunction as a result of the fall. She has a CT scan of temporal bones that does not show any abnormality and audiovestibular testing that demonstrates unilateral hearing loss and unilateral vestibular loss. The patient claims the hearing loss and balance dysfunction occurred immediately after the fall. It would be easy to concur that the fall caused this patient's problem but for the MRI scan that shows a 3 cm acoustic neuroma in the affected ear. Yes, the hearing loss COULD have occurred when she fell, but it seems unlikely. Even if it did, the fact that she has a 3 cm acoustic neuroma in that ear certainly changes the complexion of the entire case. Prognosis for hearing and vestibular loss in a patient with an acoustic neuroma is already poor. Any award would be reduced because of this fact.

REVIEW OF MEDICAL RECORDS

A review of medical records should be performed whenever possible. We find that the most helpful information is anything having to do with testing that gives objective results, information from the event, and almost any information prior to the event that is being litigated. Review of the police accident report, EMT report, ER report, and initial hospitalization can provide information that many patients may not remember. These can also be used to corroborate the patient's history as well as corroborating any information that is provided by the attorneys. An important point to identify on the initial report is whether the patient complained of dizziness/vertigo and/or loss of consciousness—both of which are usually recorded in the ER or EMT record. It is probably wise to do an exhaustive review of the pertinent medical records prior to any courtroom testimony.

MALINGERING

Malingering is the false and fraudulent simulation or exaggeration of disease, performed in order to obtain money, drugs, evade duty or criminal responsibility or other reasons readily understood from the individual's circumstances, rather than learning the individual's psychology.[5]

Although you may suspect a patient of malingering, malingering is only part of the differential diagnosis in such cases. Remember that nonphysiologic test results can also be otherwise explained. Alternative explanations include technical malfunction of equipment, poor understanding of the test requirements (as would be seen in young children and the mentally handicapped), and anxiety/panic disorder. In your capacity as an expert witness, it is probably better not to formally make the diagnosis of malingering, but rather, expound on whether the patient meets the DSM-IV criteria for malingering. After that, it will be the job of the judge and jury to decide whether malingering is an appropriate explanation of the plaintiff's behavior.

DSM IV Criteria for Malingering[6]

Malingering is suspected if any combination of the following are observed:
1. Medicolegal context of presentation.
2. Marked discrepancy between the person's claimed stress of disability and the objective findings.
3. Lack of cooperation during the diagnostic evaluation and in complying with the prescribed treatment regimen.
4. The presence of antisocial personality disorder.

Malingering by Imputation

Probably the most difficult form of malingering to deal with is malingering by imputation. This is the case where a plaintiff has a legitimate pathology and is very consistent, cooperative, and honest in their dealings with the clinicians, that is, with the exception of one or two details leading to the causation of the pathology. Generally, the only way to identify this is by thorough review of prior medical records. Even so, the plaintiff, being aware that this is a liability, may have worked hard to conceal any prior records identifying the pathology as a premorbid condition. If such a condition eventually is identified of which the plaintiff had not been forthcoming, then this is a good indicator of malingering by imputation. The expert witness needs to be able to change their opinion when new information like this arises.

On the other hand, a plaintiff who is forthright about a prior condition and claims worsening of this condition by the event that is being litigated presents a situation that is not so straightforward. The question then becomes whether the alleged incident did indeed cause worsening of the pathology and then becomes a judgment call by the clinician dictated by the specifics of the case. Of course, admission of the premorbid condition may likely reduce monetary rewards on behalf of the plaintiff.

Red Flags

Certain findings should be red flags for the clinician to raise suspicion of malingering or symptom exaggeration among plaintiffs complaining of dizziness. Obviously, this includes the finding of nonphysiologic test results, but there are also subtler issues to consider. The patient who either refuses or is unable to complete testing should raise your suspicion. Rarely do we ever encounter a nonlitigating patient who cannot complete testing, and in general, the more severely affected the patient, the more motivated they are to complete testing. When the symptoms seem too severe for the disorder identified, one must consider whether symptom exaggeration could be present. Frequent falls should raise suspicion of malingering or exaggeration. Although falls are a concern of patients with dizziness, vertigo, and poor balance, frequent falls in the absence of neurodegenerative disease are uncommon in patients with no potential for secondary gain. Patients may have one or two falls and then generally recognize this tendency. Subsequently, they adapt to their situation by either avoiding situations likely to cause falls or take other measures such as the use of a cane or walker to aid in their balance. Similarly, patients with vertigo spells will typically place themselves in a position so as to avoid a fall at the onset of a vertigo spell. Inability to easily categorize the plaintiff's complaints with a diagnosis should also cause some unease among clinicians. Patients who malinger or exaggerate tend to defy diagnostic categorization. And, of course, behavior inconsistencies such as lies, obvious exaggerations, and poor cooperation should certainly raise the specter of malingering in the mind of the clinician. Remember that those who will lie to you over small things will certainly lie to you over big things. There could be legitimate explanations for all of the above findings, but if any of these are present, a good explanation for their presence is warranted.

THE "NORMAL EVALUATION" PATIENT

Another vexing situation is the "normal patient"—a cooperative, reliable patient with a plausible history, but normal findings on all of the objective tests performed. As there are no objective findings on testing or physical examination, the entire case rests on the credibility of the patient. In our experience, patients in this group are more likely to represent true pathology. We must remember that all of the vestibular testing currently available only tests a small portion of the vestibular system. Consequently, it is reasonable to envision a patient who has pathology outside of the bounds of conventional testing. Vestibular function and symptoms can also fluctuate. Remember that test findings are a snapshot in time of that patient's vestibular status, allowing for the possibility of a normal evaluation in a patient with a vestibulopathy. If one doubts this, consider the case of BPPV. One of the major characteristics of BPPV is fatigability—the phenomenon in which positive results become negative on repeat testing. If a patient has an abnormal result from the Dix-Hallpike test, you can be sure they have BPPV. However, you cannot say for sure that a patient with a normal result from the Dix-Hallpike test does not have BPPV. In the latter scenario, the patient may have BPPV that has already "fatigued." For someone with characteristic symptoms of BPPV and a normal Dix-Hallpike test result, repeat testing is recommended. Our recommendation for the "normal patient" is similar—repeat testing.

ASSUMPTIONS/PEARLS

Your Work and Your Credentials Will Be Scrutinized

As an expert witness, you must be prepared to explain your findings and conclusions, knowing that the opposing attorney has hired an expert who will be reviewing your work. Alternative explanations of your findings will be brought forth, and you will need to expound on whether these alternative explanations are more or less likely than your conclusions. Many clinicians find it unsettling for their diagnosis/conclusions to be questioned. However, this is the rule rather than the exception when litigation is involved. Many experts will have prior scientific publications in the area being litigated. Rest assured that a good opposing legal team will have reviewed your prior publications, and any deviation from your prior opinions will make your testimony look suspect. You may have to explain excerpts from your prior papers that are placed out of context. In addition, your qualifications as an expert will routinely be examined and scrutinized by the attorney who hired you (usually before you are hired) and by the opposing counsel (at your deposition). Again, although this is unsettling for some, this is routine for expert witness work.

Never Assume Any Prior Diagnosis Is Correct

Frequently, a prior diagnosis is assumed to be correctly made and is used as a short-cut to treat the patient. While this is not a good practice in general, it is a big mistake in face of litigation. Physicians who examined and diagnosed the patient prior to your encounter with

the patient may not have been aware of any potential for secondary gain and accepted the patient at their word rather than objectively documenting any pathology. Consequently, their prior diagnosis may have been clouded by faulty information.

Cannot Assume a Normal Premorbid State

As mentioned earlier, you cannot assume a normal premorbid state. A review of old records is important in this regard, looking for the history of ear-related problems, dizziness, and associated testing. Only if there is no prior documentation can one infer that no prior pathology existed. Even in this scenario, however, many patients will have pathology of which they may not have been aware. We have found that the most common of these is noise-induced hearing loss. Easily identified by the 4 kHz notch on the audiogram, this pathology evolves slowly and in its early phases may not be noticeable to the patient. If noise-induced hearing loss has no reasonable association with the alleged injury, then it is likely a premorbid state.

Appropriate Referrals

Pathology outside of our areas of expertise should be evaluated by the appropriate professional. You should be very careful in giving expert opinions in areas outside of your specific field. One common complaint among closed head injury patients is cognitive dysfunction. Referral for neuropsychological evaluation is often helpful in objectively quantifying this issue and separating organic pathology from nonorganic causes. Similarly, patients with symptoms of anxiety and panic disorder should be referred for appropriate evaluation/treatment.

Financial Incentives Obscure the Picture

It is helpful to understand the financial motivation of all parties involved in litigation. The easiest to understand is the plaintiff. They will receive monetary recompense for the alleged injury. The expert witness should always keep this bias in mind and how it may result in exaggerating or malingering symptoms. The defense obviously wants to avoid any payout to the plaintiff and is in direct conflict with the plaintiff. The defense attorneys, while wanting to make a good defense, are usually paid on an hourly basis and have an incentive to drag out the proceedings as long as possible regardless of the outcome. The plaintiff attorneys are more interested in a shorter proceeding because they typically "invest" their own money into the case and do not have unlimited resources for protracted litigation. In fact, unless a case can win a certain sum of money, regardless of the case's merits, a plaintiff attorney may either refuse a case or become very passive in its prosecution. For example, litigation for a possible $5000 award is not attractive to an attorney who may have expenses for the pursuit of the case in excess of $5000. In any event, many more cases settle out of court rather than proceed to trial.

Litigation May Become Protracted

If you are going to be an expert witness, you need to prepare yourself for the possibility that your services may be required for one case many years after the fact. We have both been involved in cases that have taken beyond 10 years to resolve. It is not unusual for litigation to spawn additional litigation or repeat lawsuits. It seems that some litigants become "frequent flyers" in the court system.

Be Prepared to Change Your Opinion as New Evidence Arises

Sometimes when you are evaluating a patient in the context of litigation, you are not privy to all of the information concerning the plaintiff. Because of inevitable bias of either side in litigation, your opinion may be swayed by information informally relayed to you that you eventually find out is not exactly correct. Consequently, a change in your opinion during the course of evaluation may be warranted. There is no reason that an expert witness cannot change their opinion as new evidence surfaces. In fact, reevaluation of the merits of the case should be performed and a new opinion be produced when any new pertinent evidence arises. This situation is more common than many realize. Furthermore, we have witnessed patients change over time. Sometimes their symptom complex changes as the course of litigation unfolds. If this is the case, the patient needs to be reevaluated with the same scrutiny as the very first evaluation.

CONCLUSIONS

Evaluation of the dizzy patient involved in ongoing litigation is a challenging endeavor. Recognizing the challenges and appropriate management of these patients along with the legal entanglements associated with them can lead to a fruitful endeavor. Remember that the goal of the physician in this situation is not to be a patient advocate, but rather an agent of the court in pursuit of a truthful, unbiased analysis of disability, causation, and prognosis.

REFERENCES

1. McLemore T, Delozier J. 1985 National ambulatory medical care survey. In: *National Center for Health Statistics (Hyattsville, MD) Advance Data from Vital Statistics. No 128*. Washington, DC: Government Printing Office; 1987. DHHS Publication No. (PHS) 87-1250.
2. Statement on the physician acting as an expert witness. *Bull Am Coll Surg.* 2007;92(12):24–25.
3. Gianoli G, McWilliams S, Soileau J, Belafsky P. Posturographic performance in patients with the potential for secondary gain. *Otolaryngol Head Neck Surg.* 2000;122:11–18.
4. Jung J, Suh M, Kim S. Discrepancies between video head impulse and caloric tests in patients with enlarged vestibular aqueduct. *Laryngoscope.* 2017;127(4):921–926.
5. Gorman WF. Defining malingering. *J Forensic Sci.* 1982;27: 401–407.
6. DSM-IV-TR. American Psychiatric Association, 2000. In: Halligan PW, Bass C, Oakley DA, eds. *Malingering and Illness Deception*. UK: Oxford University Press; 2003.

CHAPTER 8

The Video Head Impulse Test

KRISTAL M. RISKA, AUD, PHD • OWEN D. MURNANE, PHD

INTRODUCTION

Many techniques are available for the assessment of the vestibular system, particularly the assessment of horizontal semicircular canal (SCC) function. The head impulse test (HIT) was first described by Halmagyi and Curthoys in 1988[1] and is the most widely used bedside test of SCC function. Since that time, a relatively limited number of vestibular research laboratories have used the magnetic field scleral search coil technique, the gold standard for recording eye movements, to record three-dimensional (3D) eye movement during the HIT to validate its use as a test of SCC function and to better understand the clinical utility of the test. The search coil technique is generally considered too invasive, expensive, and time-intensive for routine clinical use, and those limitations were the impetus for the development of two-dimensional (2D) eye-movement recording via high-speed video cameras. The initial studies using high-speed digital video cameras to record eye movement during the HIT (now referred to as the video head impulse test or vHIT) were published by several independent research laboratories,[2–4] with the critical experiments demonstrating comparable results for simultaneous video and scleral search coil recordings for head impulses in horizontal and vertical planes in normal controls and in selected patients with well-defined vestibular losses.[3,5,6] Since those initial studies, at least four vHIT devices have been developed, and the routine clinical use of the vHIT has expanded rapidly. The purpose of this chapter is to provide an overview of the HIT with an emphasis on the vHIT. The reader is also directed to Halmagyi et al.[7] for a comprehensive review of this topic.

BACKGROUND OF THE HEAD IMPULSE TEST

The angular vestibulo-ocular reflex (VOR) ensures gaze stability during head rotations by generating eye movements that are equal and opposite to head rotation. The gain of the VOR (eye velocity divided by head velocity) for natural head movements, therefore, approaches unity in healthy individuals. The VOR has three main anatomic components: (1) the SCCs and the superior vestibular nerve and inferior vestibular nerve afferents

in the peripheral vestibular system, (2) the vestibular and ocular motor nuclei in the brainstem, and (3) the extraocular muscles. The SCCs are positioned in three nearly orthogonal planes within the head, allowing for the detection of head rotation in 3D space. The SCCs function as angular accelerometers in a push-pull fashion with two coplanar canals on each side of the head working together, i.e., the left and right horizontal SCCs, the right anterior and left posterior SCCs or "RALP," and the left anterior and right posterior SCCs or "LARP." For example, during rightward head rotation in the horizontal plane, the discharge rate of the right horizontal SCC afferents increases and, at the same time, the discharge rate of the left horizontal SCC afferents decreases relative to the resting discharge rate. The difference in output between the right and left horizontal SCCs drives the leftward compensatory eye movement of the VOR so that the eyes remain still in space during head rotation and enable stable vision. The observation or measurement of eye movement, therefore, can aid in the detection and localization of vestibular pathology because of the relationship between the function of vestibular sensory receptors in the inner ear and the compensatory eye movements produced by the VOR. The majority of bedside and laboratory tests of vestibular function involve the observation or measurement of horizontal eye movements (i.e., horizontal VOR) produced by stimuli that activate the horizontal SCCs and the superior vestibular nerve.

The HIT is used to assess dynamic function of the SCCs and was initially described as a bedside test used to measure the function of each horizontal SCC.[1] The HIT is based on two principles or laws (Ewald's laws) in vestibular physiology: (1) eye movements evoked by stimulation of a single SCC occur in the plane of that canal, and (2) excitatory responses have a larger dynamic range than inhibitory responses.[8–13] Specifically, because the three SCC pairs (horizontal, RALP, and LARP) are nearly orthogonal to each other, a head impulse delivered in the plane of one pair will stimulate mainly that pair and not the other two SCC pairs. In addition, the VOR during a canal-plane impulse toward a particular SCC is driven largely by that SCC and not by its coplanar counterpart because of the asymmetric response (excitatory > inhibitory) of primary vestibular afferents (see Fig. 8.1). The HIT, therefore, can assess the function of each SCC separately and, in a patient with unilateral vestibular hypofunction, the gain of the VOR during ipsilesional head impulses (i.e., head rotation toward the side of the vestibular loss) will be lower than the gain during contralesional head impulses.

BEDSIDE HEAD IMPULSE TEST

The bedside HIT is the most widely used bedside test of SCC function and has largely been used to assess the function of horizontal SCCs. To perform the bedside HIT, the clinician sits in front of the patient, holds the patient's head, and instructs the patient to keep staring at an earth-fixed target (e.g., the clinician's nose). The

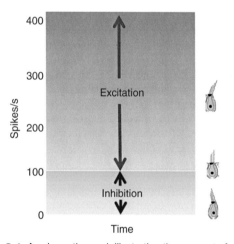

FIG. 8.1 A schematic graph illustrating the concept of Ewald's second law that states (in its general form) that semicircular canal (SCC) afferent output produced by excitation exceeds the output produced by inhibition (i.e., SCC afferent output is asymmetric). For example, when the head is rotated to the right, there is ampullopetal endolymph flow in the right horizontal SCC and an increase in the firing rate (excitation) of the right horizontal SCC afferents; as the acceleration of the head rotation increases, the firing rate continues to increase with little or no saturation. In contrast, there is a simultaneous ampullofugal endolymph flow in the left horizontal SCC and a decrease in the firing rate (inhibition) of the left horizontal SCC afferents; as the acceleration of the head rotation increases, the firing rate continues to decrease but can only decrease to zero (firing rate saturates). The asymmetric response of SCC afferents that occurs at high angular head accelerations dictates that the vestibulo-ocular reflex during a canal-plane impulse toward a particular SCC is driven largely by that SCC and not by its coplanar counterpart. Therefore, the head impulse test is capable of measuring the function of each SCC separately.

clinician turns the patient's head abruptly and unpredictably to the left or right, through a small angle (10–20 degrees). Patients with normal VOR function will be able to maintain their gaze on the target during head rotation to either side (i.e., the head rotation produces a short-latency compensatory eye movement [the VOR] that is equal and opposite of the head rotation). In contrast, patients with unilateral vestibular loss (UVL) will be unable to maintain their gaze on the target during ipsilesional head rotation. Instead, the eyes will move with the head (because of the reduction in VOR gain) and are taken off target so that at the end of the head rotation the patient must make a voluntary corrective saccade back to the target. The corrective or "catch-up" saccade is visible to the clinician and is, therefore, called an *overt* saccade. The observation of an overt saccade is an indirect sign of horizontal SCC hypofunction on the side toward which the head was rotated. The bedside HIT depends on the timing and size of the corrective saccades and on the ability of the clinician to accurately observe the corrective saccades. Corrective saccades are observed at the end of both rightward and leftward head impulses in patients with bilateral vestibular loss (BVL).

Advantages of the bedside HIT include the ability to detect UVL and BVL, no equipment cost, short test time, portability, and the ability to assess horizontal SCC function at frequencies of head rotation that are representative of head movements that occur during activities of daily living.[14,15] In addition, the bedside HIT is less likely to elicit the vertigo and occasional nausea associated with caloric stimulation.

There are, however, a number of significant limitations related to the bedside HIT. Specifically, the bedside HIT is a subjective test, and there is no objective measure of the corrective saccades or VOR gain; the outcome of the test is based on the clinician's subjective visual observation of the presence or absence of overt saccades; and the interpretation of the bedside HIT depends on the experience of the clinician.[16] Furthermore, during the bedside HIT, the magnitude of the head acceleration is unknown and likely varies within a single clinician/patient and between individual clinicians/patients. Corrective saccades that occur *during* the head rotation are called *covert* saccades, and these cannot be observed by the clinician.

The false-negative rate of the bedside HIT in patients with peripheral vestibular disorders has been estimated at 14% based on the rate of occurrence of isolated covert saccades detected with the vHIT.[17] The clinical application of the bedside HIT has been limited to the evaluation of horizontal SCC function and has not been used routinely for the assessment of vertical SCCs.

MAGNETIC FIELD SCLERAL SEARCH COIL HEAD IMPULSE TEST

The magnetic field scleral search coil technique[18] has been used to record 3D eye movement during the HIT,[19,20] and has demonstrated that covert saccades occur during the HIT in patients with UVL and BVL and that the presence of covert saccades can produce false-negative results for the bedside HIT even in patients with total UVLs.[21] The 3D search coil technique has also been used to measure the function of individual vertical SCCs using head impulses delivered in the vertical plane.[22,23] Importantly, it was shown that 3D and 2D (horizontal and vertical eye movement) scleral search coil techniques were equally accurate in detecting isolated hypofunction in horizontal and vertical SCCs, indicating that 2D methods (i.e., video pupil tracking) are capable of assessing all six SCCs independently.[24]

VIDEO HEAD IMPULSE TEST

Based on the bedside HIT first described by Halmagyi and Curthoys,[1] the vHIT is a relatively new clinical test of dynamic SCC function that uses high-speed digital video camera(s) to record eye movement during and immediately after head impulses in horizontal and vertical planes. The stimulus for the vHIT is the same stimulus used for the bedside HIT and consists of manual, passive (clinician moves patient's head), unpredictable, brisk head rotations with peak angular velocity of ~100 to ~400 degrees/second and a peak angular acceleration of ~1000 to ~4000 degrees/second.[2] The vHIT instrumentation consists of high-speed (~250 frames/second) monocular or binocular digital infrared video camera(s), a laptop computer, and software. The video camera uses pupil detection methods to record 2D eye movements. The vHIT detects and records abnormal eye movements (i.e., overt and covert saccades) and provides measures of VOR gain. Depending on the vHIT device, the camera is either embedded in head-worn goggles[2,3] or mounted on a tripod facing the patient.[4,25] Head movement is recorded by an inertial measurement unit (triaxial linear accelerometer and gyroscopes) mounted on the head-worn goggles or by the change in the angle of head position during the head impulse as recorded by an external camera. Notably, prototypes of at least two commercially available vHIT devices have been validated with comparable results obtained for simultaneous video and magnetic field scleral search coil recordings for head impulses in horizontal and vertical planes in normal controls and in selected patients with well-defined vestibular losses.[3,5,6,26]

VIDEO HEAD IMPULSE TEST TECHNIQUE

To perform the horizontal vHIT, patients are seated and eye position is calibrated immediately before testing. Patients are then instructed to maintain their gaze on an earth-fixed visual target located at a distance of ~1 meter straight ahead at eye level. The clinician stands behind the patient and manually rotates the head abruptly and unpredictably to the left or right through a small angle (10–20 degrees) in the horizontal plane to stimulate the left or right horizontal SCC (see Fig. 8.2). In general, two different hand placements have been used to perform horizontal head impulses: (1) hands on top of the patient's head or (2) hands placed on each side of the face at the jaw line. In a sample of 40 healthy adults, higher average VOR gain values were obtained for the hands-on-head technique than for the hands-on-jaw technique. In contrast, higher average head velocities were obtained for the hands-on-jaw technique than for the hands-on-head technique[27]; and the jaw technique was associated with more frequent vHIT artifacts than the head technique in a group of patients with acute vestibular syndrome.[28]

The effect of initial head position on the vHIT has also been examined (i.e., initial head position at midline with impulses directed laterally [outward impulses] vs. initial eccentric head position with impulses directed toward the midline [inward impulses]). In healthy subjects, there were no differences in either peak head velocity or amplitude for outward and inward head impulses, whereas there was a small but significant VOR gain difference noted, with higher VOR gain for outward impulses than for inward impulses.[29] There was no difference in ipsilesional VOR gains for inward and outward head impulses in patients with acute UVL.[30] Patients are probably less likely to anticipate the direction of the head impulse when the initial head position is at midline with impulses directed laterally.

To test either of the coplanar vertical canal pairs, the patient's head is first turned either to the right (LARP) or to the left (RALP) ~30–40 degrees relative to the trunk (i.e., ~30–40 degrees relative to the central earth-fixed visual target), which aligns the vertical canal pair with the sagittal plane of the trunk.[24] The patient is instructed to maintain gaze on the central target by "looking out" of the left corner (LARP) or right corner (RALP) of the eye. The clinician places one hand on top of the head and the other hand under the chin and rotates the head either forward and down toward the central fixation target (stimulates the anterior canal) or back and away from the fixation target (stimulates the posterior canal) (see Fig. 8.2). Alternatively, *both* the head and body can be turned ~30–40 degrees relative to the central fixation target (gaze remains on the central

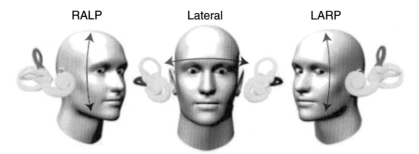

FIG. 8.2 Initial head position and head impulse directions (*arrows*) for RALP (right anterior-left posterior), LARP (left anterior-right posterior), and lateral canal stimulation as viewed from the earth-fixed visual target. Before testing the vertical canals, the head is rotated ~30–40 degrees relative to the trunk and the head impulse is a pitch movement either downward (*red vertical arrows*) to stimulate the anterior canals or upward (*blue vertical arrows*) to stimulate the posterior canals. For testing the lateral canals, the head impulse is a rotation of the head in the horizontal plane either to the right (*blue horizontal arrow*) to stimulate the right lateral canal or to the left (*red horizontal arrow*) to stimulate the left lateral canal. The desired amplitude of head rotation used to stimulate each canal is ~10–20 degrees. (screen shot from the free i-phone application (AVOR) developed by Dr. Hamish G. MacDougall, Vestibular Research Laboratory, School of Psychology, University of Sydney, Sydney, NSW, Australia.)

target) before delivering the head impulses, and this position may minimize patient discomfort and neck strain relative to turning only the head.[31,32] McGarvie et al.[31] demonstrated the importance of maintaining gaze along the plane of the stimulated SCC during the vertical canal vHIT. Specifically, they showed a substantial decrease in VOR gain as the direction of horizontal gaze shifted from 40° (gaze direction aligned with the plane of the stimulated vertical canal) to 0° (gaze direction is straight ahead and not aligned with the plane of the vertical canal so the response is a combined vertical and torsional eye movement).

VIDEO HEAD IMPULSE TEST AND VESTIBULO-OCULAR REFLEX GAIN

vHIT VOR gain is usually quantified as either position gain or velocity gain that is measured over a wide response interval or over limited time intervals usually associated with peak head velocity or peak head acceleration. Specifically, at least one vHIT device quantifies gain over a wide response interval, from 60 ms before the peak head velocity to the next zero-crossing of head velocity; position gain is then calculated as the ratio of the area under the desaccaded eye velocity waveform to the area under the head velocity waveform during the same time interval.[6] Quantifying VOR gain over a wide response interval increases the likelihood that camera movement artifacts (e.g., goggle slippage) in the eye velocity traces will be reduced if the artifact is biphasic.[6] In contrast, another commercially available vHIT device uses an interval of 100 ms post-head impulse onset, and

gain is calculated over a ±20 ms interval around fixed head velocity times of 40, 60, 80, and 100 ms; gain is also calculated as the slope of the regression between eye and head velocities over the first 100 ms.[33] A recent study has shown no difference in the mean gain and variance obtained with two different commercially available vHIT devices when the same gain calculation technique was used; however, lower variances were obtained for area gain than for regression gain.[34]

VIDEO HEAD IMPULSE TEST ARTIFACTS

Current commercially available vHIT devices provide the examiner with immediate visual and/or audio feedback regarding the adequacy of each head impulse. If the head impulse and eye movement response meet the criteria of the manufacturer's data collection/processing algorithm, then the eye movement response is accepted and the gain of the VOR is calculated. In general, vHIT data collection/processing algorithms include a minimum velocity/acceleration for the head impulse and maintenance of eye tracking during the head impulse. It is important, however, for clinicians to manually inspect the "accepted" waveforms for the presence of artifacts.

Mantokoudis et al.[28] used laboratory simulations in a healthy subject to deliberately induce artifacts that were reliably reproduced and "accepted" by the data collection/processing algorithm used by a commercially available vHIT device. The simulations were used to develop a classification scheme of horizontal vHIT artifacts: (1) delay/phase shift, e.g., eye movement

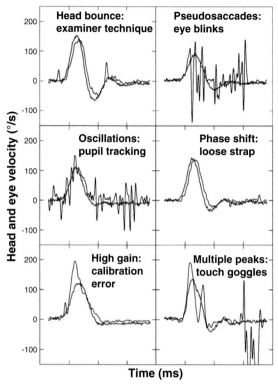

FIG. 8.3 Video head impulse test artifacts obtained from a sample of clinic patients. Head impulses are shown in red and eye movement traces are shown in black. The artifacts were identified using the artifact classification scheme developed by Mantokoudis et al.[28] All recordings were "accepted" by the manufacturer's algorithm.

leads head movement (caused by loose goggle strap); (2) high gain (calibration error); (3) pseudosaccades (eye blinks); (4) double peaks in eye trace (examiner touching goggles or mini eye blinks); (5) head impulse overshoot or bounce (examiner error produced by head direction reversal following deceleration of the head impulse); (6) eye trace goes in wrong direction (patient inattention); and (7) eye trace oscillations (loss of pupil tracking). Fig. 8.3 illustrates vHIT artifacts obtained from a sample of clinic patients according to the classification scheme of Mantokoudis et al.[28]

Mantokoudis and colleagues[28] used the artifact classification scheme to evaluate vHIT records obtained from a group of patients with acute vestibular syndrome and found that 44% of the vHIT records contained at least one artifact. The two most common artifacts that resulted in uninterpretable recordings were noisy eye movement traces with multiple peaks and eye movement traces with oscillations due to loss of pupil tracking. In a subsequent study that used the same data set,

however, there was no clinically relevant difference between the unfiltered (artifacts included) and filtered (artifacts removed) VOR gain values in terms of sensitivity and specificity for the detection of posterior inferior cerebellar artery stroke.[35]

Recently, Halmagyi et al.[7] described artifacts caused by the eyelid briefly obscuring the pupil image during the vertical canal vHIT. The artifactual eye movement response during the anterior SCC head impulse is characterized by a biphasic eye movement trace, whereas the eye movement artifact during posterior SCC impulses has the appearance of a covert saccade that overlays the vertical eye velocity trace. The eyelid artifact is observed more frequently during anterior SCC impulses than during posterior SCC impulses, and it is generally recommended that the eyelids are taped up using medical-grade tape in order to avoid this artifact.

VIDEO HEAD IMPULSE TEST RESULTS FROM HEALTHY SUBJECTS AND THE EFFECTS OF AGE

Several recent studies have reported normative VOR gain data for the horizontal vHIT[32,36-39] and the vertical vHIT[32] in relatively large samples of healthy community-dwelling individuals across a wide age span (~10–90+ years of age) and over a range of peak head velocities (~70 to ~250 degrees/second). Overall, results of these studies indicated that VOR gain was constant through 70–80 years of age, and that there was a small decrease in VOR gain at relatively high peak head velocities at all ages. The average VOR gains collapsed across age ranged from ~0.94 to 1.06 for horizontal SCCs with slightly lower average VOR gain values for vertical SCCs. The lower limit for normal VOR gain (mean VOR gain minus 2 SD) was ~0.7 to ~0.80 for horizontal canals and ~0.60 to ~0.70 for vertical canals. Fig. 8.4 shows the vHIT head and eye velocity waveforms obtained from a normal adult subject.

In addition to VOR gain, the effect of age on corrective saccades has been examined using vHIT. A greater frequency of corrective saccades was observed with increasing age, and nearly 50% of older adults generated a corrective saccade.[37] Furthermore, older healthy adults (average age of 76 years) had significantly larger corrective saccades than younger healthy adults (average age of 45 years), and there was a significant positive association between age and the amplitude of the initial corrective saccade that was independent of VOR gain; there was no effect of age on corrective saccade latency and the saccades were predominantly overt.[40] In a retrospective study, Rambold[41] found that the frequency

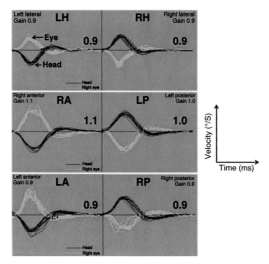

FIG. 8.4 Representative video head impulse test recordings obtained from a normal adult subject by a single examiner for head impulses in the horizontal and vertical planes. The mean vestibulo-ocular reflex gain is indicated within each panel (green tracings correspond to eye movements; black tracings correspond to head movement). *LA*, left anterior; *LH*, left horizontal; *LP*, left posterior; *RA*, right anterior; *RH*, right horizontal; *RP*, right posterior.

of occurrence of overt saccades increased as a function of age in a group of patients that had been referred for vestibular assessment but had normal caloric and vHIT results. In addition, the amplitude of the overt saccades was significantly lower in patients with normal caloric and vHIT results compared with patients with unilateral vestibular hypofunction. In aggregate, these studies suggest that both the prevalence and amplitude of corrective saccades is greater in healthy older adults than in younger adults, and that the corrective saccades observed in patients with UVL are significantly larger than those of healthy older adults.

ABNORMAL VIDEO HEAD IMPULSE TEST

In general, UVL will produce normal contralesional vHIT responses, whereas ipsilesional responses are characterized by reduced VOR gain and the presence of corrective saccades. Fig. 8.5 shows the head velocity and corresponding eye velocity waveforms for multiple head impulses in the horizontal plane obtained from two patients with UVL (see the figure legend for a detailed description). In patients with BVL, the vHIT reveals low gain and the presence of corrective saccades, bilaterally. The vHIT waveforms obtained from two patients with BVL are illustrated in Fig. 8.6 (see the figure legend for a detailed description). A brief summary of typical vHIT findings in some of the common vestibular disorders/etiologies is provided in the following sections.

Vestibular Neuritis

Vestibular neuritis (VN) is the most common peripheral vestibular disorder that results in UVL. Patients with VN generally show unilaterally reduced VOR gain (and corrective saccades) of the horizontal and anterior SCCs and normal posterior SCC function. When vHIT is used in conjunction with cervical and ocular vestibular evoked myogenic potentials (cVEMPs and oVEMPs), it is possible to differentiate among VN of the superior branch of the vestibular nerve, VN of the inferior branch, VN involving both branches of the vestibular nerve, and ampullary VN.[42-44] The vHIT is also an effective tool in monitoring the time course of recovery from VN, as it provides information regarding the absolute level of SCC function; recovery has been demonstrated as an increase or normalization of VOR gain and/or changes in corrective saccades (disappearance of saccades or decrease in saccade latency).[45-48]

Meniere's Disease

Meniere's disease (MD) is an inner ear disorder characterized by symptoms of episodic vertigo with associated hearing loss, tinnitus, and aural fullness that may last for hours. The pathophysiology of MD is unclear, but the generally accepted hypothesis is that the disease results in a hydropic condition within the labyrinth because of abnormal endolymph homeostasis.[49] The vHIT results obtained in patients with MD often indicate normal horizontal SCC function in the

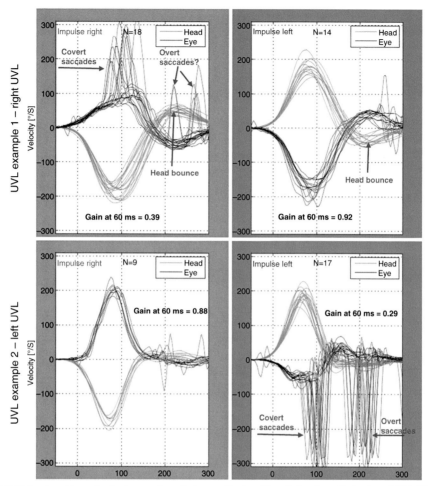

FIG. 8.5 Video head impulse test recordings in two patients with unilateral vestibular loss (UVL). The patient in the top row has UVL (right ear) due to a vestibular schwannoma (untreated), and the patient in the bottom row has UVL (left ear) secondary to vestibular neuritis. Both patients have normal contralesional vestobulo-ocular reflex (VOR) gain and abnormally low ipsilesional gain. In addition, the ipsilesional eye velocity recordings have both covert and overt corrective saccades. It should be noted that the head impulse recordings for the patient in the top row are characterized by "head bounce"; instead of the head coming to a complete stop at the end of the head rotation to the right (velocity ~0 degree/second), the head continues to move in the opposite (leftward) direction reaching velocities of ~70 degrees/second. Therefore, it is difficult to determine whether the overt saccades to the right were generated to compensate for the reduced VOR gain on the right side or were compensatory for the head rotation to the left.

presence of reduced caloric responses.[50–53] The disassociation between the results of the two tests is not surprising given the substantial difference between the stimuli used to activate the horizontal SCC during each test. McGarvie and colleagues[52] hypothesized that the hydrostatic mechanism that drives caloric responses (i.e., thermally induced differences in endolymph density across the horizontal SCC) is altered in patients with MD and that these changes in mechanical properties that reduce the caloric response would result in

minimal changes to the VOR when activated by the high-acceleration head impulse stimuli used for vHIT. The vHIT has also been used successfully to monitor SCC function following intratympanic gentamicin treatment in cases of intractable MD.[54,55]

Vestibular Schwannoma

The prevalence of vHIT abnormalities in patients with untreated vestibular schwannoma ranges from 33% to 62%[56–58] and is 90% after vestibular schwannoma

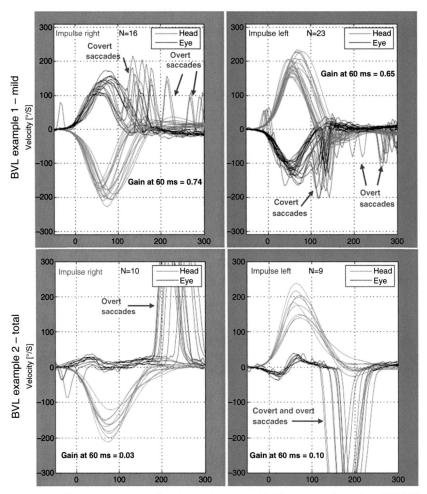

FIG. 8.6 Video head impulse test recordings in two patients with bilateral vestibular loss (BVL). The patient in the top row has a "mild" BVL (vestibulo-ocular reflex [VOR gain] <0.8 and both covert and overt corrective saccades, bilaterally) and the patient in the bottom row has almost a total BVL, with VOR gain values approaching 0 and the corrective saccades are almost all overt and substantially larger than the corrective saccades for the patient with the "mild" BVL.

surgery.[59] Mantokoudis et al.[60] performed vHIT testing preoperatively and postoperatively in five patients after unilateral vestibular deafferentation from vestibular schwannoma resection. The vHIT results revealed a postoperative decrease in ipsilesional horizontal VOR gain that remained low through a 5-day postoperative period. In contrast, contralesional VOR gain returned to the preoperative baseline by day 4. On postoperative days 1–3, corrective saccades were exclusively overt with an average latency of approximately 193 ms; however, by day 5, the average latency had decreased significantly to 134 ms (covert saccades). These authors hypothesized that patients who do not demonstrate similar decreases

in saccade latencies following unilateral vestibular deafferentation may benefit from gaze-stabilizing vestibular rehabilitation and that the persistence of low ipsilesional VOR gain justifies vestibular adaptation exercises and balance and gait training to reduce fall risk in the postoperative period. Batuecas-Caletrio et al.[59] examined corrective saccades recorded during vHIT in 49 patients one year following vestibular schwannoma surgery. Patients were classified into two groups according to the latency distribution of corrective saccades: (1) thirty-eight patients with a relatively narrow latency distribution and (2) eleven patients with a relatively wide latency distribution. There was no significant group difference in ipsilesional or contralesional horizontal VOR gain. The patients in group 2 had significantly higher scores on the Dizziness Handicap Inventory than group 1, and a significantly lower preoperative caloric weakness (i.e., less caloric asymmetry). In addition, patients in group 2 were significantly older than patients in group 1 by an average of 10 years. Notably, none of the patients in this study had undergone vestibular rehabilitation. These findings suggest an association between the latency characteristics of corrective saccades and self-perceived dizziness handicap. There may also be an age effect in which older patients show a relatively wide latency distribution of corrective saccades and may take longer to compensate after UVL.

Acute Vestibular Syndrome

There has been growing interest in the use of vHIT to assess patients who report to the emergency department (ED) with symptoms of acute vestibular syndrome (acute persistent vertigo with nystagmus, nausea and/or vomiting, gait instability, and head motion intolerance) with the goal of differentiating patients with VN from patients with brainstem or cerebellar strokes (stroke patients are more likely to have normal VOR gain on the vHIT).[61–64] Specifically, the HIT has been used in a small battery of tests that also includes assessment for direction-changing, gaze-evoked nystagmus and skew deviation; hence, the use of the acronym HINTS (*Head Impulse, Nystagmus* and *Test of Skew*) to describe the test battery.[65] The HINTS has been shown to perform well compared to other screening batteries for stroke risk. Newman-Toker and colleagues[62] reported HINTS stroke sensitivity of 96.8% and specificity of 98.5% in 190 patients who reported to the ED with acute vestibular syndrome. Mantokoudis et al.[66] reported that the use of the vHIT alone had a stroke sensitivity of 88% and a specificity of 92% for patients with posterior inferior cerebellar artery stroke; however, the use of vHIT VOR gain alone increased the risk of misclassification of patients with anterior inferior cerebellar artery stroke.

VIDEO HEAD IMPULSE TEST AND CALORICS

Following the introduction of the vHIT, there was interest in determining whether the horizontal vHIT could replace the caloric test in the vestibular test battery, as both are tests of horizontal SCC function. Using the caloric test outcome as the gold standard, the sensitivity of the vHIT in detecting UVL ranged from 29% to 79% and the specificity ranged from 86% to 100%.[50,53,67–70] The relatively low sensitivity reported for the vHIT is likely related, at least

in part, to the substantial difference between the acceleration/frequency profiles of stimuli used to activate the horizontal SCC for the caloric and vHIT, as well as differences in the underlying mechanisms that drive responses to the two stimuli. It has been suggested, therefore, that the use of the caloric test outcome as the reference test for evaluating the performance of vHIT is misguided and, rather, the test performance of the vHIT should be evaluated in patients following surgical vestibular deafferentation.[7] Recently, both the sensitivity and specificity of the vHIT have been reported to be 100% in a group of 37 normal subjects and a group of 37 patients following surgical section of the vestibular nerve.[71]

Results of a number of studies that have evaluated the test performance of the horizontal SCC vHIT using the caloric test as the reference test have recommended that the vHIT should be administered before the caloric test, and that the caloric test is only administered for patients with *normal* vHIT findings.[53,72,73] This recommendation is based on the vHIT's low negative and high positive predictive values: when the vHIT is normal, the likelihood that the caloric is abnormal is unacceptably high. In contrast, when the vHIT is abnormal, the caloric test is almost always abnormal. Results of these studies suggest that the routine inclusion of the vHIT in the vestibular test battery and the performance of the vHIT before caloric testing have the potential to decrease test time, decrease costs, increase patient comfort, and decrease the overall testing burden imposed on a relatively substantial proportion of patients referred for vestibular assessment.

VIDEO HEAD IMPULSE TEST IN CHILDREN

The vHIT has been used successfully in the vestibular assessment of children as young as 3 years of age.[74–78] Some challenges and observations reported in these studies are that longer test times are needed for children than adults (~20 min for the horizontal vHIT); children required 10%–49% more trials than adults to obtain a fixed number of valid responses; the calibration procedure had to be adapted for very young children; there is difficulty obtaining head impulse velocities >100 degrees/second; and there is inability to adequately fit the goggles in children <3 years of age or in smaller 3- and 4-year-olds. It should be noted that the issue of poorly fitting goggles in young children would be eliminated by the use of a commercially available vHIT system that uses an external camera (no goggles) to record eye movement.[25] It has been suggested that a new vHIT protocol, the suppression head impulse or SHIMP (described in the following section),

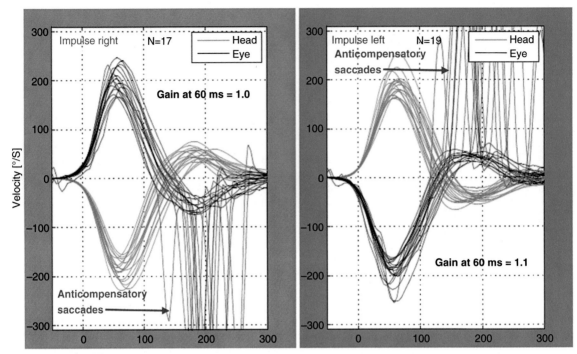

FIG. 8.7 Video head impulse test (vHIT) recordings for horizontal head impulses obtained from a normal individual using the suppression head impulse (SHIMP) protocol. The SHIMP protocol uses the same head impulse stimulus as the conventional vHIT, but uses a head-fixed (rather than an earth-fixed) visual fixation target. Similar to the conventional vHIT in normal individuals, normal vestibulo-ocular reflex gain values are observed with leftward and rightward head impulses. In contrast to the conventional vHIT, normal individuals generate a large anticompensatory saccade (a saccade that is in the same direction as the head impulse) near the end of the head rotation. Patients with unilateral vestibular loss (not shown) produce an ipsilesional anticompensatory saccade that is small (smaller than those produced by normal) or no anticompensatory saccade is generated.

may be particularly suited for children, as the visual fixation task is simpler and easier to understand than the fixation task associated with the conventional vHIT.[71]

SUPPRESSION HEAD IMPULSE PROTOCOL

Recently, MacDougall and colleagues[79] introduced a variation on the conventional vHIT protocol called the SHIMP. The SHIMP protocol uses the same head impulse stimulus as the conventional vHIT protocol, but, rather than using an earth-fixed target, patients are instructed to maintain their gaze on a *head-fixed* target (i.e., the target moves with the head during the head impulse) that is projected from a head- or goggle-mounted laser. The results obtained with the SHIMP protocol are complementary to those of the conventional vHIT protocol. That is, during the SHIMP protocol, individuals with normal horizontal VOR generate large anticompensatory saccades (a saccade that is in the *same* direction as

the head impulse) near the end of the head rotation (see Fig. 8.7) and patients with UVL produce an ipsilesional anticompensatory saccade that is small (partial UVL) or no anticompensatory saccade is generated (total UVL); BVL patients produce either small or no anticompensatory saccades at the end of head impulses to both sides.[79,80] Two distinct patterns of corrective saccades in BVL patients during the SHIMP protocol were recently reported by de Waele et al.,[81] and these patterns were correlated with the presence or absence of patient-reported oscillopsia during rapid head movements: (1) small or no anticompensatory saccades at the end of the head impulse (patients with oscillopsia) and (2) covert compensatory saccades followed by large anticompensatory saccades (patients without oscillopsia). These authors suggest that the unusual occurrence of covert compensatory saccades in conjunction with large anticompensatory saccades during SHIMP may have implications for vestibular rehabilitation.

CONCLUSION

Peripheral vestibular loss can occur in one or both labyrinths, in one or both branches of the vestibular nerve, and in one or more vestibular sensory organs. It has been demonstrated that otolith abnormalities do not always correlate with SCC involvement.[82,83] That is, vestibular pathology can affect otolith organs and spare the SCCs, or vice versa; a vestibular pathology may also affect both otolith and SCC function. The vHIT is capable of assessing the function of all six SCCs, and when combined with cVEMPs and oVEMPs, it is possible to evaluate the function of all the vestibular sensory organs and to potentially differentiate vestibular end organ from vestibular nerve dysfunction.

ACKNOWLEDGEMENT

This work was supported by a Merit Review (F1540-R) and by the Auditory and Vestibular Research Enhancement Award Program (C4339-F), both sponsored by the Rehabilitation Research and Development Service, Department of Veterans Affairs, Washington, D.C. The contents of this chapter do not represent the views of the Department of Veterans Affairs or the United States Government.

REFERENCES

1. Halmagyi GM, Curthoys IS. A clinical sign of canal paresis. *Arch Neurol.* 1988;45(7):737–739.
2. Bartl K, Lehnen N, Kohlbecher S, Schneider E. Head impulse testing using video-nystagmography. *Ann N Y Acad Sci.* 2009;1164:331–333.
3. MacDougall HG, Weber KP, McGarvie LA, Halmagyi GM, Curthoys IS. The video head impulse test: diagnostic accuracy in peripheral vestibulopathy. *Neurology.* 2009;73:1134–1141.
4. Ulmer E, Chays A. Curthoys and Halmagyi head impulse test: an analytical device [article in French]. *Ann Otolaryngol Chir Cervicofac.* 2005;122(2):84–90.
5. MacDougall HG, McGarvie LA, Halmagyi GM, Curthoys IS, Weber KP. Application of the video head impulse test to detect vertical semicircular canal dysfunction. *Otol Neurotol.* 2013;34(6):974–979.
6. MacDougall HG, McGarvie LA, Halmagyi GM, Curthoys IS, Weber KP. The video head impulse test (vHIT) detects vertical semicircular canal dysfunction. *PLoS One.* 2013;8(4):e61488.
7. Halmagyi GM, Chen L, MacDougall HG, Weber KP, McGarvie LA, Curthoys IS. The video head impulse test. *Front Neurol.* 2017;8(258):1–23.
8. Baloh RW, Honrubia V, Konrad HR. Ewald's second law re-evaluated. *Acta Otolaryngol.* 1977;83(5–6):475–479.
9. Cohen B, Suzuki JI, Shanzer S, Bender MB. Semicircular canal control of eye movements. *The Oculomotor System.* 1964:163–172.
10. Estes MS, Blanks RH, Markham CH. Physiologic characteristics of vestibular first-order canal neurons in the cat: I. Response plane determination and discharge characteristics. *J Neurophysiol.* 1975;38(5):1232–1249.
11. Ewald R. *Physiologische Untersuchungen ueber das Endorgan des Nervus Octavus.* Wiesbaden: Bergmann; 1892.
12. Goldberg JM, Fernandez C. Physiology of peripheral neurons innervating semicircular canals of squirrel monkey: I. Resting discharge and response to constant angular accelerations. *J Neurophysiol.* 1971;34(4):635–660.
13. Halmagyi GM, Curthoys IS, Cremer PD, Henderson CJ, Staples M. Head impulses after unilateral vestibular deafferentation validate Ewald's second law. *J Vestib Res.* 1990;1(2):187–197.
14. Grossman GE, Leigh RJ. Instability of gaze during locomotion in patients with deficient vestibular function. *Ann Neurol.* 1990;27(5):528–532.
15. Grossman GE, Leigh RJ, Abel LA, Lanska DJ, Thurston SE. Frequency and velocity of rotational head perturbations during locomotion. *Exp Brain Res.* 1988;70(3):470–476.
16. Jorns-Häderli M, Straumann D, Pall A. Accuracy of the bedside head impulse test in detecting vestibular dysfunction. *J Neurol Neurosurg Psychiatry.* 2007;78:1113–1118.
17. Blödow A, Pannasch S, Walther LE. Detection of isolated covert saccades with the video head impulse test in peripheral vestibular disorders. *Auris Nasus Larynx.* 2013;40:348–351.
18. Robinson DA. A method of measuring eye movement using a scleral search coil in a magnetic field. *IEEE Trans Biomed Eng.* 1963;10(4):137–145.
19. Aw ST, Haslwanter T, Halmagyi GM, Curthoys IS, Yavor RA, Todd MJ. Three-dimensional vector analysis of the human vestibuloocular reflex in response to high-acceleration head rotations: I. Responses in normal subjects. *J Neurophysiol.* 1996;76(6):4009–4020.
20. Aw ST, Halmagyi GM, Haslwanter T, Curthoys IS, Yavor RA, Todd MJ. Three-dimensional vector analysis of the human vestibuloocular reflex in response to high-acceleration head rotations. II. Responses in subjects with unilateral vestibular loss and semicircular canal occlusion. *J Neurophysiol.* 1996;76(6):4021–4030.
21. Weber KP, MacDougall HG, Halmagyi GM, Curthoys IS. Impulsive testing of semicircular-canal function using video-oculography. *Ann N Y Acad Sci.* 2009;1164(1):486–491.
22. Aw ST, Halmagyi GM, Black RA, Curthoys IS, Yavor RA, Todd MJ. Head impulses reveal loss of individual semicircular canal function. *J Vestib Res.* 1999;9(3):173–180.
23. Cremer PD, Halmagyi GM, Aw ST, et al. Semicircular canal plan head impulses detect absent function of individual semicircular canals. *Brain.* 1998;121:699–716.
24. Migliaccio AA, Cremer PD. The 2D modified head impulse test: a 2D technique for measuring function in all six semi-circular canals. *J Vestib Res.* 2011;21(4):227–234.
25. Ulmer E, Bernard-Demanze L, Lacour M. Statistical study of normal canal deficit variation range. Measurement using the head impulse test video system. *Eur Ann Otorhinolaryngol Head Neck Dis.* 2011;128(5):278–282.

26. Agrawal Y, Schubert MC, Migliaccio AA, et al. Evaluation of quantitative head impulse testing using search coils versus video-oculography in older individuals. *Otol Neurotol.* 2014;35(2):283–288.

27. Patterson JN, Bassett AM, Mollak CM, Honaker JA. Effects of hand placement technique on the video head impulse test (vHIT) in younger and older adults. *Otol Neurotol.* 2015;36(6):1061–1068.

28. Mantokoudis G, Saber Tehrani AS, Kattah JC, et al. Quantifying the vestibulo-ocular reflex with video-oculography: nature and frequency of artifacts. *Audiol Neurotol.* 2015;20(1):39–50.

29. Nyström A, Tjernström F, Magnusson M. Outward versus inward head thrusts with video-head impulse testing in normal subjects: does it matter? *Otol Neurotol.* 2015;36(3):87–94.

30. Schubert MC, Mantokoudis G, Xie L, Agrawal Y. Acute VOR gain differences for outward vs. inward head impulses. *J Vestib Res.* 2014;24(5–6):397–402.

31. McGarvie LA, Martinez-Lopez M, Burgess AM, MacDougall HG, Curthoys IS. Horizontal eye position affects measured vertical VOR gain on the video head impulse test. *Front Neurol.* 2015;17(6):58.

32. McGarvie LA, MacDougall HG, Halmagyi GM, Burgess AM, Weber KP, Curthoys IS. The video head impulse test (vHIT) of semicircular canal function–age-dependent normative values of VOR gain in healthy subjects. *Front Neurol.* 2015;6:154. http://dx.doi.org/10.3389/fneur.2015.00154.

33. Interacoustics. Gain calculation methods in vHIT 2017. https://www.youtube.com/watch?v=OYs_gi1ca2E. Accessed August 31, 2017.

34. Cleworth TW, Carpenter MG, Honeggerd F, Allum JHG. Differences in head impulse test results due to analysis techniques. *J Vestib Res.* 2017;27:163–172.

35. Mantokoudis G, Saber Tehrani AS, Wozniak A, et al. Impact of artifacts on VOR gain measures by video-oculography in the acute vestibular syndrome. *J Vestib Res.* 2016;26(4):375–385.

36. Li C, Layman AJ, Geary R, et al. Epidemiology of vestibulo-ocular reflex function: data from the Baltimore Longitudinal Study of Aging. *Otol Neurotol.* 2015;36(2):267–272.

37. Matiño-Soler E, Esteller-More E, Martin-Sanchez JC, Martin-Sanchez JM, Perez-Fernandes N. Normative data on angular vestibulo-ocular responses in the yaw axis measured using the video head impulse test. *Otol Neurotol.* 2014;36:466–471.

38. Mossman B, Mossman S, Purdie G, Schneider E. Age dependent normal horizontal VOR gain of head impulse test as measured with video-oculography. *J Otolaryngol Head Neck Surg.* 2015;44(1):1–8.

39. Yang CJ, Lee JY, Kang BC, Lee HS, Yoo MH, Park HJ. Quantitative analysis of gains and catch-up saccades of video-head-impulse testing by age in normal subjects. *Clin Otolaryngol.* 2016;41(5):532–538.

40. Anson ER, Bigelow RT, Carey JP, et al. Aging increases compensatory saccade amplitude in the video head impulse test. *Front Neurol.* 2016;7:113.

41. Rambold HA. Age-related refixating saccades in the three-dimensional video-head-impulse test: source and dissociation from unilateral vestibular failure. *Otol Neurotol.* 2016;37(2):171–178.

42. Magliulo G, Gagliardi S, Ciniglio Appiani M, Iannella G, Gagliardi M. Selective vestibular neurolabyrinthitis of the lateral and superior semicircular canal ampulla and ampullary nerves. *Ann Otol Rhinol Laryngol.* 2012;121(10):640–644.

43. Magliulo G, Gagliardi S, Ciniglio Appiani M, Iannella G, Re M. Vestibular neurolabyrinthitis: a follow-up study with cervical and ocular vestibular evoked myogenic potentials and the video head impulse test. *Ann Otol Rhinol Laryngol.* 2014;123(3):162–173.

44. Walther LE, Blödow A. Ocular vestibular evoked myogenic potential to air conducted sound stimulation and video head impulse test in acute vestibular neuritis. *Otol Neurotol.* 2013;34(6):1084–1089.

45. Allum JH, Cleworth T, Honegger F. Recovery of vestibulo-ocular reflex symmetry after an acute unilateral peripheral vestibular deficit: time course and correlation with canal paresis. *Otol Neurotol.* 2016;37(6):772–780.

46. Manzari L, Burgess AM, MacDougall HG, Curthoys IS. Vestibular function after vestibular neuritis. *Int J Audiol.* 2013;52(10):713–718.

47. Roberts HN, McGuigan S, Infeld B, Sultana RV, Gerraty RP. A video-oculographic study of acute vestibular syndromes. *Acta Neurol Scand.* 2015. http://dx.doi.org/10.1111/ane.12536.

48. Zellhuber S, Mahringer A, Rambold HA. Relation of video-head-impulse test and caloric irrigation: a study on the recovery in unilateral vestibular neuritis. *Eur Arch Otorhinolaryngol.* 2014;271(9):2375–2383.

49. Salt AN, Plontke SK. Endolymphatic hydrops: pathophysiology and experimental models. *Otolaryngol Clin North Am.* 2010;43(5):971–983.

50. Blödow A, Heinze M, Bloching MB, von Brevern M, Radtke A, Lempert T. Caloric stimulation and video-head impulse testing in Ménière's disease and vestibular migraine. *Acta Otolaryngol.* 2014;134(12):1239–1244.

51. McCaslin DL, Rivas A, Jacobson GP, Bennett ML. The dissociation of video head impulse test (vHIT) and bithermal caloric test results provide topological localization of vestibular system impairment in patients with "definite" Ménière's disease. *Am J Audiol.* 2015;24(1):1–10.

52. McGarvie LA, Curthoys IS, MacDougall HG, Halmagyi GM. What does the dissociation between the results of video head impulse versus caloric testing reveal about the vestibular dysfunction in Ménière's disease? *Acta Otolaryngol.* 2015;135(9):859–865.

53. Rambold HA. Economic management of vertigo/dizziness disease in a county hospital: video-head-impulse test vs. caloric irrigation. *Eur Arch Otorhinolaryngol.* 2015;272(10):2621–2628.

54. Marques P, Manrique-Huarte R, Perez-Fernandez N. Single intratympanic gentamicin injection in Ménière's disease: VOR change and prognostic usefulness. *Laryngoscope.* 2015;125(8):1915–1920.

55. Walther LE, Huelse R, Blättner K, Bloching MB, Blödow A. Dynamic change of VOR and otolith function in intratympanic gentamicin treatment for Ménière's disease: case report and review of the literature. *Case Rep Otolaryngol.* 2013;2013:168391.

56. Blödow A, Blödow J, Bloching MB, Helbig R, Walther LE. Horizontal VOR function shows frequency dynamics in vestibular schwannoma. *Eur Arch Otorhinolaryngol.* 2015;272(9):2143–2148.

57. Taylor RL, Kong J, Flanagan S, et al. Prevalence of vestibular dysfunction in patients with vestibular schwannoma using video head-impulses and vestibular-evoked potentials. *J Neurol.* 2015:1–10.

58. Tranter-Entwistle I, Dawes P, Darlington CL, Smith PF, Cutfield N. Video head impulse in comparison to caloric testing in unilateral vestibular schwannoma. *Acta Otolaryngol.* 2016;136(11):1110–1114.

59. Batuecas-Caletrio A, Santacruz-Ruiz S, Munoz-Herrera A, Perez-Fernandez N. The vestibule-ocular reflex and subjective balance after vestibular schwannoma surgery. *Laryngoscope.* 2014;124(6):1431–1435.

60. Mantokoudis G, Schubert MC, Tehrani ASS, Wong AL, Agrawal Y. Early adaptation and compensation of clinical vestibular responses after unilateral vestibular deafferentation surgery. *Otol Neurotol.* 2014;35(1):148–154.

61. Newman-Toker DE, Kattah JC, Alvernia JE, Wang DZ. Normal head impulse test differentiates acute cerebellar strokes from vestibular neuritis. *Neurology.* 2008;70(24, Part Pt 2):2378–2385.

62. Newman-Toker DE, Kerber KA, Hsieh YH, et al. HINTS outperforms ABCD2 to screen for stroke in acute continuous vertigo and dizziness. *Acad Emerg Med.* 2013;20(10):986–996.

63. Newman-Toker DE, Tehrani ASS, Mantokoudis G, et al. Quantitative video-oculography to help diagnose stroke in acute vertigo and dizziness toward an ECG for the eyes. *Stroke.* 2013;44(4):1158–1161.

64. Tsang BKT, Chen ASK, Paine M. Acute evaluation of the acute vestibular syndrome–differentiating posterior circulation stroke from acute peripheral vestibulopathies. *Intern Med J.* 2017. http://dx.doi.org/10.1111/imj.13552.

65. Kattah JC, Talkad AV, Wang DZ, Hsieh YH, Newman-Toker DE. HINTS to diagnose stroke in the acute vestibular syndrome: three-step bedside oculomotor examination more sensitive than early MRI diffusion-weighted imaging. *Stroke.* 2009;40(11):3504–3510.

66. Mantokoudis G, Tehrani ASS, Wozniak A, et al. VOR gain by head impulse video-oculography differentiates acute vestibular neuritis from stroke. *Otol Neurotol.* 2015;36(3):457–465.

67. Bartolomeo M, Biboulet R, Pierre G, Mondain M, Uziel A, Venail F. Value of the video head impulse test in assessing vestibular deficits following vestibular neuritis. *Eur Arch Otorhinolaryngol.* 2014;271(4):681–688.

68. Bell SL, Barker F, Heselton H, MacKenzie E, Dewhurst D, Sanderson A. A study of the relationship between the video head impulse test and air calorics. *Eur Arch Otorhinolaryngol.* 2015;272(5):1287–1294.

69. Mahringer A, Rambold HA. Caloric test and video-head-impulse: a study of vertigo/dizziness patients in a community hospital. *Eur Arch Otorhinolaryngol.* 2014;271(3):463–472.

70. McCaslin DL, Jacobson GP, Bennett ML, Gruenwald JM, Green AP. Predictive properties of the video head impulse test: measures of caloric symmetry and self-report dizziness handicap. *Ear Hear.* 2014;35(5):185–191.

71. Curthoys IS, Manzari L. Clinical application of the head impulse test of semicircular canal function. *Hear Balance Commun.* 2017. http://dx.doi.org/10.1080/21695717.2017.1353774.

72. Eza-Nuñez P, Fariñas-Alvarez C, Fernandez NP. Comparison of three diagnostic tests in detecting vestibular deficit in patients with peripheral vestibulopathy. *J Laryngol Otol.* 2016;130(2):145–150.

73. van Esch BF, Nobel-Hoff GE, van Benthem PP, van der Zaag-Loonen HJ, Bruintjes TD. Determining vestibular hypofunction: start with the video-head impulse test. *Eur Arch Otorhinolaryngol.* 2016;273(11):3733–3739.

74. Hamilton SS, Zhou G, Brodsky JR. Video head impulse testing (VHIT) in the pediatric population. *Int J Pediatr Otorhinolaryngol.* 2015;79(8):1283–1287.

75. Hülse R, Hörmann K, Servais JJ, Hülse M, Wenzel A. Clinical experience with video head impulse test in children. *Int J Pediatr Otorhinolaryngol.* 2015;79(8):1288–1293.

76. Khater AM, Afifi PO. Video head-impulse test (vHIT) in dizzy children with normal caloric responses. *Int J Pediatr Otorhinolaryngol.* 2016;87:172–177.

77. Nassif N, Balzanelli C, Redaelli de Zinis LO. Preliminary results of video head impulse testing (vHIT) in children with cochlear implants. *Int J Pediatr Otorhinolaryngol.* 2016;88:30–33.

78. Ross LM, Helminski JO. Test-retest and interrater reliability of the video head impulse test in the pediatric population. *Otol Neurotol.* 2016;37(5):558–563.

79. MacDougall HG, McGarvie LA, Halmagyi GM, et al. A new saccadic indicator of peripheral vestibular function based on the video head impulse test. *Neurology.* 2016;87(4):410–418.

80. Shen Q, Magnani C, Sterkers O, et al. Saccadic velocity in the new suppression head impulse test: a new indicator of horizontal vestibular canal paresis and of vestibular compensation. *Front Neurol.* 2016;23(7):160.

81. de Waele C, Shen Q, Magnani C, Curthoys IS. A novel saccadic strategy revealed by suppression head impulse testing of patients with bilateral vestibular loss. *Front Neurol.* 2017;8:419. http://dx.doi.org/10.3389/fneur.2017.00419A.

82. Ernst A, Basta D, Seidl RO, Todt I, Scherer H, Clarke A. Management of posttraumatic vertigo. *Otolaryngol Head Neck Surg.* 2005;132(4):554–558.

83. Iwasaki S, Fujimoto C, Kinoshita M, Kamogashira T, Egami N, Yakisoba T. Clinical characteristics of patients with abnormal ocular/cervical vestibular evoked myogenic potentials in the presence of normal caloric responses. *Ann Otol Rhinol Laryngol.* 2015;124(6):458–465.

CHAPTER 9

Positional Vertigo: As Occurs Across All Age Groups

EDWARD I. CHO, MD • JUDITH A. WHITE, MD, PHD

INTRODUCTION

Benign paroxysmal positional vertigo (BPPV) is one of the most common vestibular disorders with an estimated lifetime prevalence of 2.4% in the general adult population.[1] Out of the 5.6 million clinic visits in the United States for dizziness per year, it is estimated that 17%–42% of patients with vertigo receive a diagnosis of BPPV.[2–4] Although this disorder ranges across the lifespan, it tends to disproportionately affect older individuals aged 50–70 years and therefore has some noteworthy societal burdens.[5] For example, it is estimated that $2000 is spent on average to diagnose BPPV, and that 86% of patients have interruption in their daily activities and lost workdays because of their vertigo symptoms.[1,6–8] Furthermore, older patients with BPPV have a greater incidence of falls and impairments to their daily activities. These falls can result in secondary injuries including hip fractures and can lead to additional costs from hospital and nursing home admissions.[9] Therefore, this disorder not only affects an individual's quality of life but adversely affects society as well.

The true incidence and prevalence of BPPV are difficult to accurately estimate. Older studies have looked at the incidence of BPPV. For example, a study in Japan estimated the incidence of BPPV to be 0.01%,[10] while a study in Minnesota estimated the incidence to be 0.06%, with a 38% increase in incidence with each decade of life.[11] However, it is likely that these early epidemiologic studies were underestimates, as they only included patients who presented to physicians with their acute vestibular problem and did not include those who never sought medical care for their symptoms. A more recent study done in Germany looked at the estimated prevalence and incidence of BPPV in the general adult population using a cross-sectional, nationally representative survey of the general adult population in Germany. A prevalence of 2.4% overall with 3.2% in females and 1.6% in males was reported, and the 1-year incidence was calculated at 0.6%, approximately 10 times higher than earlier estimates.[1] The 1-year prevalence was also determined as a function of age in this study. In patients aged 18–39 years, the estimated prevalence was 0.5%, whereas the 1-year prevalence for patients aged 40–59 years was 1.7%. Finally, for patients older than 60 years, the estimated prevalence was 3.4%.[1]

BENIGN PAROXYSMAL POSITIONAL VERTIGO ACROSS THE LIFESPAN

There are very few published reports of patients with BPPV younger than 18 years. However, one series of case reports by Giacomini described nine patients who developed BPPV after intense physical activity.[12] Seven of these patients were younger than 36 years. There was one 16-year-old girl who developed BPPV after an intense dolphin stroke–style swimming activity. She was diagnosed with posterior semicircular canal (PSC) BPPV on the left. Our personal communication with Giacinto Asprella-Libonati, MD, noted that in his experience, approximately 1% of BPPV patients seen per year are pediatric patients aged 3–14 years. He reports that it is important to examine these children within 24–48 hours, as the diagnosis was able to be made in only 25% of patients referred to him by pediatricians. There seems to be a higher spontaneous resolution of BPPV in children, probably due to their continuous head movements when playing games. PSC-BPPV was the most common form (about 80% of patients), followed by lateral semicircular canal (LSC) BPPV (20% of patients). The patients' BPPV was generally related to recent minor head trauma in the previous 24–48 hours (domestic injuries, sports injuries, school injuries, dental care). Interestingly, pediatric patients with recurrent BPPV usually had a family history of migraine. These patients had more episodes of typical BPPV not preceded by head injury, often with involvement of multiple canals (LSC and PSC) in subsequent episodes (Giacinto Asprella-Libonati, MD, Italy, personal communication, August 2010).

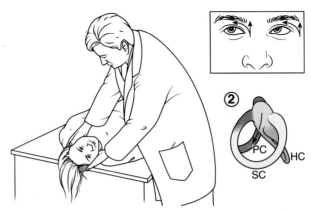

FIG. 9.1 Dix-Hallpike positioning. Lying position (head turned 45 degrees to the right). Characteristic upbeat and right torsional nystagmus is illustrated; canalith material has traveled down the long arm of the posterior semicircular canal, causing ampullofugal endolymph flow and stimulation of the cupula. (From White J. Benign paroxysmal positional vertigo: how to diagnose and quickly treat it. *Cleve Clin J Med*. 2004;9(71):722–728. Reprinted with permission. Copyright © 2004. The Cleveland Clinic Foundation. All rights reserved.)

In our experience with adults aged 18–39 years, risk factors for BPPV include certain activities such as yoga, pounding activities such as running on pavement, working underneath objects such as cars, and repetitively reaching high up for things such as books. Giacomini also found that activities such as intense aerobic activity, jogging, running on the treadmill, and swimming were associated with BPPV in individuals aged 18–39 years.[12]

Finally, in people older than 40 years, causes of BPPV include head trauma or association with other ear disorders, such as vestibular neuritis or labyrinthitis.[13-15] In adults of all ages, certain movements and head positions are likely to provoke the vertigo associated with BPPV, including lying back in bed, arising quickly, looking up, bending over, or reclining for dental or hairdressing procedures.

Recent work has suggested a correlation of recurrent episodes of positional vertigo with migraine, which is why the prevalence in females may be higher, as there is a higher incidence of migraine in women.[1] Vestibular migraine may cause episodic positional nystagmus that is difficult to differentiate from BPPV (see Chapter 11). The short duration of episodes (1–2 days) and frequent recurrence in otherwise healthy young patients with a history of migraine meeting International Headache Society criteria often aid in making this diagnosis. Particle repositioning maneuvers are usually not effective in vestibular migraine. The positional nystagmus seen with vertigo during vestibular migraine attacks may also appear atypical or have central features.

PATHOPHYSIOLOGY OF BENIGN PAROXYSMAL POSITIONAL VERTIGO

Regardless of age, the pathophysiology of BPPV does not change. BPPV is likely caused by otoconia that fall into the PSC or LSC after becoming detached from the utricle. The reasons for the detachment are many but include age, trauma, and infection. Schuknecht was the first to suggest that these basophilic deposits on the cupula of the PSC are the cause of BPPV.[16] However, further work and intraoperative observations suggest that these canalithic particles are likely to be floating in the PSC or LSC where they render the canal gravitationally sensitive.[17,18]

Approximately 94% of BPPV cases involve the PSC-BPPV.[19] Dix and Hallpike first observed this in 1952 and developed the head maneuver that produces the characteristic ipsidirectional torsional nystagmus used to identify BPPV.[20] During this maneuver, the patient's head is turned 45 degrees to one side while seated. The patient is then moved quickly to a supine position with the neck slightly extended and the head remaining turned. The characteristic ipsidirectional torsional nystagmus is seen when the undermost ear is affected. The patient is then brought back up to a sitting position, and the nystagmus is often noted to reverse direction as the canalithic particles fall back into the canal by gravity. The characteristics of BPPV nystagmus include onset after several seconds, a decline in eye speed velocity over 10–30 seconds and diminished nystagmus velocity on immediately repeating the Dix-Hallpike test (Fig. 9.1).[20,21] Although Dix-Hallpike testing needs no special equipment, visualization of nystagmus can be

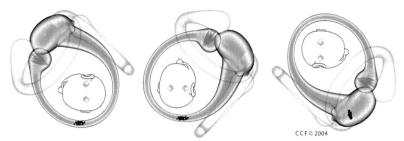

CCF© 2004

FIG. 9.2 Geotropic lateral semicircular canal (LSC) benign paroxysmal positional vertigo. The left ear is viewed from above as the patient lies supine. Head position is indicated. In the central figure, the patient is supine and canalith material is in the distal LSC. On the left side of the figure, the patient has rolled onto the left ear and the canalith material moves toward the left LSC cupula, causing an ampullopetal endolymph current that is excitatory. On the right of the figure, the patient has rolled onto the right ear and the canalith material moves away from the cupula, causing an ampullofugal endolymph flow that is inhibitory. Nystagmus beats toward the undermost ear. (Courtesy of the Cleveland Clinic Foundation 2004, Cleveland, OH; with permission.)

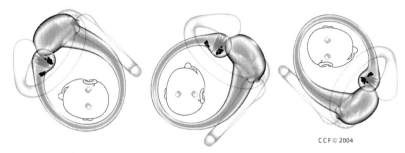

CCF© 2004

FIG. 9.3 Apogeotropic lateral semicircular canal benign paroxysmal positional vertigo. The left ear is viewed from above, as the patient lies supine. Head position is indicated. In the central figure, the patient is supine, and canalith material is in the proximal lateral semicircular canal, possibly adherent to the cupula. On the left side of the figure, the patient has rolled onto the left ear, causing an ampullofugal endolymph current that is inhibitory. On the right of the figure, the patient has rolled onto the right ear, causing an ampullopetal endolymph flow that is excitatory. Nystagmus beats away from the undermost ear. (Courtesy of the Cleveland Clinic Foundation 2004, Cleveland, OH; with permission.)

aided by the use of infrared video or optical Frenzel lenses, which eliminate visual fixation.

Lateral (horizontal) canal involvement is the next most common variant of BPPV, constituting 5%–15% of BPPV cases.[22,23] LSC-BPPV was first described by McClure in 1985 and is characterized by nystagmus provoked by supine bilateral head turns beating toward the undermost ear.[24] Two distinct subtypes of LSC-BPPV based on the direction of horizontal nystagmus during supine head turns are geotropic and apogeotropic. Geotropic LSC-BPPV beats toward the undermost ear on supine positional testing. The horizontal nystagmus has a short latency and prolonged duration with poor fatigability. This is thought to be caused by canalithic particles moving under the influence of gravity within the long arm of the LSC, which in turn causes the stimulation of utriculopetal endolymph flow when the affected ear is undermost (Fig. 9.2). Apogeotropic LSC-BPPV is characterized by a similar short latency and prolonged duration of horizontal nystagmus, but the direction beats away from the undermost ear, during supine positional testing. Apogeotropic LSC-BPPV was reported by Pagnini and Baloh in 1995.[25] Factors likely responsible for apogeotropic LSC-BPPV include otoconial debris that adheres to the cupula of the lateral canal, causing the cupula to become gravity sensitive (cupulolithiasis), or otoconia trapped in the proximal segment of the lateral canal near the cupula (Fig. 9.3).[24–27]

DIAGNOSIS AND TREATMENT

Initially, BPPV treatments were exercise based and emphasized compensation and habituation.[28] However, specific canalith repositioning maneuvers based on

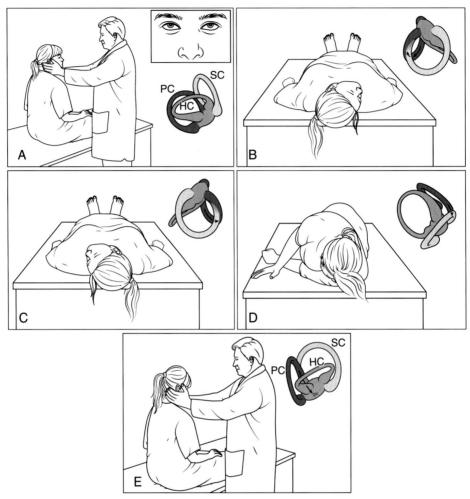

FIG. 9.4 Canalith repositioning procedure for right posterior semicircular canal benign paroxysmal positional vertigo. **(A)** The patient begins in the seated position with the head turned 45 degrees toward the examiner. **(B)** The patient is placed in the right Dix-Hallpike position and the characteristic nystagmus may be observed. **(C)** The patient remains supine and the head is slowly rotated toward the opposite ear. **(D)** The patient rolls onto the opposite shoulder and directs the head into a nose-down position. **(E)** After any nystagmus subsides, the patient is assisted in returning to the original position. (From White J. Benign paroxysmal positional vertigo: how to diagnose and quickly treat it. *Cleve Clin J Med*. 2004;9(71):722–728. Reprinted with permission. Copyright © 2004. The Cleveland Clinic Foundation. All rights reserved.)

an improved understanding of the pathophysiology of BPPV have been developed in the last 20 years and are now the standard of treatment. Canalith repositioning maneuvers for PSC-BPPV include the Semont,[29] the Epley,[30] and a modified Epley maneuver performed without mastoid vibration (Fig 9.4).[18] There is good evidence that vestibular suppressant medication is not as effective as repositioning maneuvers and vestibular therapy for treatment of BPPV.[31,32]

Although Dix-Hallpike testing is highly sensitive to PSC-BPPV, it lacks sensitivity in LSC-BPPV. For this reason, testing patients suspected of having BPPV should include Dix-Hallpike positioning to head hanging right and left positions and supine position testing in the head center, right ear down, and left ear down positions. The Dix-Hallpike test was entirely negative in case reports of two patients whose horizontal nystagmus with lateral supine head turns reached 12 and

16 degrees/second.[33] In four other patients, the horizontal nystagmus observed in Dix-Hallpike positions appeared to beat in the contralateral direction to that observed during supine positional testing (one geotropic and three apogeotropic). Furthermore, in most of the other patients with LSC-BPPV, the nystagmus that occurred during Dix-Hallpike testing had a lower velocity than that seen on supine positional testing.[33]

Identification of the involved ear in LSC-BPPV can be especially difficult because the semicircular canals are coplanar, and nystagmus is seen in both lateral supine positions. Order effect and head tilt may also affect the direction of nystagmus.[34] In geotropic LSC-BPPV, the nystagmus velocity is highest with the affected ear down. Treatment for geotropic LSC-BPPV consists of full-body 360-degree roll maneuvers toward the unaffected ear at 90-degree increments every 30–60 seconds, beginning with the patient in the supine position with the head flexed to 30 degrees and laterally rotated toward the affected ear.[35] The Gufoni maneuver is also highly effective and is performed with the patient beginning in the sitting position and lying quickly to the unaffected side and then rotating the head 45 degrees downward, maintaining this position for 2 to 3 minutes as described in Casani.[27]

Treatment for apogeotropic LSC-BPPV consists of a variety of maneuvers because none is universally effective. Identification of the affected ear can be more challenging in apogeotropic LSC-BPPV. Nystagmus velocity is usually higher with the affected ear uppermost, and spontaneous nystagmus (which usually beats toward the involved side) is occasionally seen in the supine position. The Lempert 360-degree roll maneuver toward the unaffected ear may be used first. The modified Gufoni maneuver can also be performed with the patient beginning in the sitting position and lying quickly to the affected side and then rotating the head 45 degrees upward, maintaining this position for 2–3 minutes, as described by Appiani.[36] Vannucchi-Asprella maneuvers are performed by briskly moving the patient from the sitting to the supine position and turning the head rapidly to the unaffected side, and then returning to sitting and moving the head back to midline. This maneuver is repeated five to eight times in rapid succession.[37]

Finally, anterior semicircular canal BPPV is a controversial entity. Some investigators suggest that the paroxysmal nystagmus has a pure or torsional downbeat component in contrast to posterior canal, which has a vertical upbeat component. Because the same maneuvers used to treat PSC-BPPV appear effective for suspected anterior canal involvement (although they may be performed on the contralateral side in some reports), the question may have more theoretical than clinical relevance.

EFFICACY OF TREATMENT

Multiple studies have investigated efficacy of treatment by comparing subjective assessment of patient self-reported vertigo frequency and severity and an objective assessment using repeated Dix-Hallpike testing. These studies have noted a poor correlation between self-report and Dix-Hallpike test results. Studies by Pollack,[38] Dornhoffer,[39] and Ruckenstein[40] found that 22%–38% of patients continue to report symptoms despite negative Dix-Hallpike test results, whereas Sargent[41] noted reports of subjective improvement despite persistent positive Dix-Hallpike test results in his study sample. Lynn suggested that objective Dix-Hallpike testing should be considered the gold standard of outcome measures in BPPV.[42] Controlled trials performed without Dix-Hallpike testing are generally excluded from evidence-based reviews.[43]

The impact of canalith repositioning on the quality of life in patients with BPPV has been demonstrated using the Medical Outcomes Study 36-item Short Form (SF-36)[44] and the Dizziness Handicap Inventory Short Form (DHI-S).[45] In one study, patients with active BPPV scored worse than population norms on both measures and had improved scores 1 month after canalith repositioning maneuvers were performed (DHI-S mean decrease 8.1 [$P < .001$, $n = 40$][46]; SF-36 subscales normalized [$P < .05$]).[47]

Recurrence is common after successful canalith repositioning for BPPV. One or two treatments are commonly effective in eliminating the current episode in greater than 90% of cases; however, treatment does not prevent future episodes.[48] Although the average recurrence rate is approximately 15% per year,[30,48,49] reported rates have ranged from 5% per year[50] to 45% at 30 weeks.[51]

Conversion between the PSC and LSC can occasionally occur when Dix-Hallpike testing is repeated after canalith repositioning has been performed. When this occurs, the patient develops brisk horizontal nystagmus that responds well to a 360-degree supine roll maneuver toward the unaffected side. In a study done by our group, we found that 241 cases of PSC-BPPV resulted in 15 LSC conversions, a rate of 6.2%. Repeat Dix-Hallpike testing after repositioning increases the diagnostic sensitivity for lateral canal conversions, allowing for rapid identification and immediate management (Fig. 9.5).[52]

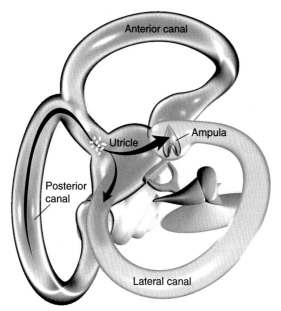

FIG. 9.5 Conversion of posterior to lateral canal benign paroxysmal positional vertigo. Canalith material leaves the posterior semicircular canal and can move onto the cupula of the lateral semicircular canal or into the long arm of the lateral semicircular canal. In the first instance, the nystagmus on supine positioning is apogeotropic horizontal; in the latter instance, it is geotropic horizontal. (Courtesy of the Cleveland Clinic Foundation 2004, Cleveland, OH; with permission.)

The use of postural restrictions after repositioning has declined in recent years. Patients were initially advised to keep their head elevated for 24–48 hours after canalith repositioning and avoid lying on the affected side for 5 days, all of which theoretically allowed the free-floating otolithic particles to settle into the utricle rather than return to the semicircular canal. However, several studies have suggested that these instructions do not increase treatment efficacy.[53–55] Massoud studied outcomes for particle repositioning maneuvers in patients ($n = 46$) who were randomized to postprocedure restrictions or control (i.e., no restrictions), with follow-up at 1 week.[54] Of patients in the control group, 93% had resolution of BPPV, compared with 88% of patients who received postprocedure restrictions. This difference did not reach statistical significance, possibly owing to the small sample size. Some centers continue to observe postprocedure restrictions based on anecdotal experience.

Other complications of canalith repositioning include an isolated report of fainting, sweating, pallor,

and hypotension during maneuvers accompanied by severe vertigo, possibly reflecting a vasovagal response.[56]

In an evidence-based review published in 2005, White found that the efficacy for a single treatment session for PSC-BPPV was 78% (range = 53%–99%, including 22 studies).[57] The treatment efficacy increased with repeated sessions and usually reached at least 90%. Overall, nine placebo controlled trials consisting of 505 patients were evaluated in this metaanalysis. The risk of persistent BPPV without treatment was 69% versus the risk of persistent BPPV after a single canalith repositioning treatment was 28%, a statistically significant difference ($Z = 9.09$; $P < .00001$). Therefore, the relative risk (risk of BPPV in the treatment group compared with the control group) was 39% (95% CI 0.32–0.48), representing a relative risk reduction of 61% (1 minus relative risk). The absolute risk reduction was 41%, which is used to estimate the treatment effect considering the actual frequency of the disorder in both groups. The number needed to treat was 2 (whole number rounded from 2.38), meaning that two patients would need to be treated to achieve a favorable outcome compared with no treatment. Typically, a number needed to treat value within the range of 2–3 indicates that a treatment is very effective.[58]

The efficacy of canalith repositioning for LSC-BPPV depends on whether the nystagmus is geotropic or apogeotropic. For geotropic nystagmus (nystagmus beating toward the undermost ear on supine positional testing), treatment can alleviate symptoms in 75%–100% of patients.[27,33,37] These same maneuvers are also used to treat the apogeotropic variant (nystagmus beating away from the undermost ear on supine positional testing). The apogeotropic variant is more difficult to treat, however, because the treatment depends on mobilization of the otoconial debris. When the otoconial debris can be mobilized from near the cupula into the posterior portion of the LSC by repositioning maneuvers, the apogeotropic nystagmus can be converted to geotropic nystagmus, which is predictive of an excellent treatment response.[37] Casani used the Gufoni procedure in nine patients with apogeotropic LSC-BPPV with a 44% success rate.[27] Asprella has described related techniques of rapid supine head turns in the Vannucchi-Asprella technique with somewhat better results,[37] and White et al.[33] reported a 50% success rate. Therefore, cupulolithiasis of the horizontal semicircular canal explains many of the features of apogeotropic LSC-BPPV, including its persistence and resistance to treatments that have demonstrated success with canalithiasis, such as roll maneuvers.

In addition, it is possible that some apogeotropic LSC-BPPV cases represent a subtype of vestibular neuritis, which is a more central lesion. The superior vestibular nerve innervates the LSC crista, superior canal crista, macula utriculi, and dorsum of the macula sacculi. Nadol[59] showed that superior division vestibular neuritis may cause degeneration of the lateral canal crista. The neuritis could also affect the utricular nerve, thus removing otolith inhibition from the LSC efferents at the level of the vestibular nuclei. Animal experiments have demonstrated that apogeotropic horizontal nystagmus develops in cats after unilateral utricular nerve inactivation.[60] Gacek theorizes that a loss of inhibitory otolith input is responsible for some cases of PSC-BPPV, a model that can also be considered in apogeotropic LSC-BPPV.[61] Otolith-canal mismatch or neural degeneration may also be a factor in the persistence of apogeotropic LSC-BPPV, despite aggressive therapy aimed at particle repositioning or liberation.

In our published series, treatment resolved the geotropic LSC-BPPV in all 10 patients.[33] The affected ear was identified as the side provoking the highest velocity nystagmus in the supine head turn, and roll maneuvers were performed toward the unaffected ear in each patient during the initial office visit. Symptoms resolved immediately in 7 of the 10 patients. Symptoms resolved in two additional patients with roll maneuvers in physical therapy. One patient required additional treatment in physical therapy, including repeated roll procedures and modified Brandt-Daroff habituation exercises to achieve symptom resolution.

Only 5 of the 10 patients in the apogeotropic group experienced complete resolution of their vertigo and nystagmus. One of these five patients responded to treatment in the first session, which consisted of vigorous 120 degrees horizontal head shaking for 1 min. This treatment was used because the patient was unable to roll or engage in a physical therapy program following a traumatic fall with orthopedic injuries. Subsequent follow-up with supine head turn testing demonstrated complete resolution of nystagmus. In the four additional successfully treated apogeotropic patients, roll maneuvers were effective. The remaining five apogeotropic LSC-BPPV patients continued to experience persistent nystagmus. One patient reported substantial symptomatic improvement but continued to show apogeotropic positional nystagmus and was treated with roll maneuvers and modified Brandt-Daroff habituation exercises in physical therapy before declining further treatment. The other four patients continued in physical therapy with mildly persisting symptoms. Treatment included roll maneuvers, modified Brandt-Daroff habituation exercises, Gufoni maneuvers, Vanucchi-Asprella maneuvers, and vestibular rehabilitation. Chi-square testing revealed that the outcome was statistically significantly poorer in the apogeotropic group than the geotropic group (Chi-square = 7.3; df = 1; $P < .007$).[33]

Finally, there is an association between BPPV and postural control, as patients often experience postural instability while BPPV is present. Increased anterior-posterior sway has been documented on computerized dynamic posturography (CDP).[62–65] Some residual postural instability has been observed even after the successful treatment of BPPV.[63,64] Theories regarding this persistent postural instability include receptor sensitivity alteration, residual scant debris in the semicircular canal, otolith dysfunction, or dysfunctional central adaptation.[64]

The elderly may be more affected by residual postural instability after successful BPPV treatment. Blatt suggested that younger subjects were more likely to show recovery of postural stability after successful BPPV treatment.[63] Their study sample size was small (33 patients aged 38–91 years) and did not specifically report data on the number and outcome of the elderly patients. Conditions more common in the elderly, including orthopedic problems, deconditioning, and medical conditions such as diabetes, neuropathy, and neurologic disorders, may complicate the assessment of postural control in this age-group. To examine the recovery of the elderly from BPPV, follow-up is necessary to compare postural stability before and after successful BPPV treatment.

Our personal experience has revealed a significant improvement in postural control after canalith repositioning for PSC-BPPV in elderly patients (Judith White, MD, PhD, Cleveland, OH, unpublished observations, July 2005.) In these observations, we found that the most sensitive measure was the Dynamic Gait Index (DGI) ($P = .011$), particularly the horizontal head turn condition ($P = .02$). The improvement in baseline to posttreatment scores of 3.4 points exceeds the 3-point criterion for clinically significant improvement suggested in other published studies using the DGI to assess fall risk reduction.[66] This improvement suggests that canalith repositioning for BPPV reduces fall risk in elderly patients with BPPV.

CDP results were consistent with DGI findings and with previously published reports noting impaired postural stability in patients with active PSC-BPPV.[62–65] Total CDP score and vestibular subscale scores showed a trend toward improvement after treatment, although significance may have been limited by small sample size. Improvement after canalith repositioning was also reflected in a significant change in DHI scores ($P = .027$).

SURGICAL TREATMENT

Plugging of the involved semicircular canal may be a consideration in patients with BPPV with unquestionable localization to the affected semicircular canal and persistent symptoms and has been used successfully in patients with refractory PSC-BPPV.[67] Challenges in definitively identifying the affected side make the surgical option less appealing in LSC-BPPV compared with PSC-BPPV. Horii reported a case of LSC-BPPV that did not improve when treated with plugging of the LSC, and the patient required additional treatment on the unoperated side.[68]

CONCLUSIONS

BPPV is one of the most common causes of vertigo. As our world population continues to age, it is expected that societal burdens from BPPV will increase. This is due to the higher risk of falls and fall-related injury in the elderly that occur owing to vertigo and associated postural instability. BPPV does occur across the lifespan, but there are very few published reports of its occurrence in children. However, when it does occur in the age-group of 3–14 years, it is typically associated with minor traumatic activities or migraine. Regardless of age, the pathophysiology of BPPV is thought to be caused by otoconia that fall into the PSC or LSC after detaching from the utricle. This can occur secondary to trauma, infection, old age, or other factors. Approximately 94% of BPPV occurs in the PSC and can be diagnosed with Dix-Hallpike testing. Approximately 5%–15% of BPPV involves the LSCs. This can be diagnosed with supine bilateral head turns. The geotropic form, which is characterized by displaced otolithic particles moving under the influence of gravity within the long arm of the LSC, can be effectively treated with a 360-degree log roll or the Gufoni maneuver. The apogeotropic form, on the other hand, is more difficult to treat because it is due to either adherence of otoconia to the cupula or a more central cause such as a subtype of vestibular neuritis.

Strong evidence exists for the efficacy of canalith repositioning procedures. Efficacy for treatment of PSC-BPPV is estimated to be up to 90% after one or two sessions. Treatment efficacy for LSC-BPPV depends on whether the nystagmus is geotropic or apogeotropic. For geotropic forms, the efficacy of canalith repositioning is estimated to be 75%–100%. The efficacy of canalith repositioning for apogeotropic LSC-BPPV, on the other hand, is approximately 44%–50%, because some forms may represent cupulolithiasis, other vestibular dysfunction, or central disorder.

If canalith repositioning procedures do not provide relief, surgery may be an option for PSC-BPPV. Plugging of the involved semicircular canal has been used successfully in cases of resistant PSC-BPPV. However, this option has been more difficult for LSC-BPPV due to the challenges in identifying the affected side.

Ideally, successful management of patients with BPPV involves an interdisciplinary team, including otolaryngologists, audiologists, physical therapists, family practice providers, and in some cases may also include neurologists. Ultimate goals of BPPV management are resolution of symptoms, improved postural control with reduction of fall risk, and decreased societal burden of BPPV.

REFERENCES

1. von Brevern M, Radtke A, Lezius F, et al. Epidemiology of benign paroxysmal positional vertigo: a population based study. *J Neurol Neurosurg Psychiatry.* 2007;78(7):710–715.
2. Schappert SM. National ambulatory medical care survey: 1989 summary. *Vital Health Stat.* 1992;13(110):1–80.
3. Katsarkas A. Benign paroxysmal positional vertigo (BPPV): idiopathic versus post-traumatic. *Acta Otolaryngol.* 1999;119(7):745–749.
4. Hanley K, O'Dowd T, Considine N. A systematic review of vertigo in primary care. *Br J Gen Pract.* 2001;51(469):666–671.
5. Baloh RW, Honrubia V, Jacobson K. Benign positional vertigo: clinical and oculographic features in 240 cases. *Neurology.* 1987;37(3):371–378.
6. Nedzelski JM, Barber HO, McIlmoyl L. Diagnoses in a dizziness unit. *J Otolaryngol.* 1986;15(2):101–104.
7. Neuhauser HK. Epidemiology of vertigo. *Curr Opin Neurol.* 2007;20(1):40–46.
8. Li JC, Li CJ, Epley J, Weinberg L. Cost-effective management of benign positional vertigo using canalith repositioning. *Otolaryngol Head Neck Surg.* 2000;122(3):334–339.
9. Oghalai JS, Manolidis S, Barth JL, Stewart MG, Jenkins HA. Unrecognized benign paroxysmal positional vertigo in elderly patients. *Otolaryngol Head Neck Surg.* 2000;122(5):630–634.
10. Mizukoshi K, Watanabe Y, Shojaku H, Okubo J, Watanabe I. Epidemiological studies on benign paroxysmal positional vertigo in Japan. *Acta Otolaryngol Suppl.* 1988;447:67–72.
11. Froehling DA, Silverstein MD, Mohr DN, Beatty CW, Offord KP, Ballard DJ. Benign positional vertigo: incidence and prognosis in a population-based study in Olmsted County, Minnesota. *Mayo Clin Proc.* 1991;66(6):596–601.

12. Giacomini PG, Ferraro S, Di Girolamo S, Villanova I, Ottaviani F. Benign paroxysmal positional vertigo after intense physical activity: a report of nine cases. *Eur Arch Otorhinolaryngol.* 2009;266(11):1831–1835. Epub 2009 Mar 1814.

13. Schuknecht HF. Mechanism of inner ear injury from blows to the head. *Ann Otol Rhinol Laryngol.* 1969;78(2):253–262.

14. Barber HO. Positional nystagmus, especially after head injury. *Laryngoscope.* 1964;74:891–944.

15. Barber HO. Head injury audiological and vestibular findings. *Ann Otol Rhinol Laryngol.* 1969;78(2):239–252.

16. Schuknecht HF. Cupulolithiasis. *Arch Otolaryngol.* 1969;90(6):765–778.

17. Hall SF, Ruby RR, McClure JA. The mechanics of benign paroxysmal vertigo. *J Otolaryngol.* 1979;8(2):151–158.

18. Parnes LS, Price-Jones RG. Particle repositioning maneuver for benign paroxysmal positional vertigo. *Ann Otol Rhinol Laryngol.* 1993;102(5):325–331.

19. Honrubia V, Baloh RW, Harris MR, Jacobson KM. Paroxysmal positional vertigo syndrome. *Am J Otol.* 1999;20(4):465–470.

20. Dix MR, Hallpike CS. The pathology symptomatology and diagnosis of certain common disorders of the vestibular system. *Proc R Soc Med.* 1952;45(6):341–354.

21. Baloh RW, Sakala S, Honrubia V. The mechanism of benign paroxysmal positional nystagmus. *Adv Otorhinolaryngol.* 1979;25:161–166.

22. Cakir BO, Ercan I, Cakir ZA, Civelek S, Sayin I, Turgut S. What is the true incidence of horizontal semicircular canal benign paroxysmal positional vertigo? *Otolaryngol Head Neck Surg.* 2006;134(3):451–454.

23. Parnes LS, Agrawal SK, Atlas J. Diagnosis and management of benign paroxysmal positional vertigo (BPPV). *CMAJ.* 2003;169(7):681–693.

24. McClure JA. Horizontal canal BPV. *J Otolaryngol.* 1985;14(1):30–35.

25. Baloh RW, Yue Q, Jacobson KM, Honrubia V. Persistent direction-changing positional nystagmus: another variant of benign positional nystagmus? *Neurology.* 1995;45(7):1297–1301.

26. Fife TD. Recognition and management of horizontal canal benign positional vertigo. *Am J Otol.* 1998;19(3):345–351.

27. Casani AP, Vannucci G, Fattori B, Berrettini S. The treatment of horizontal canal positional vertigo: our experience in 66 cases. *Laryngoscope.* 2002;112(1):172–178.

28. Brandt T, Daroff RB. Physical therapy for benign paroxysmal positional vertigo. *Arch Otolaryngol.* 1980;106(8):484–485.

29. Semont A, Freyss G, Vitte E. Curing the BPPV with a liberatory maneuver. *Adv Otorhinolaryngol.* 1988;42:290–293.

30. Epley JM. The canalith repositioning procedure: for treatment of benign paroxysmal positional vertigo. *Otolaryngol Head Neck Surg.* 1992;107(3):399–404.

31. McClure JA, Willett JM. Lorazepam and diazepam in the treatment of benign paroxysmal vertigo. *J Otolaryngol.* 1980;9(6):472–477.

32. Fujino A, Tokumasu K, Yosio S, Naganuma H, Yoneda S, Nakamura K. Vestibular training for benign paroxysmal positional vertigo. Its efficacy in comparison with antivertigo drugs. *Arch Otolaryngol Head Neck Surg.* 1994;120(5):497–504.

33. White JA, Coale KD, Catalano PJ, Oas JG. Diagnosis and management of lateral semicircular canal benign paroxysmal positional vertigo. *Otolaryngol Head Neck Surg.* 2005;133(2):278–284.

34. Bisdorff AR, Debatisse D. Localizing signs in positional vertigo due to lateral canal cupulolithiasis. *Neurology.* 2001;57(6):1085–1088.

35. Lempert T, Tiel-Wilck K. A positional maneuver for treatment of horizontal-canal benign positional vertigo. *Laryngoscope.* 1996;106(4):476–478.

36. Appiani GC, Catania G, Gagliardi M, Cuiuli G. Repositioning maneuver for the treatment of the apogeotropic variant of horizontal canal benign paroxysmal positional vertigo. *Otol Neurotol.* 2005;26(2):257–260.

37. Asprella Libonati G, Gagliardi G, Cifarelli D, Larotonda G. "Step by step" treatment of lateral semicircular canal canalolithiasis under videonystagmoscopic examination. *Acta Otorhinolaryngol Ital.* 2003;23(1):10–15.

38. Pollak L, Davies RA, Luxon LL. Effectiveness of the particle repositioning maneuver in benign paroxysmal positional vertigo with and without additional vestibular pathology. *Otol Neurotol.* 2002;23(1):79–83.

39. Dornhoffer JL, Colvin GB. Benign paroxysmal positional vertigo and canalith repositioning: clinical correlations. *Am J Otol.* 2000;21(2):230–233.

40. Ruckenstein MJ. Therapeutic efficacy of the Epley canalith repositioning maneuver. *Laryngoscope.* 2001;111(6):940–945.

41. Sargent EW, Bankaitis AE, Hollenbeak CS, Currens JW. Mastoid oscillation in canalith repositioning for paroxysmal positional vertigo. *Otol Neurotol.* 2001;22(2):205–209.

42. Lynn S, Pool A, Rose D, Brey R, Suman V. Randomized trial of the canalith repositioning procedure. *Otolaryngol Head Neck Surg.* 1995;113(6):712–720.

43. Blakley BW. A randomized, controlled assessment of the canalith repositioning maneuver. *Otolaryngol Head Neck Surg.* 1994;110(4):391–396.

44. Ware Jr JE, Sherbourne CD. The MOS 36-item short-form health survey (SF-36). I. Conceptual framework and item selection. *Med Care.* 1992;30(6):473–483.

45. Jacobson GP, Newman CW. The development of the dizziness handicap inventory. *Arch Otolaryngol Head Neck Surg.* 1990;116(4):424–427.

46. Lopez-Escamez JA, Gamiz MJ, Fernandez-Perez A, Gomez-Finana M, Sanchez-Canet I. Impact of treatment on health-related quality of life in patients with posterior canal benign paroxysmal positional vertigo. *Otol Neurotol.* 2003;24(4):637–641.

47. Gamiz MJ, Lopez-Escamez JA. Health-related quality of life in patients over sixty years old with benign paroxysmal positional vertigo. *Gerontology.* 2004;50(2):82–86.

48. Nunez RA, Cass SP, Furman JM. Short- and long-term outcomes of canalith repositioning for benign paroxysmal positional vertigo. *Otolaryngol Head Neck Surg.* 2000;122(5):647–652.

49. Furman JM, Cass SP. Benign paroxysmal positional vertigo. *N Engl J Med.* 1999;341(21):1590–1596.

50. Sakaida M, Takeuchi K, Ishinaga H, Adachi M, Majima Y. Long-term outcome of benign paroxysmal positional vertigo. *Neurology.* 2003;60(9):1532–1534.

51. Beynon GJ, Baguley DM, da Cruz MJ. Recurrence of symptoms following treatment of posterior semicircular canal benign positional paroxysmal vertigo with a particle repositioning manoeuvre. *J Otolaryngol.* 2000;29(1):2–6.

52. White JA, Oas JG. Diagnosis and management of lateral semicircular canal conversions during particle repositioning therapy. *Laryngoscope.* 2005;115(10):1895–1897.

53. Marciano E, Marcelli V. Postural restrictions in labyrintholithiasis. *Eur Arch Otorhinolaryngol.* 2002;259(5):262–265. Epub 2002 Mar 2019.

54. Massoud EA, Ireland DJ. Post-treatment instructions in the nonsurgical management of benign paroxysmal positional vertigo. *J Otolaryngol.* 1996;25(2):121–125.

55. Nuti D, Nati C, Passali D. Treatment of benign paroxysmal positional vertigo: no need for postmaneuver restrictions. *Otolaryngol Head Neck Surg.* 2000;122(3):440–444.

56. Yimtae K, Srirompotong S, Sae-Seaw P. A randomized trial of the canalith repositioning procedure. *Laryngoscope.* 2003;113(5):828–832.

57. White J, Savvides P, Cherian N, Oas J. Canalith repositioning for benign paroxysmal positional vertigo. *Otol Neurotol.* 2005;26(4):704–710.

58. Smeeth L, Haines A, Ebrahim S. Numbers needed to treat derived from meta-analyses–sometimes informative, usually misleading. *BMJ.* 1999;318(7197):1548–1551.

59. Nadol Jr JB. Vestibular neuritis. *Otolaryngol Head Neck Surg.* 1995;112(1):162–172.

60. Fluur E. Positional and positioning nystagmus as a result of utriculocupular integration. *Acta Otolaryngol.* 1974;78(1–2):19–27.

61. Gacek RR. Pathology of benign paroxysmal positional vertigo revisited. *Ann Otol Rhinol Laryngol.* 2003;112(7): 574–582.

62. Black FO, Nashner LM. Postural disturbance in patients with benign paroxysmal positional nystagmus. *Ann Otol Rhinol Laryngol.* 1984;93(6 Pt 1):595–599.

63. Blatt PJ, Georgakakis GA, Herdman SJ, Clendaniel RA, Tusa RJ. The effect of the canalith repositioning maneuver on resolving postural instability in patients with benign paroxysmal positional vertigo. *Am J Otol.* 2000;21(3):356–363.

64. Di Girolamo S, Paludetti G, Briglia G, Cosenza A, Santarelli R, Di Nardo W. Postural control in benign paroxysmal positional vertigo before and after recovery. *Acta Otolaryngol.* 1998; 118(3):289–293.

65. Voorhees RL. The role of dynamic posturography in neurotologic diagnosis. *Laryngoscope.* 1989;99(10 Pt 1): 995–1001.

66. Hall CD, Schubert MC, Herdman SJ. Prediction of fall risk reduction as measured by dynamic gait index in individuals with unilateral vestibular hypofunction. *Otol Neurotol.* 2004;25(5):746–751.

67. Parnes LS. Update on posterior canal occlusion for benign paroxysmal positional vertigo. *Otolaryngol Clin North Am.* 1996;29(2):333–342.

68. Horii A, Imai T, Mishiro Y, et al. Horizontal canal type BPPV: bilaterally affected case treated with canal plugging and Lempert's maneuver. *ORL J Otorhinolaryngol Relat Spec.* 2003;65(6):366–369.

CHAPTER 10

Vestibular Neuritis

JOHN C. GODDARD, MD • JOSE N. FAYAD, MD

Case study: L.R. is a 40-year-old female referred by her primary care physician with a chief complaint of acute, severe, room-spinning vertigo. She stated that she awoke at 4 a.m. when the sensation of vertigo came on very suddenly, was quite violent, and was accompanied by nausea and vomiting. She recalled having to crawl on the floor to make it to the bathroom and felt that the room continued to spin any time she opened her eyes. She eventually made it back to her bed and had to lie still, without moving her head, to minimize the waves of nausea and episodes of vomiting. She felt a "heavy" sensation in her head for several days afterward. Although it was difficult to remember the details, she did not recall a loss of hearing or any associated ringing in her ears with the episode. The patient felt a bit nauseated the day before the vertigo began but otherwise had been in good health. The patient was ultimately taken to the emergency room by her spouse, where she was hydrated intravenously and given vestibular suppressants and antiemetics. Several days after the onset of the vertigo, the patient described feeling quite unsteady, especially with any rapid movement of her head or body.

INTRODUCTION

Vestibular neuritis is characterized by the acute onset of vertigo with associated nausea, vomiting, and generalized imbalance. The acute phase is often severe and can last from a few hours to several days. A sense of imbalance and unsteadiness, exacerbated by motion, may linger for weeks to months. Auditory symptoms are uncommon, although patients may occasionally report ear fullness and tinnitus. Patients with accompanying hearing loss are believed to have a slightly different pathophysiologic entity termed acute labyrinthitis.

The precise etiology of vestibular neuritis remains elusive. Several theories have been postulated and supported, at least partially, within the literature. Dix and Hallpike[1] in the 1950s suggested that an infectious process affecting Scarpa's ganglion or the vestibular nerve might be responsible. Lindsay and Hemenway[2] felt that an ischemic process might be responsible, although they found no direct evidence of vascular occlusion. More recent efforts have suggested that a viral agent may be the underlying cause.[3–7] While individual

studies have demonstrated the presence of herpes simplex virus DNA within vestibular nerve fibers and Scarpa's ganglion, others have demonstrated histologic changes within the vestibular nerve suggestive of viral-induced atrophy and inflammation.[6–8] Anatomic studies have also demonstrated that the superior vestibular nerve, which supplies the utricle, superior, and horizontal semicircular canals, is more likely to be involved in cases of vestibular neuritis.[2,9] Goebel and colleagues have shown an anatomic basis for this observation related to the increased length, reduced diameter, and increased bony trabeculae of the bony canal housing the superior vestibular nerve (and its divisions) as compared with the inferior vestibular nerve.[10]

In clinics specializing in vestibular disorders, vestibular neuritis accounts for between 3% and 10% of diagnoses.[11] An annual incidence of vestibular neuritis approximating 3.5 cases per 100,000 persons was reported by Sekitani and colleagues, but further literature on the subject is lacking.[12] In this same report, which was based on a large Japanese population, the peak age distribution for vestibular neuritis was between 30 and 50 years, with a range of 3–88 years. Furthermore, approximately 12% of patients in this study were more than 65 years.[12] Dix and Hallpike, in their review of 100 cases of vestibular neuritis, found that 94% of cases occurred among patients between the ages of 20 and 59 years.[1] While middle-aged individuals do seem to be more commonly affected, the authors' experience would suggest that vestibular neuritis likely accounts for a larger percentage of vestibular diagnoses than outlined in these reports. This may be a consequence of differences in geographic referral patterns, variations in health care access, and a general lack of follow-up in patients achieving rapid resolution of symptoms.

CLINICAL CHARACTERISTICS

Despite an inability to clearly identify the cause of vestibular neuritis, a thorough understanding of its clinical course and management has been established. The typical onset is one of intense vertigo, often noted on awakening. Patients may have a tendency to fall toward the involved side and will frequently demonstrate spontaneous nystagmus with direction being constant despite changes in gaze. Head or body movements exacerbate the symptoms, and patients will often try to minimize any such movements by lying completely still. Although the initial vertigo symptoms often subside over a period of days, patients may have a longer period of continued imbalance. This imbalance may manifest as difficulty making quick movements or turns, slight swaying during walking, or a generalized feeling of unsteadiness. Patients also often complain of a heavy feeling in their head or simply feeling "off" for days to weeks after the initial episode. Benign paroxysmal positional vertigo (BPPV) is common in patients who have had vestibular neuritis and can occur at varying intervals after the acute attack. The cause of frequent occurrence of BPPV in these patients is not known, although Schuknecht suggested that utricular otoconia might be loosened with the initial neuritis.[13] Repeated bouts of vestibular neuritis have also been described, which many contend lends evidence toward a possible viral reactivation process as seen in herpes zoster oticus.[5] Another theory to account for recurrent vertigo seen following acute vestibular neuritis is that stepwise compensation or periodic decompensation of unilateral vestibular loss causes reemergence of dizziness that eventually fully compensates. Some patients will be left with unilateral vestibular loss.

DIAGNOSIS AND DIFFERENTIATION FROM CENTRAL INSULT/STROKE

As with most vestibular disorders of peripheral origin, a diagnosis of vestibular neuritis is primarily reached through a complete and thorough history and physical examination. A history of chronic ear disease should be elicited, as complications of chronic otitis media are quite common and may present with vertigo (e.g., labyrinthine fistula or cerebellar abscess). The duration of the vertigo attack is a critical component in the history of any patient with a complaint of dizziness and is particularly helpful in diagnosing vestibular neuritis. However, variability in the duration of the initial attack of vertigo is possible (i.e., from several hours to several days), while recurrent episodes of intense vertigo may occur with years of time between individual events. The presence of any other neurologic symptoms is as important as the duration of the vertigo attack. As there are several potentially dangerous causes of dizziness, a high degree of suspicion for a central cause must always be maintained (Box 10.1). Directed questioning regarding associated symptoms is of paramount importance in

---

> **BOX 10.1**
> **Differential Diagnosis of Acute Vertigo/Acute Vestibular Syndrome**
>
> | | |
> |---|---|
> | Cerebellar hemorrhage or ischemia | Multiple sclerosis |
> | Brainstem hemorrhage or ischemia | Labyrinthitis |
> | Vertebral artery dissection | Traumatic disruption of otic capsule |
> | Inner ear decompression sickness | Meniere's disease |
> | Otic capsule violating temporal bone fracture | |

---

ruling out vertigo resulting from a stroke syndrome (see Chapter 16). In particular, clinicians should ask about any weakness or change in sensation (pain, temperature, or numbness) of the limbs or face, slurred speech, vision changes including diplopia, dysphagia, change in voice, memory loss, or ataxia. These symptoms are indicative of a central insult and require a distinctly different management paradigm than that used in patients with vestibular neuritis. Brainstem/cerebellar infarct (e.g., Wallenberg syndrome) or hemorrhage may present with some form of dizziness but will invariably be accompanied by other neurologic signs and symptoms (see Chapter 2). These patients often will be unable to stand or walk. Physical examination findings highly suggestive of central neurologic insult include direction changing or vertical nystagmus, skew deviation, Horner's syndrome (ptosis, miosis [constricted pupil], anhidrosis [decreased sweating], possible enophthalmos), and loss of pain and temperature sensation on the contralateral side of the body. The head impulse test will be *normal* with vertebrobasilar stroke.[14] In fact, Newman-Toker et al. reported that the presence of normal horizontal head impulse test, direction-changing nystagmus in eccentric gaze, or skew deviation (vertical ocular misalignment) was 100% sensitive and 96% specific for stroke in the first 48 h of symptom onset.[14] In patients in whom a central neurologic deficit is identified or suspected, imaging is diagnostic, with magnetic resonance imaging (MRI) being the preferred modality. Although rare, compromise of the posterior cerebral circulation may manifest with neck pain (from trauma or vertebral artery dissection) and associated dizziness and requires prompt neurosurgical consultation.

Physical examination should be performed to confirm the absence or presence of neurologic involvement. In addition to a complete head and neck examination with an otoscopic examination and testing of all cranial nerves, tuning fork testing, cerebellar testing, gait assessment, and a full neurologic examination should be performed. Chronic ear disease and any associated complications are usually discernible from a combination of history and physical examination including a careful microscopic otoscopic examination. Both high-resolution computed tomography (CT) and MRI of the temporal bones should be obtained if intracranial pathology or complication of otologic origin such as brain abscess is suspected, and the appropriate treatment should be instituted accordingly. Any neurologic abnormalities on physical examination (e.g., Horner's syndrome, loss of facial sensation, skew deviation, direction changing, or vertical nystagmus) should prompt further investigation into a central cause with dedicated imaging of the brain, preferably in the form of MRI. Patients with vestibular neuritis may sway toward the side of the involved ear while standing, but an inability to stand without assistance (i.e., postural dyscontrol) is indicative of a central lesion and demands dedicated imaging.

Patients with vestibular neuritis present with characteristic spontaneous nystagmus that may have both horizontal and torsional components and a fast phase directed toward the uninvolved ear and that improves with visual fixation. Head thrust testing (i.e., head impulse testing) toward the affected ear will often demonstrate compensatory "catch-up" or refixation saccades indicating a peripheral vestibular insult.[15] Formal vestibular testing, although not performed in practice in the acute setting, has been performed in research settings and typically demonstrates reduced caloric responses.[1] Imaging studies are not required in classic cases of vestibular neuritis, but as outlined previously, the presence of any additional or unusual signs or symptoms demands an assessment for the presence of a central lesion.

In addition, vestibular neuritis can mimic other conditions, including migraine-associated vertigo (MAV). MAV is most often seen in patients having a history of headaches or a family history of migraine[16] (see Chapter 11). In patients with MAV, the headache itself may occur before or after the onset of dizziness, whereas the sensation of dizziness may represent true vertigo or merely a sense of disequilibrium. The variability of symptom duration in patients with MAV, with dizziness lasting from several hours to even a whole day, may explain why there might be some difficulty in distinguishing between this entity and cases of vestibular neuritis.

MAV occurs in both adults and children, although in pediatric cases it is commonly referred to as benign paroxysmal vertigo of childhood[16] (see Chapter 3 and Chapter 5). Although pediatric patients with vestibular neuritis have been reported, this diagnosis remains uncommon in children.[17,18] Reasons for this apparent predilection for middle-aged individuals are not known, and further investigation into the etiology of vestibular neuritis, viral or otherwise, is likely to aid in understanding this disease process.

A vestibular neuritis-like presentation may be the initial symptom complex of a patient with Meniere's disease. The acute vertigo lasts longer in vestibular neuritis (>5 hours to days) compared with the acute vertigo in Meniere's disease (usually fewer than 5 hours). Meniere's disease is also accompanied by hearing loss, fullness, and tinnitus in the affected ear; patients with vestibular neuritis do not have acute hearing loss or change in hearing.

MANAGEMENT: ACUTE PHASE

Management of patients with acute vestibular neuritis is primarily supportive. The acute phase is best managed with vestibular suppressants, antiemetics, and, in some patients, intravenous hydration. Common medications used in this acute phase, including meclizine, diazepam, and ondansetron, have been extensively reviewed elsewhere.[15] Patients who are more susceptible to dehydration, including children, the elderly, and individuals with underlying systemic disorders, may require hospitalization for a brief period. It has been suggested that the early administration of steroids may improve the rate and extent of recovery of vestibular function, although controversy remains as to the best method of assessing vestibular recovery and whether there is truly an improvement in clinical symptomatology.[19-22] The use of antiviral medications has also been proposed as an adjunctive treatment; however, evidence supporting their effectiveness is lacking.[20]

MANAGEMENT: CHRONIC PHASE

Once the acute phase of vestibular neuritis has passed, treatment efforts are aimed at improving central compensation through vestibular rehabilitation (see Chapter 19). In addition to minimizing the use of vestibular suppressants, early exercise is encouraged, and patients are instructed regarding vestibular exercises designed to enhance gaze stability and postural control and improve the tolerance of head and body movements. A major goal of vestibular rehabilitation is to improve the vestibulo-ocular reflex (VOR), which stabilizes visual images during head movement. Video head impulse testing has been increasingly used to assess the VOR in the setting of vestibular dysfunction, with a recent study demonstrating that VOR results were no different in patients who felt they had recovered and those who felt they had not recovered following an episode of vestibular neuritis.[23] These data support the notion that compensation requires more than VOR resolution and recovery. The degree of compensation is somewhat variable and likely depends on a number of factors, including patient age and underlying functional status, degree of initial vestibular injury (and any subsequent end-organ recovery), and patient motivation. Although many patients may be able to compensate with the help of self-directed vestibular exercise programs, others may require formal vestibular rehabilitation under the supervision of a certified vestibular therapist (see Chapter 19). Elderly individuals and patients with prolonged recovery would likely be excellent candidates for such a course of treatment.

In rare instances, when prolonged vestibular therapy is not effective and patients are debilitated by their symptoms, medical or even surgical intervention may be warranted. In such patients, the authors suggest that an MRI of the brain and videonystagmography and other objective vestibular testing should be performed to document the absence of an eighth nerve or central lesion and to determine the degree of peripheral vestibular dysfunction. Medical options are centered around the use of central nervous system suppressants. Chemical labyrinthectomy with intratympanic gentamicin may completely denervate an incomplete loss of peripheral vestibular dysfunction seen during the acute phase of vestibular neuritis. The complete ablation may allow a more functional compensation. Surgical options in the setting of chronic vestibular neuritis include vestibular nerve section if hearing is present or labyrinthectomy in cases of a dead or unserviceable ear. Although surgical intervention is considered a solution of last resort, it can be quite effective in improving patient symptoms.[24,25]

CONCLUSION

In summary, vestibular neuritis is characterized by the acute onset of severe vertigo, nausea, and imbalance; an absence of other neurologic deficits; and the presence of normal (i.e., recently unchanged) hearing. History and physical examination alone are usually adequate for diagnosis, although one must ensure that a central insult is not present. Imaging is generally not required if the history and physical examination support a diagnosis of vestibular neuritis. However, CT imaging should be considered in the setting of chronic ear disease with

MRI reserved for patients with suspected complications of acute or chronic ear disease or patients with signs and symptoms suggestive of a central (i.e., brainstem or cerebellar) etiology. Management of the acute phase of vestibular neuritis is primarily medical and supportive, while long-term treatment is designed to improve vestibular compensation.

REFERENCES

1. Dix M, Hallpike C. The pathology, symptomatology, and diagnosis of certain common disorders of the vestibular system. *Proc R Soc Med.* 1952;45(6):341–354.
2. Lindsay JR, Hemenway WG. Postural vertigo due to unilateral partial vestibular loss. *Ann Otol Rhinol Laryngol.* 1956;65:692–708.
3. Furata Y, Takasu T, Fukuda S, et al. Latent herpes simplex virus type 1 in human vestibular ganglia. *Acta Otolaryngol Suppl.* 1993;503:85–89.
4. Hirata Y, Gyo K, Yanagihara N. Herpetic vestibular neuritis: an experimental study. *Acta Otolaryngol Suppl.* 1995;519(suppl):S93–S96.
5. Gacek R, Gacek M. The three faces of vestibular ganglionitis. *Ann Otol Rhinol Laryngol.* 2002;111(2):103–114.
6. Theil D, Arbusow V, Deurfuss T, et al. Prevalence of HSV-1 LAT in human trigeminal, geniculate, and vestibular ganglia and its implication for cranial nerve syndromes. *Brain Pathol.* 2001;11(4):408–413.
7. Baloh RW, Ishiyama A, Wackym P, et al. Vestibular neuritis: clinical–pathological correlation. *Otolaryngol Head Neck Surg.* 1996;114:586–592.
8. Schuknecht HF, Kitamura K. Vestibular neuronitis. *Ann Otol Rhinol Laryngol.* 1981;78:1–19.
9. Nadol JB. Vestibular neuritis. *Otolaryngol Head Neck Surg.* 1995;112:162–172.
10. Goebel J, O'Mara W, Gianoli G. Anatomic considerations in vestibular neuritis. *Otol Neurotol.* 2001;22:512–518.
11. Neuhauser H. Epidemiology of vertigo. *Curr Opin Neurol.* 2007;20:40–46.
12. Sekitani T, Imate Y, Noguchi T, et al. Vestibular neuronitis: epidemiological survey by questionnaire in Japan. *Acta Otolaryngol Suppl.* 1993;503:9–12.
13. Schuknecht HF. Positional vertigo: clinical and experimental observations. *Trans Am Acad Ophthalmol Otolaryngol.* 1962;66:319–331.
14. Newman-Toker D, Kattah J, Talkad A, Wang D, Ys-Hsiang H. HINTS to diagnose stroke in the acute vestibular syndrome – three-step bedside oculomotor exam more sensitive than early MRI DWI. *Stroke.* 2009;40(11):3504–3510.
15. Baloh R. Vestibular neuritis. *N Engl J Med.* 2003;348:1027–1032.
16. Reploeg MD, Goebel JA. Migraine-associated dizziness: patient characteristics and management options. *Otol Neurotol.* 2002;23(3):364–371.
17. Wiener-Vacher SR. Vestibular disorders in children. *Int J Audiol.* 2008;47:578–583.

18. Bower CM, Cotton RT. The spectrum of vertigo in children. *Arch Otolaryngol Head Neck Surg.* 1995;121:911–915.
19. Kitahara T, Kondoh K, Morihana T, et al. Steroid effects on vestibular compensation in humans. *Neurol Res.* 2003;25:287–291.
20. Strupp M, Zingler V, Arbusow V, et al. Methylprednisolone, valacyclovir, or the combination for vestibular neuritis. *N Engl J Med.* 2004;351(4):354–361.
21. Shupak A, Issa A, Golz A, et al. Prednisone treatment for vestibular neuritis. *Otol Neurotol.* 2008;29:368–374.
22. Goudakos J, Markou K, Franco-Vidal V, et al. Corticosteroids in the treatment of vestibular neuritis: a systematic review and meta-analysis. *Otol Neurotol.* 2010;31:183–189.
23. Patel M, Arshad Q, Roberts RE, et al. Chronic symptoms after vestibular neuritis and the high-velocity vestibulo-ocular reflex. *Otol Neurotol.* 2016;37:179–184.
24. Benecke JE. Surgery for non-Meniere's vertigo. *Acta Otolaryngol Suppl.* 1994;513:37–39.
25. Pappas D, Pappas D. Vestibular nerve section: long-term follow up. *Laryngoscope.* 1997;107:1203–1209.

CHAPTER 11

Migraine-Associated Vertigo

TIMOTHY C. HAIN, MD • MARCELLO CHERCHI, MD, PHD

INTRODUCTION

The clinical association of migraine and vertigo or dizziness has been given many names in the literature, including migraine-associated vertigo, migraine-associated dizziness, vestibular migraine, migrainous vertigo, migraine-related vestibulopathy, basilar artery migraine, and others. According to Stewart and associates, 17% of the female population and 6% of males experience severe migraine headaches.[1] Because about one-third of persons with migraine experience dizziness,[2] the prevalence of migraine combined with vertigo or dizziness is expected to be about 3% of the population. "Vestibular migraine" is the most recent nomenclature for the combination of migraine and vertigo. If the criteria for vestibular migraine recommended by the International Headache Society are used, prevalence has been estimated to be roughly 1% of the population.[3] It is clear that the combination of migraine and dizziness is common in the general population.

Research studies concerning "vestibular migraine" usually employ criteria proposed by Neuhauser and Lempert,[3] which entail a complex decision tree. These criteria are well suited to research endeavors. In this review we will use a looser definition better suited to practicing clinicians—namely, headaches with migrainous characteristics combined with dizziness or vertigo, and refer to this more pragmatically defined entity as "migraine-associated vertigo" or MAV.

The literature concerning migraine in general is immense and even that regarding MAV is substantial; therefore, an exhaustive review is impractical. In addition, other reviews have been published recently.[3,4] Here we will focus on the salient features of MAV, concentrating on points of interest to the clinician.

It is important to understand that the diagnosis of "migraine" means only that the patient endorses a particular set of symptoms, as delineated by the International Headache Society. There is no biomarker for migraine, and the diagnosis of migraine is not nearly as specific or certain as diagnosing a brain tumor with imaging, or a hypothyroid state with blood testing. It is to be hoped that as we better understand the molecular biology and genetics of migraine symptoms, we will be able to categorize migraine into headache variants, associated with objective markers and individualized treatments.

PATHOPHYSIOLOGY OF MIGRAINE-ASSOCIATED VERTIGO

The pathophysiology of migraine remains poorly understood and probably is variable as well. In this discussion, we will use the mechanistic framework that migraine sufferers are more sensitive to many types of sensory input, and that when there is an overload of sensory input, a threshold is surpassed, triggering a cortical event followed by brainstem events causing even more sensory signaling to occur, generally resulting in a severe headache and a transient "shutdown" of the individual.

There is good evidence that the brain of many persons with migraine is hyperexcitable.[5] Persons with migraine are generally more likely to experience discomfort from bright light, loud sound, smells, motion, and many other sensory inputs that are not disturbing to nonmigraineurs. Migraine sufferers are frequently extraordinarily sensitive to sensory stimuli during their headaches[6] but also are often more sensitive at baseline, independent of their migraine headaches. As an example, patients with migraines often give a history of motion sickness. Studies find that 45% of children with migraines[7] and 50% of adults with migraines[8] report a history of being highly susceptible to motion sickness. In other words, sensory sensitivity accompanying migraines may be "hardwired."

If we attempt to become more specific about mechanism, research and clinical data suggest involvement of many processes—vascular, electrical, and biochemical processes. Research on migraine aura, such as the "cortical spreading depression of Leão"[9,10] and changes in blood flow in the occipital cortex demonstrated in migraines with certain visual auras,[11] implicates both vascular dysregulation and abnormal electrical activity. The response of migraine to serotonin agonists such as triptans implicates biochemical dysfunction of trigeminal brainstem circuits.[12] The vasodilator peptide, calcitonin gene-related peptide (CGRP), is found in cell bodies of trigeminal neurons. CGRP probably modulates vascular nociception and has been heavily implicated in the headache of migraine. There may be a positive feedback loop in which sensory overload triggers cortical circuitry that causes release of CGRP, which increases painful input.[13] Triptans, acting as 5-HT1B/D agonists, block these responses.

In MAV the same general mechanisms have been proposed. The fact that patients with MAV often have nystagmus[14] implicates dysfunction at the level of the brainstem (particularly the vestibular nuclei), although another obvious possibility is cortical dysfunction affecting the purported vestibular cortex.

COMMON HISTORICAL FEATURES OF MIGRAINE-ASSOCIATED VERTIGO

MAV, by any name, is broadly defined and almost "anything goes" with respect to symptoms and timing, as long as one combines a "migrainous" headache and dizziness. A study of MAV found that the most common vestibular symptom was rotational vertigo (70%), followed by intolerance of head motion (48%) and positional vertigo (42%).[15] Less common symptoms include a sensation of motion sickness, floating, rocking, tilting, a sensation of walking on an uneven surface, and lightheadedness. The chronology is similarly variable. Neuhauser[15] found the most common duration to be 5–60 minutes (33%), followed by 1–24 hours (21%), seconds to 5 minutes (18%) and more than 24 hours (2%). There are also reports of symptoms lasting months to years.[16] Onset can be gradual or abrupt. Cutrer proposed that the mechanism of short vertigo attacks was aura, while longer attacks were due to processes resembling central sensitization.[17]

Vertigo or dizziness and migraine headaches need not be simultaneous for patients to qualify for a potential diagnosis of MAV. Neuhauser reported that during symptoms of MAV, 45% of patients consistently have migraine headache, 48% of patients sometimes have migraine headache, and 6% of patients never have migraine headache.[15] During an MAV incident, 70% of patients have photophobia and 64% have phonophobia.[15]

Some patients identify triggers for MAV that are similar to triggers for other migraines, including dietary factors (caffeine, chocolate, alcohol, aged cheeses, monosodium glutamate, nitrites), weather-related triggers (low pressure, storm fronts, changes of season), and internal states (physical exertion, dehydration, sleep deprivation, menses). The time lapse between trigger exposure and symptom onset is usually on the order of minutes to hours but is occasionally more delayed.

Patients with MAV commonly report unusual discomfort from motion and visual input including both bright light and "busy" visual environments. "Motion sickness" symptoms, punctuated by dizziness attacks, may occur with or without headache.

Patients with migraine or MAV can have hearing complaints, especially tinnitus and phonophobia, but these are almost always transient and nonprogressive.[18] Transient synchronous bilateral reduction of hearing is unusual but almost unique to migraine. One study of patients with both migraine and dizziness reported that 66% describe phonophobia, 63% describe tinnitus, 32% describe hearing loss, and 11% describe fluctuating hearing loss and aural fullness.[19] In patients with MAV and hearing symptoms, hearing often fluctuates in both ears at the same time. This, of course, differentiates MAV from Meniere's disease or labyrinthitis.

DEMOGRAPHICS AND RISK FACTORS OF MIGRAINE-ASSOCIATED VERTIGO

The prevalence of MAV has been reported to be 0.98%,[3] but as mentioned in the introduction, looser criteria for MAV would support a higher prevalence of about 3%. Using the narrower criteria in the clinic might result in many patients—2% of the population—with a potentially treatable illness being excluded. Similar to migraine in general,[1,20] MAV affects women about three times more frequently than men. Migraine in women is particularly common in their 30s and also at the perimenopausal transition (usually early 50s).[1,21]

Migraine occurs with greater than chance frequency in association with several important otologic disorders. First, approximately 15% of the general population has migraine (most of these are women). About one-third of patients with benign paroxysmal positional vertigo (BPPV), twice the general prevalence, have migraines,[22] with a higher percentage in females (43%) than in males (21%).[23] Radke reported that 56% of patients with Meniere's disease also have symptoms meeting criteria for migraines.[24] The mechanism for the association between these otologic entities and MAV remains unclear.

PHYSICAL EXAMINATION IN MIGRAINE-ASSOCIATED VERTIGO

A patient who has MAV and no other illnesses typically has a normal physical examination. One exception to this is that patients with migraine (including MAV) may have nystagmus[8,25] that, while not typically observable on direct inspection in the light, may be discernible on video Frenzel goggle examination[14] or more detailed testing by videonystagmography.[14,25,26]

PARACLINICAL TESTING FOR MIGRAINE-ASSOCIATED VERTIGO

Because MAV is defined entirely by symptoms, it is a diagnosis of exclusion. Usually, the most significant overlap is with otologic disorders, and for this reason, a screening otologic and vestibular workup is advisable. The most useful tests include audiometry (to exclude Meniere's disease and labyrinthitis), videonystagmography, rotary chair testing, and video head impulse testing (to exclude vestibular neuritis). Patients with MAV generally have normal audiograms. Although studies of other otovestibular functions may suggest abnormality, these are exceptions to the general rule that otologic testing is normal in migraine.

In patients where doubt about the diagnosis remains, and especially where symptoms are not transient or are unresponsive to migraine medication, brain imaging is warranted. For the most part, imaging is normal; however, a modestly increased occurrence of white matter hyperintensities has been documented on MRI in patients with migraine with aura, compared with age-matched controls.[27] These imaging findings, which can resemble those of multiple sclerosis, are generally not accompanied by any clinical correlates.

Oculomotor testing, especially at the bedside (see Chapter 2), can be helpful to exclude other conditions. No oculomotor abnormalities are diagnostic of MAV, but the finding of subtle oculomotor abnormalities is compatible with the diagnosis. By subtle, we mean that these abnormalities generally are found through viewing the patient's eyes in total darkness, using video Frenzel goggles. Von Brevern and colleagues[25] reported that there are minor oculomotor abnormalities in 70% of patients with acute MAV. In our experience with these patients, there may be weak spontaneous nystagmus with horizontal or vertical components. The nystagmus can be positional as well, again generally with a horizontal or vertical vector, but on occasion there is a "bitorsional" pattern resembling bilateral BPPV, lacking the upbeating component.

Although the tests described above can exclude other disorders, there are no tests that can be relied on to confirm a diagnosis of MAV. This is unsurprising since patients with MAV function normally during most of their lives.

DIFFERENTIAL DIAGNOSIS OF MIGRAINE-ASSOCIATED VERTIGO

When headache and dizziness coincide, MAV is by far the most likely diagnosis. MAV is more challenging to diagnose in persons who have headaches and dizziness at different times, or in persons who have no headaches at all. An additional complication to the differential diagnosis is the fact that migraines may be triggered by vertigo.[28]

Other causes of combined dizziness and headache include structural lesions of the brain, and the chance occurrence of headache, possibly migrainous, and another source of vertigo.

Structural lesions of the brain are rare but potentially life-threatening. Prominent examples include brain tumors and the Chiari-1 malformation. Brain tumors are most easily distinguished from migraine by their timing (gradually progressive rather than the typical fluctuation of MAV), lack of sensory amplification (i.e., sensitivity to light, sound, etc.), lack of response to triptan medications, and, of course, abnormal imaging. In the Chiari malformation, the headache is generally posterior, there is downbeating nystagmus, and again, imaging is abnormal.

The main difficulty in Meniere's disease patients with headache is allocating symptoms between Meniere's disease per se and potential migraine. Approximately 50% of patients diagnosed with Meniere's disease also meet criteria for migraine.[24] This can be a particular problem when a destructive treatment for Meniere's disease such as intratympanic gentamicin is being considered, because to our knowledge, MAV does not respond to either gentamicin or vestibular nerve section. Practically, we think it is best to simply make a reasonable attempt to treat MAV (see following section).

Vertebrobasilar insufficiency (VBI) can often but not always be distinguished from MAV based on the history and lack of headache. A typical VBI patient will also be older and usually will have multiple vascular risk factors (see Chapter 16). VBI will typically cause multiple cranial nerve symptoms (e.g., visual abnormalities, diplopia or oscillopsia, dizziness, dysphagia) and may culminate in frank syncope, although dizziness also can be the only presenting symptom.[29] Usually, the ultimate diagnosis of VBI is based on the magnetic resonance angiogram that shows narrowing of the posterior circulation.

TREATMENT OF MIGRAINE-ASSOCIATED VERTIGO

Treatment of MAV involves a bit of detective work, but also incorporates both abortive and prophylactic therapies. First the patient should keep a log of symptoms. Patients whose symptoms are infrequent and

TABLE 11.1
Most Common Prophylactic Medications for Migraine-Associated Vertigo

Group	Medication	Initial Dose		Target Dose
Antidepressant	Venlafaxine	1/3 of a capsule of 37.5 XL QAM, increased by another 1/3 every week		37.5–75 XL
Anticonvulsant	Topiramate	25 mg HS, increase by 25 mg every week		50–100 mg QHS
	Sodium valproate	250 HS, increase to 500 HS after 1 week		500–1000 mg daily
β-Blocker	Propranolol LA	60 mg QHS		60–120 mg QHS
Calcium channel blocker	Verapamil SR	120 mg HS		1 mg/lb

have consistent triggers are fortunate in that trigger avoidance may be the only treatment necessary. Even if a trigger cannot be altered (e.g., weather changes), its recognition can at least provide some predictability to symptoms. Some patients do much better when they avoid certain foods (such as monosodium glutamate or red wine), or large amounts of caffeine. Most patients are also pleased to be told that management starts with lifestyle modifications rather than medication. The diet is supplemented with magnesium as well (about 500 mg/day), which has a mild positive effect on migraine.[30] Although vitamins such as CoQ-10 and riboflavin are also reported to be helpful in migraine, in general, we have not found them to be especially useful in MAV.

If no triggers are found, or if trigger avoidance is not possible, then MAV can be treated pharmacologically. There are only a few published randomized trials of medications specifically for MAV; therefore, in clinical practice MAV is managed similarly to other migraines.[31] The choice of abortive versus prophylactic therapy depends on the frequency, duration, and severity of the episodes. In a patient whose episodes are rare, abortive therapy is often adequate. Prophylactic strategies are favored when attacks are very abrupt in onset (e.g., making driving dangerous), frequent (i.e., more than once per week), severe, or of very long duration. Patients using a prophylactic approach can still use abortive therapy for breakthrough symptoms.

The three main groups of prophylactic medications used are anticonvulsants, antihypertensives, and antidepressants (see Table 11.1). Agents from each group can be combined in refractory cases. It is critical to start with very low doses of any chosen medication, because the sensory hypersensitivity of migraine often also extends to medications.

Medication trials usually are performed over 4–6 weeks and are terminated by either significant side effects or attainment of the target dose for 1 month without symptom control.

In our practice we most commonly start with the antidepressant venlafaxine, followed by the anticonvulsant topiramate, and then β-blockers (e.g., propranolol). Numerous detailed reviews of migraine prophylactic strategies[32–35] and abortive strategies[36] are available. A practical algorithm for prevention is provided in Fig. 11.1, and relevant dosing is provided in Table 11.1.

It is absolutely necessary to know about and communicate with patients the usual side effects of these drugs. Tricyclic antidepressant medications (amitriptyline, nortriptyline) have very strong tendencies to increase the patient's weight, which is often going to be unacceptable to the typical woman of childbearing age experiencing migraine. Several of these medications (e.g., topiramate, sodium valproate) have high risk of birth defects when taken by pregnant women, and patients need to be informed about this as well. Medications that are best tolerated by cognitive workers such as teachers or fellow professionals are venlafaxine, verapamil, and sodium valproate. Both the β-blockers and verapamil are antihypertensives and may not be suitable for young women with blood pressures on the lower side of normal.

There has been considerable recent interest in the use of onabotulinumtoxinA injections for migraine. This therapy has been approved in the United States for treatment of chronic migraine headache. Although its overall efficacy is not impressive, its main clinical utility is in patients who have failed to respond to, or failed to tolerate, multiple oral therapies.[37] There are no published studies on the use of onabotulinumtoxinA for MAV. Our own clinical experience suggests

Migraine prevention

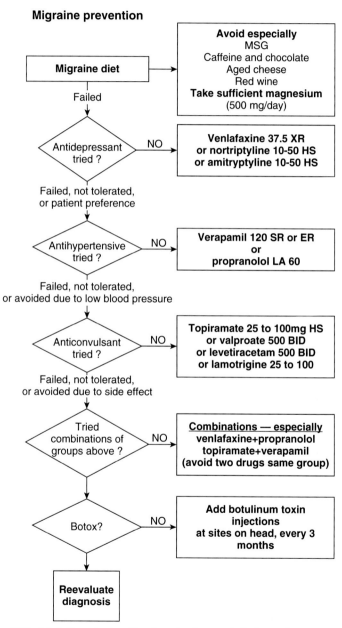

FIG. 11.1 Sample algorithm for migraine prophylaxis medications.

that in patients with chronic migraines who also have MAV and who are treated with onabotulinumtoxinA, only about 20%–30% of patients experience improvement in the vertiginous component of their symptoms. Given the otherwise refractory nature of these patients' symptoms, onabotulinumtoxinA probably deserves formal and systematic study as a treatment for MAV.

PROGNOSIS OF MIGRAINE-ASSOCIATED VERTIGO

The prognosis of MAV is probably similar to that of migraines in general, although no study has specifically explored this. In the general population, women can expect migraines to persist during their childbearing years but decrease in frequency and severity after menopause is complete.[1,21]

With respect to medical management, most patients with MAV are able to bring symptoms under a reasonable degree of control, meaning that the frequency will be significantly reduced, and breakthrough symptoms can be diminished with migraine abortive therapies.

REFERENCES

1. Stewart W, Shechter A, Rasmussen B. Migraine prevalence. A review of population based studies. *Neurology*. 1994;44(suppl 4):S17–S23.
2. Selby G, Lance JW. Observations on 500 cases of migraine and allied vascular headache. *J Neurol Neurosurg Psychiatry*. 1960;23:23–32.
3. Neuhauser H, Lempert T. Vestibular migraine. *Neurol Clin*. 2009;27(2):379–391.
4. Eggers SD. Migraine-related vertigo: diagnosis and treatment. *Curr Neurol Neurosci Rep*. 2006;6(2):106–115.
5. Aurora SK, Wilkinson F. The brain is hyperexcitable in migraine. *Cephalalgia*. 2007;27(12):1442–1453.
6. Burstein R, Yarnitsky D, Goor-Aryeh I, Ransil BJ, Bajwa ZH. An association between migraine and cutaneous allodynia. *Ann Neurol*. 2000;47(5):614–624.
7. Barabas G, Matthews WS, Ferrari M. Childhood migraine and motion sickness. *Pediatrics*. 1983;72(2):188–190.
8. Kayan A, Hood JD. Neuro-otological manifestations of migraine. *Brain*. 1984;107(Pt 4):1123–1142.
9. Leão AAP. Spreading depression of activity in the cerebral cortex. *J Neurophysiol*. 1944;7:359–390.
10. Leão AAP, Morison RS. Propagation of spreading cortical depression. *J Neurophysiol*. 1945;8:33–46.
11. Olesen J, Friberg L, Olsen TS, et al. Timing and topography of cerebral blood flow, aura, and headache during migraine attacks. *Ann Neurol*. 1990;28(6):791–798.
12. Welch KM. Concepts of migraine headache pathogenesis: insights into mechanisms of chronicity and new drug targets. *Neurol Sci*. 2003;24(suppl 2):S149–S153.
13. Ramadan NM. Targeting therapy for migraine: what to treat? *Neurology*. 2005;64(10 suppl 2):S4–S8.
14. Polensek SH, Tusa RJ. Nystagmus during attacks of vestibular migraine: an aid in diagnosis. *Audiol Neurootol*. 2010;15(4):241–246.
15. Neuhauser H, Leopold M, von Brevern M, Arnold G, Lempert T. The interrelations of migraine, vertigo, and migrainous vertigo. *Neurology*. 2001;56(4):436–441.
16. Waterston J. Chronic migrainous vertigo. *J Clin Neurosci*. 2004;11(4):384–388.
17. Cutrer FM, Baloh RW. Migraine-associated dizziness. *Headache*. 1992;32(6):300–304.
18. Battista RA. Audiometric findings of patients with migraine-associated dizziness. *Otol Neurotol*. 2004;25(6):987–992.
19. Dash AK, Panda N, Khandelwal G, Lal V, Mann SS. Migraine and audiovestibular dysfunction: is there a correlation? *Am J Otolaryngol*. 2008;29(5):295–299.
20. Lipton RB, Bigal ME, Diamond M, Freitag F, Reed ML, Stewart WF. Migraine prevalence, disease burden, and the need for preventive therapy. *Neurology*. 2007;68(5):343–349.
21. MacGregor EA. Migraine headache in perimenopausal and menopausal women. *Curr Pain Headache Rep*. 2009;13(5):399–403.
22. Uneri A. Migraine and benign paroxysmal positional vertigo: an outcome study of 476 patients. *Ear Nose Throat J*. 2004;83(12):814–815.
23. von Brevern M, Radtke A, Lezius F, et al. Epidemiology of benign paroxysmal positional vertigo: a population based study. *J Neurol Neurosurg Psychiatry*. 2007;78(7):710–715.
24. Radtke A, Lempert T, Gresty MA, Brookes GB, Bronstein AM, Neuhauser H. Migraine and Meniere's disease: is there a link? *Neurology*. 2002;59(11):1700–1704.
25. von Brevern M, Zeise D, Neuhauser H, Clarke AH, Lempert T. Acute migrainous vertigo: clinical and oculographic findings. *Brain*. 2005;128(Pt 2):365–374.
26. Celebisoy N, Gokcay F, Sirin H, Bicak N. Migrainous vertigo: clinical, oculographic and posturographic findings. *Cephalalgia*. 2008;28(1):72–77.
27. Hougaard A, Amin FM, Ashina M. Migraine and structural abnormalities in the brain. *Curr Opin Neurol*. 2014;27(3):309–314.
28. Murdin L, Davies RA, Bronstein AM. Vertigo as a migraine trigger. *Neurology*. 2009;73(8):638–642.
29. Fife TD, Baloh RW, Duckwiler GR. Isolated dizziness in vertebrobasilar insufficiency: clinical features, angiography, and follow-up. *J Stroke Cerebrovasc Dis*. 1994;4(1):4–12.
30. Holland S, Silberstein SD, Freitag F, Dodick DW, Argoff C, Ashman E. Evidence-based guideline update: NSAIDs and other complementary treatments for episodic migraine prevention in adults: report of the Quality Standards Subcommittee of the American Academy of Neurology and the American Headache Society. *Neurology*. 2012;78(17):1346–1353.

31. Obermann M, Strupp M. Current treatment options in vestibular migraine. *Front Neurol.* 2014;5:257.

32. Buchanan TM, Ramadan NM. Prophylactic pharmacotherapy for migraine headaches. *Semin Neurol.* 2006;26(2):188–198.

33. Ramadan NM. Prophylactic migraine therapy: mechanisms and evidence. *Curr Pain Headache Rep.* 2004;8(2):91–95.

34. Ramadan NM, Silberstein SD, Freitag FG, Gilbert TT, Frishberg BM. *Evidence-Based Guidelines for Migraine Headache in the Primary Care Setting: Pharmacological Management for Prevention of Migraine.* US Headache Consortium 2000.

35. Silberstein SD. Preventive migraine treatment. *Continuum (Minneap Minn).* 2015;21(4 Headache):973–989.

36. Silberstein SD. Practice parameter: evidence-based guidelines for migraine headache (an evidence-based review): report of the Quality Standards Subcommittee of the American Academy of Neurology. *Neurology.* 2000;55(6):754–762.

37. Aurora SK, Dodick DW, Turkel CC, et al. OnabotulinumtoxinA for treatment of chronic migraine: results from the double-blind, randomized, placebo-controlled phase of the PREEMPT 1 trial. *Cephalalgia.* 2010;30(7):793–803.

CHAPTER 12

Superior Semicircular Canal Dehiscence

GERARD J. GIANOLI, MD, FACS • JAMES S. SOILEAU, MD

INTRODUCTION

Superior semicircular canal dehiscence (SSCD) can be defined as an anatomic anomaly found (occasionally incidentally) on high-resolution temporal bone computed tomography (CT) scan or at surgical exploration (Fig. 12.1) or as a syndrome, a constellation of symptoms, that frequently accompanies this anatomic deviation. An anatomic dehiscence of bone overlying the superior semicircular canal (SSC) at its interface with the middle cranial fossa dura has been proposed to be a developmental abnormality.[1] Bone overlying the middle ear cavity and mastoid air cell system (tegmen tympani and tegmen mastoideum) separating the ear from the middle cranial fossa (a.k.a. the floor of the middle cranial fossa) thickens progressively during the first 3 years of life, such that CT findings of SSCD in a 1-year-old patient may "disappear" by the time the patient is 3 or 4 years old.[2] At this age, the incidence of an anatomic finding of SSCD is believed to be relatively stable, rendering 1%–2% of the general population at risk for developing SSCD syndrome.[3]

The calvarium initially thickens in early childhood, but then, later in life, the thickness of the calvarium and the area of the middle fossa floor in question, very slowly thins. This has also been proposed as a possible cause for development of SSCD in patients who had very thin bone covering the SSC earlier in life.[4] Additional factors that may make an individual susceptible to SSCD are erosive processes such as arachnoid granulations, cholesteatoma, other neoplastic processes, and trauma/fractures. More recently, the CDH23 gene (associated with Usher Syndrome and nonsyndromic hearing loss) has been found to be a genetic risk factor for the development of SSCD.[5]

SSCD has been called the great otologic mimicker because of the myriad of clinical presentations that are similar or identical to other major otologic disorders, such as patulous Eustachian tube, otosclerosis, Meniere's disease, benign paroxysmal positional vertigo (BPPV), perilymph fistula, sudden sensorineural hearing loss, and acute vestibular neuritis.[6] This variety of presentations gives rise to a disorder that can go undiagnosed or misdiagnosed for quite some time.

Consider the SSCD patient who presents initially with conductive hearing loss without vestibular symptoms and is diagnosed with otosclerosis. Unless the patient undergoes some investigation beyond basic audiometry, the patient can go for quite some time labeled as having "otosclerosis" before a different diagnosis is considered. Even after the patient develops vestibular symptoms, many clinicians may preserve the otosclerosis label while adding other diagnoses, such as BPPV or "otosclerosis with Meniere's disease." Clinicians must maintain a level of open-mindedness and not "pigeonhole" patients into a single diagnosis when dealing with patients with symptoms of SSCD.

To make the condition even more interesting, a patient with the absence of bone overlying the SSC may be completely asymptomatic. It has been recognized since the initial description of the problem in 1998 that a "second event" is suspected to be the root cause of the onset of the symptoms of SSCD. The leading suspected cause is head trauma or conditions that cause increased intracranial pressure. This is the presumed reason that SSCD symptoms are rarely seen in children.

INCIDENCE AND ETIOLOGY

The prevalence of SSCD has been found to be much higher in a series of analyzed CT scans than on temporal bone histology. Carey et al. identified a complete absence of bone over the superior canal histologically in 0.5% of 1000 vertically sectioned adult temporal bones.[3] There was an additional 1.4% with very thin (<0.1 mm) bone covering the SSC. Added together, the histologic prevalence of thin or dehiscent SSCs approached 2%. This study also reported that 50% of patients with SSCD had bilateral involvement. Carey and colleagues[3] also analyzed 36 infant temporal bones and concluded that the thickness of the bone overlying the superior canal was consistently thin. The thickness of the bone covering the SSC gradually increased with age, reaching adult thickness by 3 years of age.

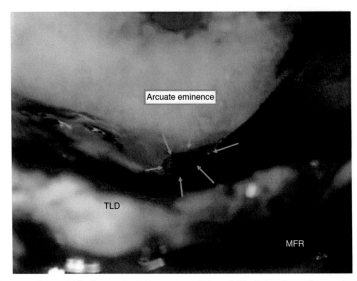

FIG. 12.1 Intraoperative, middle fossa craniotomy view of the middle fossa floor demonstrating superior semicircular canal dehiscence (SSCD) (*multiple arrows*). *MFR*, middle fossa retractor; *TLD*, temporal lobe dura.

Roberto et al.[7] used tetracycline staining to investigate the deposition of bone in a dog model at 10, 25, and 50 days of age. This study demonstrated progressive deposition of endochondral and endosteal bone over the SSC postnatally. The bone deposition decreased with age. These findings are in agreement with observations in the study by Carey et al.[3]

In a related study, Hirvonen and colleagues[8] reported a CT temporal bone study of bone thickness over the SSC in patients with SSCD and those without SSCD. Among those with SSCD, the contralateral SSC bone was thinner (or dehiscent), compared with those patients without SSCD. This finding of thin bone overlying the SSC bilaterally supports the notion of SSCD as a developmental anomaly related to bony deposition in early life.

Several observations point to SSCD as a developmental anomaly requiring a "second event" to produce symptoms:

1. Studies demonstrating development of bone over the SSC occurring later (postnatally) than other parts of the inner ear.
2. Clinical observations of asymptomatic but anatomic SSCD noted during intraoperative exploration of the middle cranial fossa for encephalocele repair.
3. Symptoms of SSCD rarely present in the pediatric population.

Thus, a second event may be required in addition to the congenital anomaly of thin or absent superior canal bone to produce clinical symptoms. Roughly half of patients with SSCD report an event they attribute to symptom onset. This "second event" is typically noted to be head trauma, a Valsalva-type episode, barotrauma, or some other type of intracranial pressure-altering event.

CLINICAL PRESENTATION

SSCD was first reported by Minor et al.[1] in eight patients who exhibited symptoms of short-lived episodic vertigo in response to certain sounds or activities that would cause transient increases in intracranial or middle ear pressure (e.g., Valsalva, coughing, sneezing, nose-blowing, auto-insufflation). These activities produce torsional nystagmus, which directly implicates SSC stimulation. Activities causing increased middle ear pressure (e.g., loud sound, positive pressure in the ear canal, autoinsufflation) induce nystagmus with the slow phase upward and the superior pole of the eye directed *away* from the affected ear. Activities causing transient elevation in intracranial pressure (e.g., Valsalva against a closed glottis, jugular venous compression) or negative pressure in the ear canal result in the slow phase of nystagmus directed downward and the superior pole of the eye directed *toward* the affected ear. The clinical findings of Tullio's phenomenon and pressure-induced nystagmus associated with SSCD has been termed "Minor's syndrome." Although the vertigo caused by SSCD is most characteristically reported as short-lived, other descriptions of vestibular symptoms have been reported as well, including more prolonged vertigo spells, chronic disequilibrium, and drop attacks.

Since the first identification of SSCD as a cause for Minor's syndrome, other symptoms and clinical presentations have been identified.[9]

Although the presentation of patients with SSCD is highly variable, the most recognizable presentation will include Tullio's phenomenon, pressure-induced vertigo with transient increases in intracranial or middle ear pressure, and autophony. While these symptoms are characteristic of SSCD, they are certainly not present in all SSCD patients, and their absence cannot be used as a means to exclude the diagnosis of SSCD. The more nonspecific symptoms of vestibulopathy such as head movement–induced disequilibrium is frequently described by patients but not particularly helpful in confirming the diagnosis of SSCD. Aural pressure and aural fullness are commonly reported, as are complaints of hearing loss, distorted hearing, pulsatile tinnitus, aural fullness, and hyperacute hearing.

There are also vague cognitive and neurobehavioral symptoms frequently reported by SSCD patients that are not specific to SSCD but should be included in the discussion during patient education. These symptoms include depression, "brain fog," short-term memory problems, and difficulty with concentration. These symptoms often improve after surgical repair of SSCD.[10]

Patients with SSCD may have been given other diagnoses prior to presentation. The biggest indicator of a misdiagnosis is nonresponse to treatment. This should always prompt the clinician to reassess the prior diagnosis.

PHYSICAL EXAMINATION

Routine head and neck examinations are typically normal in the SSCD patient. Microscopic otoscopy is normal as well, unless there has been prior surgical intervention. The vestibular component of the physical examination should include evaluation with infrared video goggles. This is typically unremarkable but may reveal spontaneous nystagmus and head thrust or head-shake abnormalities if there has been any vestibular loss. In some extreme cases, one can identify spontaneous torsional nystagmus that is synchronous with the pulse.

Tuning fork testing can also be helpful. Patients may "hear" the tuning fork in the affected (SSCD) ear when the tuning fork is placed on the ankle or some other remote bone location.

Pneumatic otoscopy can be an effective screening tool for SSCD. Symptoms of vertigo, or a feeling that the world shifts or moves, will often be reported during pneumatic otoscopy. Infrared video-oculography (VOG) cameras can be used to observe and/or record the resulting pressure-induced nystagmus. If VOG cameras are not available, a second examiner, an assistant or family member can also watch for pressure-induced nystagmus. The direction of pressure-induced nystagmus is dependent on the location of dehiscence and whether positive or negative pressure is applied.

TESTING

Much of the published literature on SSCD discusses CT imaging and vestibular evoked myogenic potential (VEMP), an electrical potential measured from the sternocleidomastoid muscle elicited by a sound stimulus to the ipsilateral ear. Relatively high-intensity sound stimulates the hair cells in the ampulla of the saccule, which in turn send afferent impulses along the inferior vestibular nerve to vestibular nuclei in the brainstem. The vestibular nuclei send efferent projections along the vestibulospinal (vestibulocollic) tract to the sternocleidomastoid muscle to facilitate head stabilization. Athough the CT scan is imperative (the "gold standard"), and VEMP testing is often helpful, we feel this limited testing is inadequate for patients presenting with symptoms of SSCD. Because SSCD is a disorder that can mimic many other otologic disorders, can cause a number of secondary pathologies, and may require invasive surgery to resolve, we feel a full audiovestibular test battery is warranted.

CT scan sections should be performed at the submillimeter level, preferably 0.24 mm thickness, but no thicker than 0.6 mm. The thinner section scan gives a more accurate portrayal of the defect. Thicker scans can be prone to both false-positive and false-negative findings.[11] Both coronal and Pöschl views will demonstrate the dehiscence, but the Pöschl view is a parasagittal view perpendicular to the petrous ridge/long axis of the temporal bone displaying the entirety of the SSC (Fig. 12.2). Because of this, Poschl views tend to only identify large dehiscences. Slices perpendicular to the SSC, such as coronal or Stenvers views, are more sensitive in detecting a dehiscence. MRI should be performed to evaluate for concomitant intracranial abnormalities. One of the more frequent findings in SSCD patients is Chiari

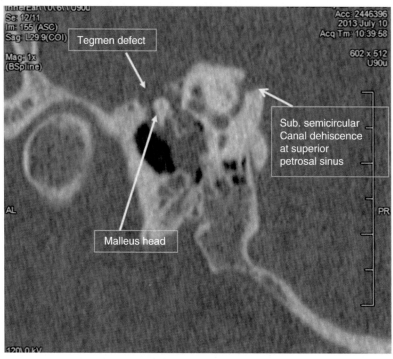

FIG. 12.2 Left temporal bone computed tomography (CT) scan in a Pöschl view demonstrating malleus impinged by overlying temporal lobe encephalocele with CSF leak and superior semicircular canal dehiscence (SSCD) at the superior petrosal sinus.

malformation.[12] Additionally, MRI findings suggestive of elevated intracranial pressure, such as empty sella, vertical tortuosity of the optic nerves, prominent arachnoid spaces around the optic nerves, flattening of the globe, slit-like ventricles, venous sinus abnormalities, and Chiari/cerebellar ectopia should also be sought.

Audiometric testing may be normal, may show some degree of sensorineural hearing loss in the affected ear, or more characteristically, may demonstrate low-frequency conductive loss, often with supranormal bone conduction thresholds. To distinguish the patient with low-frequency conductive loss who has SSCD from a patient with otosclerosis or a patient with other middle ear pathology, impedance testing is critical. The patient with SSCD typically has normal tympanograms and *intact* acoustic reflexes, whereas patients with otosclerosis will show *absent* acoustic reflexes.[13]

VEMP testing may show reduced threshold responses compared with laboratory norms or the contralateral ear. VEMP testing may show an asymmetric result in patients with unilateral SSCD or may be completely normal. Amplitude of the VEMP has not been found to be a reliable measure for SSCD. In patients with reduced vestibular function, the VEMP response may be absent.[6] Electrocochleography is frequently abnormal in SSCD patients and often normalizes after successful surgery to plug the dehiscent canal.[14]

A full vestibular evaluation should be performed on any patient who is to undergo SSCD surgery. Any identified vestibular abnormality is helpful in (1) the decision to proceed with surgery and (2) outcome expectations. Patients with SSCD have varied vestibular test profiles including severe unilateral vestibular hypofunction and occasionally severe bilateral vestibular hypofunction. Such patients will continue to experience symptoms from these vestibular deficits despite successful surgical treatment of their SSCD. Additionally, BPPV is a frequent secondary pathology that may need treatment in addition to treatment of SSCD.

Video head impulse testing (vHIT) has been introduced to clinical practice recently (see Chapter 8). However, because clinical experience with this testing methodology has not yet been widespread and has only been available for a limited time, we recommend caution when using this as a means to determine "normal" semicircular canal function. Recent studies have shown poor correlation of vHIT with caloric irrigation studies[15]; therefore, we cannot recommend using vHIT in place of caloric irrigation. However, in the context of SSCD, vHIT may prove to be invaluable in determining superior canal function preoperatively and postoperatively. In patients who have undergone SSCD occlusion, vHIT may be helpful in determining whether the posterior semicircular canal has actually been occluded and therefore hypofunctioning.

PATHOPHYSIOLOGY

The most commonly espoused theory for the pathophysiology of SSCD is the "third window" phenomenon. This theory posits that the flexible nature of the SSCD allows for possible egress of endolymph from the SSC resulting in abnormal stimulation of the cupula. Additionally, low-frequency sound energy transmitted through the inner ear is allowed to dissipate through this bony defect, resulting in the auditory conductive component noted in some SSCD patients. Merchant and Rosowski[16] proposed that SSCD could be classified among a number of anomalies that produce a third mobile window on the scala vestibuli side of the cochlea. Included among these are lateral or posterior canal dehiscence, enlarged vestibular aqueduct, dehiscence of the internal auditory canal, carotid dehiscence (into the cochlea), diffuse dehiscence (such as in Paget's disease), and other congenital abnormalities of the inner ear. The hearing loss in these patients with a pathologic third mobile window is characterized by poor air conduction thresholds and normal or supranormal bone conduction thresholds.

However, the third window theory does not completely explain all of the findings of SSCD. Among these are the existence of asymptomatic patients, the presentation of patients with only auditory and no vestibular findings or vice versa, Ménière's-type vertigo spells, and the absence of symptoms in pediatric patients who have definite dehiscence on imaging. It has been proposed that a second event such as trauma or a major pressure-altering event (Valsalva-type maneuver; barotrauma) causes a disruption of very thin bone over the superior canal, thus creating a symptomatic SSCD. However, this only explains adult onset of symptoms and not the other findings, nor does it explain a true dehiscence in an asymptomatic patient. Gianoli and Soileau[17] proposed the theory that alteration of intracranial pressure

may result in increased compliance at the round and oval windows and, if pressure changes were extreme, potential disruption of the windows resulting in a frank middle ear perilymph fistula. This theory could explain the above exceptions to the third mobile window theory and also explain why round window reinforcement has been noted to resolve SSCD symptoms (at least temporarily) in many patients. They further proposed a grading system for SSCD:

> Stage 1: Asymptomatic SSCD—anatomic dehiscence with no symptoms.
> Stage 2: Minor's syndrome—Tullio's phenomenon and Valsalva-induced vertigo, correlating with increased compliance of the cochlear windows.
> Stage 3: Meniere's syndrome—vertigo and hearing loss mimicking Meniere's disease, correlating with a frank oval or round window perilymph fistula.
> Stage 4: End stage—profound hearing loss and/or vestibular areflexia, as a result of repeated damage from stage 3.

It should be noted that BPPV is a frequent comorbidity at any of these stages.

OTHER DEHISCENCES

Among patients who present with symptoms and testing consistent with SSCD, there are some who do not have SSCD. These patients may be found to have dehiscence of labyrinthine bone in other areas. Among these are posterior semicircular canal dehiscence at the posterior fossa dura or at the jugular bulb, horizontal canal dehiscence (usually due to erosive processes such as cholesteatoma), cochlear dehiscence at the labyrinthine segment of the facial nerve, cochlear dehiscence at the carotid artery, and horizontal canal dehiscence near the second genu of the facial nerve. Each of these has minor variations from the typical presentation of SSCD, but the most common unifying symptom seems to be pressure-induced dizziness/vertigo from either internal or external sources. These dehiscences are more commonly found among SSCD patients and may be clinically identical in their presentation. Finally, patients may present with a syndrome identical to SSCD but have no radiographically visible dehiscence. The collection of patients presenting with this syndrome has been named "otic capsule dehiscence syndrome."[18]

Near Dehiscence

Many clinicians have noted patients with SSCD symptoms and no bony defect of the SSC or any other place in the labyrinthine bone. Some of these patients will have extreme thinning of SSC bone to the point where the bone itself is flexible enough to transmit pressure to the inner ear. These so-called near dehiscences share many features with definite SSCD but typically do not have reduced thresholds on VEMP testing. These patients also have a generally favorable outcome with SSCD surgery.[19]

TEGMEN DEHISCENCE AND OSSICULAR HEAD IMPINGEMENT

Among anomalies frequently seen with SSCD are multiple dehiscences of the tegmen tympani and tegmen mastoideum.[20] Usually these are of no significance unless there has been dural herniation through the dehiscence, resulting in an encephalocele and possible CSF leak (Fig. 12.2). An encephalocele with prolapse onto the ossicular heads in the epitympanum can cause a conductive hearing loss and autophony, which can accompany SSCD. Similarly, a large tegmen tympani dehiscence may allow impingement of the ossicular heads without a prolapsing encephalocele. If SSCD repair does not include repair of this type defect, symptoms of autophony and conductive hearing loss will persist.

TREATMENT: NONSURGICAL

Treatment options for SSCD have emphasized surgical intervention, but it must be kept in mind that there are considerations for nonsurgical treatment. In patients with no symptoms, surgery should be deferred. Some patients may have hearing loss as their only symptom. For these patients we advise against surgery. Surgery is most successful for patients with vestibular symptoms and for the symptom of autophony, but hearing is seldom improved with surgery. Restricted activity or vestibular rehabilitation can be very successful nonsurgical options for patients who have minimal symptoms. Lastly, for patients who have concomitant elevated intracranial pressure, measures directed at lowering CSF pressure can be immensely rewarding.

WINDOW REINFORCEMENT

Among the more minimally invasive procedures is window reinforcement surgery.[21] The technique varies among surgeons but is basically perilymph fistula repair surgery of the round window. We advocate reinforcement of both the round and the oval windows if this option is chosen. Outcomes for this procedure are initially quite good, but there is a fairly high recurrence

rate within 1 year after surgery. In general, the larger the dehiscence, the less likely this procedure seems to be adequate for long-term control of symptoms. This procedure, like the others, is most successful in controlling vestibular symptoms. It also seems to be relatively unsuccessful for alleviation of autophony. The main advantage of this approach is its minimally invasive nature and low risk for serious complications, while its main disadvantage is the low rate of long-term success. Although we still offer this minimal approach to patients, we are careful to counsel about the lower success rate. However, we will also typically include window reinforcement concomitantly with resurfacing or occlusion of the SSCD.

RESURFACING

In general, SSC resurfacing involves placing some material over the dehiscence to prevent transmission of pressure from the intracranial cavity to the inner ear.[9] Resurfacing techniques also vary quite significantly from surgeon to surgeon. Among the materials used for resurfacing are bone, bone chips, hydroxyapatite bone cement, silastic sheeting, cartilage, and glass ceramic implants. The goal of resurfacing is a rigid repair between the SSCD and the temporal lobe dura. Surgical outcomes for resurfacing are highly successful for controlling vestibular symptoms and autophony. Resurfacing to completely cover the dehiscent area is relatively easy with smaller dehiscences but more challenging with larger dehiscences that extend to the edge of the petrous ridge and into the posterior fossa. The biggest problem with resurfacing is inadequate coverage of the defect, which can be the result of slippage of the resurfacing material, incorrect placement, or inadequate curing of the hydroxyapatite cement. However, when successfully performed, this technique gives excellent results while preserving SSC patency and function.

OCCLUSION/PLUGGING

The concept of occlusion of the SSC stems from our collective experience with posterior semicircular canal occlusion for intractable BPPV. The goal is to occlude the SSC to prevent motion of the ampulla. By definition, the function of the SSC is removed. This is not significant for most patients, but in some situations the loss of SSC function can have significant untoward consequences. In particular, surgical occlusion of bilateral SSCD will result in bilateral loss of SSC function and can be problematic for some patients. Older patients, patients at risk for poor central compensation, and patients who have already lost significant vestibular function should be counseled carefully regarding plugging. Lastly, in very large defects, occlusion runs the risk of plugging the crus commune, which would effectively result in the loss of both superior and posterior semicircular canal function.

TRANSMASTOID VERSUS MIDDLE FOSSA VERSUS COMBINED APPROACH

The surgical approach for repair/resurfacing or occlusion of SSCD can be accomplished via middle fossa craniotomy, transmastoid approach, or combined middle fossa/transmastoid approach. The advantage of the middle fossa approach is the visibility of the defect. The middle fossa approach gives the best exposure of the SSCD defect, but the nature of SSCD anatomy is such that there can be multiple middle fossa defects. In some patients, tegmen defects can camouflage the SSCD. Because of this issue, some surgeons have advocated the use of navigational systems to ensure the correct defect is addressed. This point cannot be stressed enough because we have had occasion to do revision surgery on patients who had the wrong defect plugged or repaired with obvious consequences. Conversely, the middle fossa approach allows the repair of multiple tegmen defects, as long as the correct defect is also repaired! The other disadvantage of the middle fossa craniotomy is the need for a larger craniotomy defect and more extensive brain retraction than the other approaches with subsequent inpatient hospital admission.

The transmastoid approach has the advantage of minimal brain retraction, which converts the surgery into an outpatient procedure. The major disadvantage of the transmastoid approach is poor visibility of the defect. Although an experienced surgeon should have no trouble identifying the SSC in the mastoid, actual visualization of the dehiscence is usually difficult or impossible; therefore, the occlusion or repair is often done blindly, without actually seeing the defect. Fortunately, most of the time this is not necessary but may be problematic depending on the individual anatomy. Another disadvantage of the transmastoid approach relates to the "normal" anatomy of most SSCD patients. We find that most SSCD patients have a very low tegmen and, consequently, there is not much room for dissection superior to the level of the horizontal semicircular canal compared with non-SSCD patients, making dissection somewhat challenging in the area of the SSC.

The combined transmastoid/middle fossa craniotomy approach has the advantage of both approaches, and consequently, this is the one we advocate and utilize in the vast majority of surgery for SSCD. The combined approach allows for minimal brain retraction while allowing for excellent visibility of the defect and localization of the defect, obviating the need for a navigational system. The minimal brain retraction also allows this to be an outpatient procedure. The main disadvantage of the combined approach is the need for mastoid obliteration at the conclusion of the procedure to prevent future encephalocele formation.

OUTCOMES

Two large reviews comparing various surgical treatments for SSCD have been recently published.[22,23] The authors note no significant differences in outcomes for surgical treatment of SSCD, with the exception of window reinforcement surgery, with the difference attributed to limited patient numbers presented in the literature. It is noted in the reviews that individual surgical techniques vary quite considerably from one surgeon to another, that the number of reported surgeries is relatively low, and that there is little consistency between reports with regard to outcome measures, thus making the reviewers' job of comparison quite difficult. With that disclaimer, conclusions from these reviews are that surgical outcomes generally provide excellent improvement rates in vestibular symptoms and autophony. In our experience, resolution or significant improvement in vestibular symptoms occurs in over 95% of patients. Autophony is improved in more than 90% of patients. Hearing improvement is seldom seen; therefore, we do not advocate surgery if hearing loss is the sole symptom. Similarly, we do not advocate the surgery for the sole symptom of tinnitus. Tinnitus can improve, worsen, or remain unchanged postoperatively. However, one observation we have made is that tinnitus may continue to improve long after the 1-year postoperative period.

COMPLICATIONS

Complications reported following SSCD surgery include early failure with recurrence of symptoms, late failure, sensorineural hearing loss, vestibular loss, postoperative BPPV, tinnitus, infection, facial paralysis, and other complications seen with major ear surgery. Severe hearing loss is seen in approximately 4% of patients following surgical techniques directly addressing the SSCD (transmastoid and middle fossa approaches), whereas hearing loss following window reinforcement surgery does not seem to occur. There have been anecdotal reports of higher risk of hearing loss in revision surgery and patients who have undergone prior stapes surgery.

Early failure of repair/occlusion is fairly uncommon. Late failures have been reported, although it is too soon to estimate whether this is common. In our experience with over 400 SSCD surgeries since 1998, delayed failure for resurfacing is quite low and is probably in the range of 1% or so. Delayed failures seem to be somewhat more common with occlusion techniques. Some patients who have initially excellent results with occlusion procedures will have recurrence of SSCD symptoms, albeit milder than their preoperative symptoms. These patients do quite well with revision surgery. We have postulated that this may be secondary to retraction of the soft tissue plug, allowing movement in the SSC, a.k.a. "loose plug syndrome." This has led some surgeons who had advocated occlusion procedures to adopt an approach of occlusion and resurfacing concomitantly.

Other complications typically seen with major ear surgery are, of course, expected but do not seem to be any more common than other otologic procedures of similar complexity.

CONCLUSIONS

Diagnosis of SSCD requires symptoms consistent with the pathology, physiologic testing consistent with SSCD, and high-resolution CT confirming the presence of SSCD. Comprehensive evaluation should be performed to rule out concomitant pathologies or other plausible causes for the patient's symptoms. Choosing among the various treatment options for SSCD and individualizing the care for each patient can significantly improve the quality of these patients' lives. The range of treatment options includes nonsurgical strategies geared toward reducing pressure-altering episodes to the ear, or vestibular rehabilitation which may be the best options for those patients who are averse to surgery or patients for whom surgery/anesthesia represents greater risk. Minimally invasive approaches with window reinforcement procedures can be effective for patients whose main symptoms are vestibular in nature, albeit at a lower success rate and higher recurrence rate than more invasive surgical procedures. For those patients with the most severe vestibular symptoms and incapacitating autophony, more direct surgical alternatives are preferred: occlusion or resurfacing of the SSCD, through a transmastoid, middle fossa, or a combined approach. The ultimate goal of SSCD treatment is symptom alleviation/control; SSCD is not a dangerous condition; and each patient, in consultation with the specialist who presents the various treatment options, must decide how debilitating the symptoms are and whether the risks of treatment are outweighed by the benefit of alleviation of symptoms.

REFERENCES

1. Minor LB, Solomon D, Zinreich JS, Zee DS. Sound- and/or pressure-induced vertigo due to bone dehiscence of the superior semicircular canal. *Arch Otolaryngol Head Neck Surg*. 1998;124:249–258.
2. Meiklejohn DA, Corrales CE, Boldt BM, et al. Pediatric semicircular canal dehiscence: radiographic and histologic prevalence, with clinical correlation. *Otol Neurotol*. 2015;36(8):1383–1389.
3. Carey JP, Minor LB, Nager GT. Dehiscence or thinning of the bone overlying the superior semicircular canal in a temporal bone survey. *Arch Otolaryngol Head Neck Surg*. 2000;126(2):137–147.
4. Davey S, Kelly-Morland C, Phillips JS, Nunney I, Pawaroo D. Assessment of superior semicircular canal thickness with advancing age. *Laryngoscope*. 2015;125(8):1940–1945.
5. Noonan KY, Russo J, Shen J, et al. CDH23 related hearing loss: a new genetic risk factor for semicircular canal dehiscence? *Otol Neurotol*. 2016;37(10):1583–1588.
6. Zhou G, Gopen Q, Poe DS. Clinical and diagnostic characterization of canal dehiscence syndrome: a great otologic mimicker. *Otol Neurotol*. 2007;28(7):920–926.
7. Roberto M, Favia A, Lozupone E. Postnatal bone growth in the semicircular canals of the dog. *Ital J Anat Embryol*. 1998;103:27–34.
8. Hirvonen TP, Weg N, Zinreich SJ, Minor LB. High-resolution CT findings suggest a developmental abnormality underlying superior canal dehiscence syndrome. *Acta Otolaryngol*. 2003;123(4):477–481.
9. Smullen JL, Andrist EC, Gianoli GJ. Superior semicircular canal dehiscence: a new cause of vertigo. *J La State Med Soc*. 1999;151:397–400.
10. Wackym PA, Balaban CD, Mackay HT, et al. Longitudinal cognitive and neurobehavioral functional outcomes before and after repairing otic capsule dehiscence. *Otol Neurotol*. 2016;37(1):70–82.
11. Tavassolie TS, Penninger RT, Zuñiga MG, Minor LB, Carey JP. Multislice computed tomography in the diagnosis of superior canal dehiscence: how much error, and how to minimize it? *Otol Neurotol*. 2012;33(2):215–222.
12. Kuhn JJ, Clenney T. The association between semicircular canal dehiscence and Chiari type I malformation. *Arch Otolaryngol Head Neck Surg*. 2010;136(10):1009–1014.
13. Picavet V, Govaere E, Forton G. Superior semicircular canal dehiscence: prevalence in a population with clinical suspected otosclerosis-type hearing loss. *B-ENT*. 2009;5(2):83–88.
14. Arts HA, Adams ME, Telian SA, El-Kashlan H, Kileny PR. Reversible electrocochleographic abnormalities in superior canal dehiscence. *Otol Neurotol*. 2009;30(1):79–86.
15. Jung J, Suh MJ, Kim SH. Discrepancies between video head impulse and caloric test in patients with enlarged vestibular aqueduct. *Laryngoscope*. 2017;127(4):921–926.
16. Merchant SN, Rosowski JJ. Conductive hearing loss caused by third window lesions of the inner ear. *Otol Neurotol*. 2008;29:282–289.

17. Gianoli G. Superior semicircular canal dehiscence repair. In: Babu S, ed. *Practical Otology for the Otolaryngologist.* San Diego: Plural Publishing; 2013:287–296.

18. Wackym PA, Wood SJ, Siker DA, Carter DM. Otic capsule dehiscence syndrome: superior semicircular canal dehiscence syndrome with no radiographically visible dehiscence. *Ear Nose Throat J.* 2015;94(8):E8–E24.

19. Ward BK, Wenzel A, Ritzl EK, et al. Near-dehiscence: clinical findings in patients with thin bone over the superior semicircular canal. *Otol Neurotol.* 2013;34(8):1421–1428.

20. Gianoli GJ. Deficiency of the superior semicircular canal. *Curr Opin Otolaryngol Head Neck Surg.* 2001;9:336–341.

21. Silverstein H, Kartush JM, Parnes LS, et al. Round window reinforcement for superior semicircular canal dehiscence: a retrospective multi-center case series. *Am J Otolaryngol.* 2014;35(3):286–293.

22. Gioacchini F, Alicandri-Clufelli M, Kaleci S, Scarpa A, Cassandro E, Re M. Outcomes and complications in superior semicircular canal dehiscence surgery: a systematic review. *Laryngoscope.* 2016;126:1218–1224.

23. Ziylan F, Kinaci A, Beynon A, Kunst H. A comparison of surgical treatments for superior semicircular canal dehiscence: a systematic review. *Otol Neurotol.* 2017;38: 1–10.

CHAPTER 13

Meniere's Disease: A Challenging and Relentless Disorder

MAROUN T. SEMAAN, MD, FACS • SARAH E. MOWRY, MD, FACS •
NAUMAN MANZOOR, MD • CLIFF A. MEGERIAN, MD, FACS

Clinical Vignette

A.S. was a 34-year-old healthy female, without significant past medical history, who presented to the otology clinic 10 years ago for evaluation of a 3-day complaint of a "blocked" right ear: muffled hearing, aural fullness, and a low-pitched "oceanlike" sound. She denied vertigo or significant disequilibrium. She denied any recent viral illnesses. The otoscopic examination was normal. She had a similar episode 8 months earlier that spontaneously resolved. She denied a history of migraine, photophobia, phonophobia, or visual aura associated with her hearing changes. An audiogram performed 10 years ago during the first event is shown in Fig. 13.1A, which demonstrated right-sided low-frequency sensorineural hearing loss (SNHL) rising to normal with an excellent word discrimination score (WDS). Her tympanogram and stapedial reflexes (not shown) were normal. A follow-up audiogram, performed 3 weeks following the initial presentation (Fig. 13.1B), showed normal hearing thresholds bilaterally.

An audiogram performed during our next clinic visit (Fig. 13.1C) revealed moderate rising to mild low-frequency SNHL for the right ear with a WDS of 84%. The Stenger test was negative.

Additional testing was performed to aid in diagnosis. A gadolinium-enhanced magnetic resonance imaging (gadolinium-MRI) centered on the internal auditory canals was normal. Electrocochleography (ECoG) showed an elevated summating potential/action potential (SP/AP) ratio of 0.64/0.74 on the right side (Fig. 13.2), with the contralateral ear showing a normal ratio (<0.4—not shown). The presumed diagnosis was cochlear hydrops (CH). She completed a 10-day course of prednisone, and instructions were given for a low-salt diet. Her hearing returned to normal.

Six months later the patient developed a recurrence of her right-sided hearing loss, aural fullness, roaring right-sided tinnitus, and a vertigo spell that lasted approximately 3 hours and was associated with nausea and vomiting. She also described a sensation of falling backward. On examination, she had right-beating horizontal nystagmus with a slight torsional component, increasing in amplitude on right lateral gaze. The audiogram showed moderate rising to mild SNHL in the right ear (Fig. 13.1D), with a WDS of 76%. A vestibular-evoked myogenic potential (VEMP) showed an increased threshold on the right side (Fig. 13.3). She was treated with a course of steroids and started on hydrochlorothiazide and triamterene. The patient's symptoms were consistent with the diagnosis of right-sided probable Meniere's disease.

INTRODUCTION

Meniere's disease (MD) is characterized by episodic vertigo, fluctuating hearing loss, aural pressure, and tinnitus, usually in one ear. Since its description by Prosper Meniere in the Gazette médicale de Paris in 1861,[1] the pathophysiology and management of MD has been a controversial topic. Depending on the geographic location, the incidence of MD varies between 4.3 and 15.3 per 100,000.[2,3] Affected individuals are usually between the third and seventh decades of life with a female to male ratio of 1.3:1.

There have been several classification schemes to define MD.[4,5] Most recently, the Barany Society, in conjunction with numerous other international groups, including the American Academy of Otolaryngology–Head and Neck Surgery, proposed a simplified classification scheme (Table 13.1).[5] This scheme identifies two groups: definite and probable MD. Alternatively, staging systems have been proposed that are based on the residual hearing and residual vertigo after treatment (Tables 13.2 and 13.3).[4] These staging systems may be used to assess the degree of disability and help quantify treatment efficacy. Furthermore, the staging systems allow for uniform reporting of outcomes for various treatment modalities.

The diagnosis of MD, an idiopathic condition, is made after excluding other causes that may mimic the disorder. These conditions can be infectious (e.g., otosyphilis),[6] neurologic (e.g., migraine),[7] autoimmune (e.g., Cogan's syndrome, autoimmune inner ear disease),[8] and neoplastic (e.g., intralabyrinthine or vestibular schwannomas, endolymphatic sac [ELS] tumors)[9] (Table 13.4).[5]

In this chapter, we present a clinical vignette of a patient with MD who ultimately displays the full spectrum of the disease, and we discuss the clinical presentation, the diagnostic evaluation, and the different therapeutic modalities available to patients with this challenging disease.

TABLE 13.1
Definition of Meniere's Disease According to the 2015 Barany Society Consensus Statement

Definition	Symptoms
Definite Meniere's disease	• ≥2 definitive spontaneous episodes of vertigo each lasting 20 minutes to 12 hours • Audiometrically documented low to mid-frequency • Sensorineural hearing loss in one ear, defining the affected ear on at least one occasion before, during, or after one of the episodes of vertigo • Fluctuating aural symptoms in the affected ear (including hearing loss, tinnitus, and aural fullness) • Other causes excluded
Probable Meniere's disease	• One definitive episode of vertigo • Audiometrically documented hearing loss on at least one occasion • Tinnitus or aural fullness in the treated ear • Other causes excluded

TABLE 13.2
Staging of Meniere's Disease According to the 1995 Guidelines of the Committee on Hearing and Equilibrium of the American Academy of Otolaryngology and Head and Neck Surgery

Stage	Four-Tone Average (dB)
1	≤25
2	26–40
3	41–70
4	>70

TABLE 13.3
American Academy of Otolaryngology (AAO) Disability Class Associated With Meniere's Disease

Numerical Value	Class
0	A
1–40	B
41–80	C
81–120	D
>120	E
Secondary treatment initiated due to disability from vertigo	F

Reporting guidelines according to the 1995 guidelines of the Committee on Hearing and Equilibrium of the American Academy of Otolaryngology and Head & Neck Surgery. Numerical value = (X/Y) × 100. X is the average number of definitive spells per month for the 18–24 months after therapy and Y is the average number definitive spells per month for the 6 months before therapy.

TABLE 13.4
Differential Diagnosis of Meniere's Disease

Neoplastic	Vestibular schwannoma Endolymphatic sac tumor Meningioma
Genetic	Autosomal dominant sensorineural hearing loss type 9 (DFNA9) caused by *COCH* gene Autosomal dominant sensorineural hearing loss type 6/14 (DFNA6/14) caused by WSF1 gene
Autoimmune	Cogan's syndrome Autoimmune inner ear disease Susac's syndrome Vogt-Koyanagi-Harada syndrome
Infectious	Otosyphilis Neuroborreliosis
Neurologic	Vestibular migraine Cerebrovascular events/transient ischemic attack/stroke Vestibular paroxysmia (neurovascular compression syndrome)
Anatomic	Third window syndromes including superior canal dehiscence, enlarged vestibular aqueduct, perilymphatic fistula

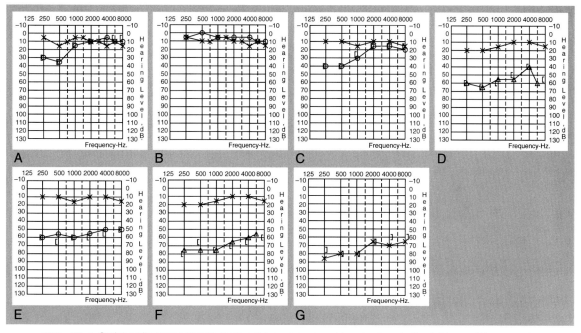

FIG. 13.1 Serial audiograms demonstrating the progression of hearing loss in the right ear of the example patient. **(A)** Initial audiogram showing normal left-sided hearing and mild low-frequency right-sided sensorineural hearing loss. The word discrimination score (WDS; not shown) was 100%. **(B)** Normal bilateral hearing. The WDS (not shown) was 100%. **(C)** Normal left-sided hearing and mild low-frequency right-sided sensorineural hearing loss. The WDS (not shown) was 84%. **(D)** Normal hearing thresholds on the left and moderate sensorineural hearing loss on the right side. The WDS (not shown) was 76%. **(E)** Normal hearing thresholds on the left and moderate sensorineural hearing loss on the right. The WDS (not shown) was 72%. **(F)** Normal hearing thresholds on the left and severe sensorineural hearing loss on the right. The WDS (not shown) was 24%. **(G)** Severe sensorineural hearing loss on the left. The WDS (not shown) was 36%.

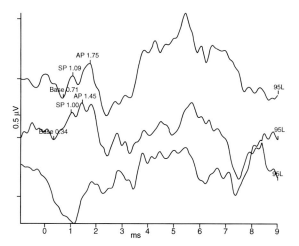

FIG. 13.2 Electrocochleography results in the affected ear. The summating potential/action potential (SP/AP) ratio was elevated (0.64/0.74).

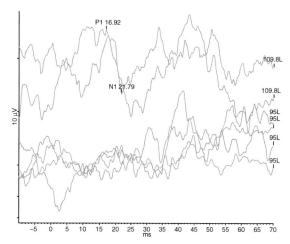

FIG. 13.3 Cervical vestibular-evoked myogenic potential (cVEMP) test. On the right, the cVEMP thresholds were elevated (109.8 dB) compared with the left side.

What Are the Diagnostic Criteria for Meniere's Disease?

The current consensus guidelines published in 2015 by the Barany Society after collaboration with an international group of experts identify two diagnostic categories for MD summarized as follows: definite and probable MD. The criteria for definite MD are "(1) two or more spontaneous episodes of vertigo each lasting 20 minutes to 12 hours; (2) audiometrically documented low- to medium-frequency SNHL in the affected ear on at least one occasion before, during, or after one of the episodes of vertigo; (3) fluctuating aural symptoms including hearing, tinnitus, or aural fullness in the affected ear; and (4) not better accounted for by another vestibular diagnosis."[5] According to these criteria, there may be nonsimultaneous onset of vertigo and hearing loss. In some patients, the hearing loss may precede the onset of vertigo by several months or years. Alternatively, episodic vertigo may precede the onset of hearing loss by weeks to months, although vestibular symptoms are usually accompanied by tinnitus and aural fullness. Some patients experience an increase in tinnitus intensity or aural fullness associated with the episodes of vertigo.

Probable MD is noted to include one or two episodes of vertigo or dizziness lasting 20 minutes to 24 hours. Patients can also experience fluctuating aural symptoms including hearing loss, tinnitus, and aural fullness in the affected ear. Patients with probable MD do not have documented low-frequency hearing loss or do not describe true vertigo symptoms.[5]

Differential Diagnosis of Meniere's Disease—Migraine and Meniere's Disease

The diagnosis of MD is one of exclusion. The practitioner must confirm that no other etiology is the likely cause of symptoms. Approximately 1% of the population suffers from vestibular migraine (see Chapter 11).[7] Early in the course of MD, before the patient manifests all symptoms of the disease, MD may be very difficult to be distinguished from vestibular migraine, as these disorders share many similar symptoms.[10] Although patients with vestibular migraine may have fluctuating hearing, tinnitus, and aural fullness with each episode, the hearing loss usually does not progress to the levels seen in MD. Furthermore, many migraine patients report that vestibular symptoms can last up to 72 hours, which is highly unusual in MD. Some patients may manifest symptoms consistent with both disorders. Diagnosis of migraine is more common in patients with a definitive diagnosis of MD.[11]

What Is the Role of Adjunctive Tests in the Diagnosis of Meniere's Disease?

A national survey showed that depending on the region (West, Midwest, Northeast, New England, and Atlantic coast), 26.9%–46.7% of treating otolaryngologists relied on history, physical examination, and audiometry only to establish the diagnosis of MD.[12] Others obtained adjunctive tests to support their diagnosis.

Electrophysiologic studies

In recent years, several diagnostic tests have been proposed to study the presence of endolymphatic hydrops (ELH) and complement the diagnosis of CH or MD. Two electrophysiologic tests merit mention: ECoG and cervical and ocular vestibular-evoked myogenic potentials (cVEMP and oVEMP).

ECoG is recorded in response to condensation and rarefaction click or tone-burst stimuli. The SP and AP of the eighth nerve are recorded via ear canal or transtympanic electrodes. An elevated SP/AP ratio (>0.4) and/or a widened AP width (>3 ms) are considered to be indicative of ELH. The alteration of SP and AP morphology in the hydropic ear is thought to result from a mechanical asymmetry in the basilar membrane (i.e., nonlinear basilar membrane vibration).[13] Reports in the literature regarding sensitivity and specificity of ECoG vary widely. Ge X et al.[14] reviewed 1549 patients with MD and found an elevated SP/AP ratio in 71.6%. They also showed that the sensitivity of ECoG increased with duration and severity of the disease. The sensitivity increases from 71% in stage 1 disease to 90% in stage 4 disease and from 43% in MD of less than 1 year duration to 100% when MD has been present for over 30 years. Others have reported combining the SP amplitude, SP area, SP/AP area ratio, and total SP/AP area to improve diagnostic accuracy.[15] Abnormal ECoG findings for MD will be present when the disease is active; if the disease is not active, ECoG results may be normal; therefore, a negative ECoG study does not rule out MD (false negative).

The cVEMP is a short latency (8 ms) inhibitory potential of the ipsilateral sternocleidomastoid muscle evoked by brief and loud (>85 dB) click or tone-burst stimuli. The cVEMP is thought to be a recording of vestibulocollic reflex activity generated in the saccule and carried via the inferior vestibular nerve. Results of cVEMP testing in patients with MD are somewhat contradictory. MD patients may have elevated or absent VEMP thresholds compared with controls.[16] These findings are more common in MD patients with Tumarkin's crisis[17] and are seen in 27% of the contralateral asymptomatic ears of affected individuals.[18] Other studies have shown no difference between MD patients and control patients with regard to either VEMP amplitude or threshold.[19,20] The sensitivity of cVEMP for a diagnosis of MD ranges from 50% to 63%.[20,21] However, the cVEMP peak to peak amplitude may be a useful measure to monitor the progression of MD, as this value decreases over time.[22]

The oVEMP reflex arc involves the contralateral orbicularis oculi and may be mediated partially by the utricle. oVEMPs are less frequently abnormal in patients with MD, particularly in early stages of the disease. Chen et al. found that only 16% of subjects had abnormal oVEMP responses, and the majority of these abnormalities were seen in patients with long-standing MD.[23]

We feel that both cVEMP and ECoG can be used to complement the clinical picture but should not be the sole basis for or against diagnosis.

Caloric testing and head thrust testing

The role of videonystagmography (VNG) in the diagnosis of MD is somewhat limited. Significant caloric weakness is present in 42%–73% of patients with MD.[24] Complete loss of function is seen in 6%–11%. Approximately 23%–29% of patients will have an abnormal angular vestibulo-ocular reflex on head thrust testing with gain asymmetry and phase lead being the most common findings.[24,25]

We feel that caloric testing is useful in the (1) assessment of contralateral function before an ablative procedure, (2) assessment of residual function after an ablative procedure, and (3) assessment of ipsilateral function—if residual function is good, we favor a nondestructive procedure.

Retrocochlear studies

When surveyed for workup of retrocochlear pathology, 57.7%–93.3% of otologists obtained retrocochlear studies.[12] One of the diagnostic criteria of MD is that other causes have been ruled out; therefore, we obtain a gadolinium-enhanced MRI of the internal auditory canals on all of our MD patients.

What Is Cochlear Hydrops? What Is Its Significance?

The term "cochlear hydrops" has been used to describe fluctuating hearing loss without associated vertigo. This may represent an earlier phase of a continuum ranging from mild cochlear involvement to full cochleovestibular dysfunction seen in MD.

House et al.[26] studied the relationship of CH and MD. In their retrospective review of 950 "hydropic"

ears, 71% were diagnosed with unilateral MD and 29% were labeled as unilateral CH. Bilateral MD (BMD) at presentation was seen in 11% with another 14% of unilateral MD becoming BMD. Of patients initially diagnosed as having unilateral CH, 33% developed MD over an average of 7.6 years of follow-up.

What Is the Pathophysiology of Cochlear Hydrops and Meniere's Disease?

Although ELH is felt to be the underlying histopathologic finding in MD, to date no histopathologic study has confirmed the presence of ELH in patients with CH. Despite the lack of direct evidence of this association, electrophysiologic studies demonstrating elevated SP/AP ratio suggest ELH.[27]

The pathophysiology of hydrops remains unknown. Several intrinsic (genetic, anatomical, autoimmune, or vascular)[28-32] and extrinsic (allergy, viral, neoplastic, or trauma)[33-35] causes can result in the disturbance of mechanisms involved in the regulation of endolymphatic fluid homeostasis.

Work to identify an underlying pathophysiology of ELH has identified several possible gene products for the disorder. Abnormal distribution of aquaporin 4 and 6, transmembrane water channels, may be the underlying cause of the ELH seen in MD patients.[36,37] Genetic polymorphisms have been identified in these genes in MD patients.[38] Other histochemical abnormalities noted in MD patients include abnormally thickened basement membranes and loss of the neuroepithelium in the saccule and semicircular canals. Whether this disturbance causes a predominant alteration in the longitudinal versus radial flow of the endolymph has been long debated.[39,40] On the other hand, it remains unclear whether the subsequent hydrops is the result of a cytochemical abnormality or an anatomical anomaly.

In fact, the relationship of ELH to the symptoms of MD has also been questioned, raising debate as to whether the observed ELH is the direct pathologic initiator of cochleovestibular dysfunction or "epiphenomena" of subtler biochemical perturbations. In a review of their temporal bone registry, Merchant et al.[41] found that all 28 patients with Meniere syndrome had evidence of ELH. However, of the 79 patients with ELH only 51 had Meniere's symptoms. Classic symptoms were absent in 9 of the 35 patients with "idiopathic hydrops" and in 42 of the 44 patients with "secondary hydrops."

In an effort to identify ELH with more certainty in vivo, Nakishima et al.[42] described visualization of ELH in MD patients using intratympanic gadolinium and delayed high-resolution (3T) MRI; however, intratympanic gadolinium administration is off-label; therefore an intravenous (IV) gadolinium protocol has been developed.[43] This MRI technique has subsequently shown higher rates of ELH in patients with MD compared with control patients, with sensitivity for diagnosis of 85%,[44] and has significant promise in diagnosing hydrops and confirming the diagnosis of MD.

During the following year, our patient had a total of five episodes of severe vertigo associated with aural fullness, fluctuating hearing, and tinnitus. Over the course of that year, she developed a progression of her hearing loss. The audiogram showed moderate low-frequency SNHL in the right ear, with a WDS of 72% (Fig. 13.1E). Three of the spells responded to a steroid taper and a regimen of antiemetics. Two episodes were treated with intratympanic injections of dexamethasone (IT-Dex) that gave temporary relief of vertigo. Her hearing remained unchanged, and she acquired a hearing aid for hearing assistance.

Nine months later, she developed a recurrence of vertigo spells occurring weekly. These spells did not respond to a combination of oral and intratympanic steroids. A Meniett (Norcross, GA) device was used without success. Her audiogram was unchanged, and she continued to use her hearing aid.

At that time, destructive and nondestructive options were discussed owing to the weekly vertigo spells. She underwent ELS decompression with placement of a shunt (endolymphatic sac surgery [ESS]). The sigmoid was noted to be farforward requiring decompression. The sac was hypoplastic and inferiorly displaced. This resulted in the complete resolution of her vertigo spells. Her hearing remained stable. Nevertheless, she continued to complain of moderate to severe roaring tinnitus and a constant sensation of aural fullness.

What Is the Role of Medical Management?

The medical management of MD includes a low-salt diet, avoidance of caffeine derivatives and alcohol, diuretics, vasodilators, and steroids.

Diuretics and low-sodium diet are effective in controlling the symptoms of MD in 71%–79% and is the preferred first-line therapy for patients with MD.[45,46] Initially described in the 1930s by Furstenburg et al., the low-sodium diet with diuretics (800–1000 mg/day and ammonium chloride) has evolved over time to a slightly more liberal sodium allowance (1500–2000 mg/day) and use of a potassium-sparing diuretic (hydrochlorothiazide with triamterene).[47,48] A Cochrane database review of all prospective randomized control trials (RCTs) between 1966 and 2005, comparing diuretics to placebo, failed to show a single trial of good enough quality to meet the standard criteria set for review.[49]

Another Cochrane database review of all RCTs comparing betahistine (a vasodilator) to placebo between 1966 and 1999 was completed. The analysis of six trials with 162 patients of good enough quality to meet the inclusion criteria failed to show any benefit of the betahistine.[50] A recently conducted RCT of betahistine versus placebo failed to find significant benefit of either a low or high dose of betahistine in terms of vertigo control when compared with placebo.[51]

Steroids, whether administered orally or intratympanically, have been used to treat acute exacerbations of MD.[52] In a series of 129 patients with unilateral MD, Boleas-Aguirre et al.[53] demonstrated that dexamethasone (12 mg/mL) administered intratympanically resulted in vertigo control in 91% of patients. Although more than half the patients responded to one or two injections, 21% required more than four injections. A meta-analysis by the Cochrane review identified significant improvement in vertigo episodes over a 24-month follow-up period with intratympanic dexamethasone (4 mg/mL) treated once daily for 5 days when compared with placebo.[54]

In a recent survey of general otolaryngologists and neurotologists, several differences in medical management were identified between the groups. Neurotologists were more likely to prescribe a low-salt diet and use intratympanic medications than their general otolaryngology counterparts, while both physician groups used diuretic therapy equally.[55]

What Is the Role of Vestibular Rehabilitation in the Acute Phase?

The role of vestibular rehabilitation in the acute phase of the disease has been questioned. Because of the fluctuating and dynamic nature of the vestibular symptoms seen in MD, most physicians feel that vestibular rehabilitation has limited benefits. Although the acute vertiginous spells are usually self-limited, chronic unsteadiness between the episodes of vertigo is a common complaint in patients with MD. Gottshall et al. showed that vestibular rehabilitation, even outside the acute care of patients with surgically ablated vestibular function, seems to improve the overall balance function in both patient-reported and objective measures (see Chapter 19).[56]

What Is the Initial Treatment if Medical Therapy Fails?

In a survey by Kim et al., 50% of otologists proceed with ESS, whereas 39% will perform an intratympanic injection of gentamicin (IT-Gent). The rest will offer a Meniett (9%) or a vestibular nerve section (VNS) (2%).[12] However, positive pressure therapy, such as the

Meniett device, has not been shown via meta-analysis to significantly impact vertigo spells.[57]

Controversies with endolymphatic sac surgery

A detailed review of this topic is beyond the scope of this chapter. The reader is referred to several more comprehensive reviews of the subject, including Sood et al. and Lim et al.[58,59] However, we will highlight some of the pertinent clinical studies.

Whether limited to sac decompression and/or placement of a shunt, the efficacy of sac surgery has been and continues to be debated. The decompression of a tight ELS, the alteration of the neovascularization in the perisaccular region, the passive diffusion of endolymph, the creation of an osmotic gradient, and the decreased production of endolymph have all been proposed as potential mechanisms of action.[39]

Is endolymphatic sac surgery better than natural history?

Many authors questioned the efficacy of this procedure when compared with natural history (NH). Others have questioned its long-term efficacy.

Quaranta et al. retrospectively evaluated 38 patients with intractable MD with a minimum of 7 years follow-up.[60] Twenty patients underwent ESS and eighteen were offered surgery but declined (NH group). In their sample, 85% of the patients in the ESS group and 74% of the NH patients had complete or substantial control of vertigo. The difference between the two groups was not significant initially; however, it was significant at 2 and 4 years follow-up. At 2 years, 65% of ESS patients had complete or substantial control of vertigo, and at 4 and 6 years 85% of patients reported satisfactory relief. Only 32% of the NH patients had complete or substantial control of vertigo at 2 years. This percentage rose to 50% at 4 years and to 74% at 6 years. Hearing results between the two groups were not significantly different.

Silverstein et al.[46] performed a retrospective study comparing patients who were offered surgery but declined (N = 50) with those who underwent surgery (N = 83). Of the nonoperated group, 57% had complete control of vertigo at 2 years; 71% had complete control after an average of 8.3 years. In the surgical ESS group, 40% had complete control of vertigo after 2 years; 70% had complete control after an average of 8.7 years. Their results suggest that ESS does not alter the long-term natural course of vertigo control in MD.

On the other hand, Telischi et al. reviewed the long-term vertigo control in 234 patients who underwent ESS followed for at least 10 years (mean, 13.5 years).[61] Among these 234 patients, 63% did not undergo any

further surgery to control vertigo, and an additional 17% required only revisions of the ELS shunt. Thus, 80% never required a destructive procedure. Of the 147 patients with only the original ESS, 93% reported no dizziness or mild to no disability. Of the group who underwent only revisions of the original shunt, 96% stated that they had no more dizziness or mild to no disability. In addition, Wick et al. described a cohort of ESS patients who received steroids intraoperatively using two different delivery methods: intratympanic only and intratympanic plus intra-ELS perfusion. Of the patients who had intratympanic steroids before postauricular incision, 83% achieved class A/B vertigo control with a mean follow-up of 95 months. Among the patients in the group who received intratympanic steroids plus intra-ELS steroid perfusion, 93% achieved class A/B vertigo control with a mean follow-up of 41 months. In contrast, 66% of patients in a control group who had shunting alone (i.e., no steroids) achieved class A and B control.[62] Kato et al., using a disease-specific quality of life questionnaire, found that quality of life was improved in 87% of 159 patients with MD who underwent ESS.[63]

Is endolymphatic sac decompression without shunt placement effective?

In a review of 94 patients with definite MD who underwent an ELS-mastoid shunt (54 patients) and ELS decompression (40 patients), Brinson et al. showed a class A or B vertigo control in 67% of the endolymphatic mastoid-shunt group and in 66% of the ELS decompression at 18–24 months follow-up.[64] In a histologic study, Chung et al. demonstrated that some patients (53%) obtained relief from vertigo after putative ESS without either having the sac exposed or having a shunt placed within the lumen.[65]

Regardless of the nuances in analyzing the outcome of ESS, the operation remains a commonly performed, nondestructive procedure.

After 2 years, our patient had a recurrence of her vertigo spells associated with a frequent sensation of disequilibrium. The disequilibrium is described as a sensation of being off-balance and unsteady, which seems to be exacerbated by sudden quick motions. This was accompanied by a constant foggy sensation in her head.

She felt quite disabled by her recurrent symptoms and decided to quit her job and stopped driving. A repeat audiogram was unchanged (Fig. 13.1E). A VNG showed reduced caloric vestibular response of 81% for the right ear and findings consistent with right peripheral vestibular hypofunction (Fig. 13.4). She was counseled regarding chemical or surgical labyrinthectomy versus VNS. Because she felt that her

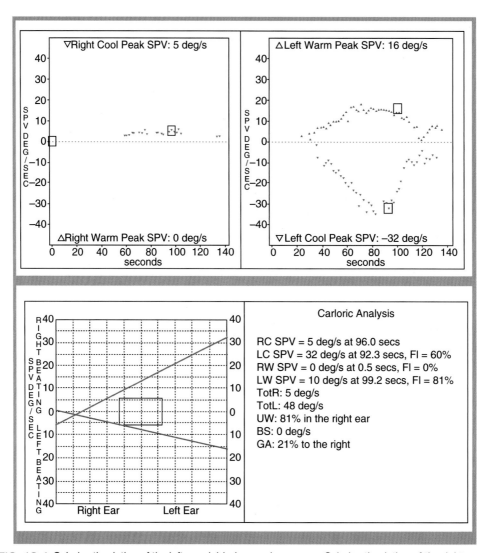

FIG. 13.4 Caloric stimulation of the left ear yielded a good response. Caloric stimulation of the right ear yielded a poor response (slow-phase eye velocity of 5 degrees/s with cold water stimulation and 0 degrees/s with warm water stimulation). The reduced vestibular response was calculated at 81%.

hearing was serviceable, she elected to have a retrosigmoid selective VNS. Her hearing was preserved and she was able to continue using her hearing aid. Even though the overall frequency of vertigo spells improved, she continued to have attacks 12 months after surgery. She noted that her episodes had changed in character, and she described what seemed like an impending sensation of falling backward; she has had two episodes of Tumarkin's crisis. A repeat VNG showed no response to standard caloric stimulation for the right ear. Ice caloric testing showed a residual response on the right side (Fig. 13.5). Her hearing deteriorated to severe SNHL (Fig. 13.1F), and the WDS dropped to 24%. A VEMP showed absent responses (Fig. 13.6). She then elected to have IT-Gent using the titration method. This too failed to completely control her vertigo, and she then had a transmastoid labyrinthectomy (TML) that resulted in the resolution of the vertigo spells. She completed 4 months of vestibular rehabilitation.

What is the best next step in management if nondestructive procedures fail to control vertigo?

When nondestructive procedures or interventions fail to control vertigo, the treating otologist will need to

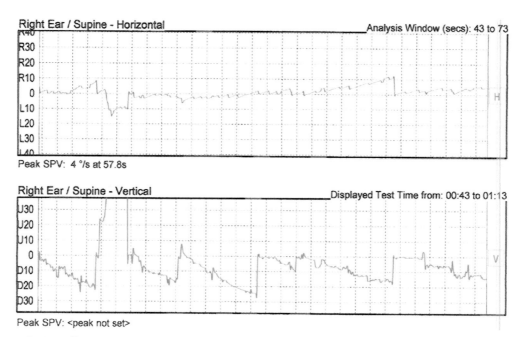

FIG. 13.5 Responses obtained with ice calorics in the right ear. The presence of low-velocity nystagmus suggests the presence of a few residual functional vestibular fibers on the side that underwent vestibular nerve section.

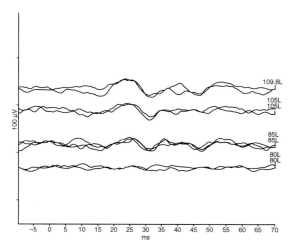

FIG. 13.6 Absent right-sided cervical vestibular-evoked myogenic potential responses indicative of severe saccular dysfunction.

resort to neural or labyrinthine destructive procedure to ablate residual vestibular function in an effort to control the ongoing vestibulopathy. These are grouped into chemical labyrinthectomy using IT-Gent, surgical labyrinthectomy (transcanal or transmastoid), and selective VNS.

Chemical labyrinthectomy. The use of chemical labyrinthectomy in the treatment of MD was introduced in the 1970s and popularized in the mid-1990s.[66,67] Gentamicin is a selective vestibulotoxic aminoglycoside antibiotic that causes apoptotic cell death of the vestibular dark cells resulting in partial or complete ablation of peripheral vestibular function.[68,69] Its cochleotoxic effects vary considerably, and hearing deterioration with this method ranges from 13% to 35% depending on the degree of vestibulopathy induced in a dose-dependent manner.[70]

The therapeutic effect of IT-Gent depends on host-dependent and host-independent factors. Host-dependent factors, such as round window permeability, diffusion along the scala tympani, and genetic susceptibility to aminoglycosides, affect the biologic response seen with IT-Gent perfusion. Furthermore, host-independent factors, such as dosage, method, and technique of administration, may influence the bioavailability and pharmacokinetics of gentamicin.

Advocates of vestibular ablation using IT-Gent cite the avoidance of surgery and general anesthesia, and the absence of surgical complications, such as meningitis, facial paralysis, and cerebrospinal fluid leak. Nevertheless, many physicians are reluctant to use IT-Gent in patients with serviceable hearing because of its unpredictable effect on hearing.

When hearing is poor, IT-Gent is a reasonable option that offers effective vertigo control with minimal morbidity. If failed, a TML can be offered.

A meta-analysis reviewed 27 published reports between 1978 and 2002 using five different administration methods: multiple daily dosages, weekly dosing technique, low-dose technique, continuous microcatheter delivery, and the titration method.[70] The titration technique (daily or weekly until the onset of nystagmus, hearing loss, or resolution of vertigo) resulted in the highest complete and effective vertigo control rate (81.7% with daily doses and 96.3% with weekly doses). The incidence of hearing loss ranged between 23.7% with the low-dose method and 34.7% with the multiple daily dosage method. The incidence of profound hearing loss was similar in all five methods and was 6%. When comparing the degree of vestibular ablation with complete vertigo control and incidence of hearing loss, the complete ablation of vestibular function resulted in 92.1% vertigo control and 36.7% incidence of hearing loss, whereas partial vestibular ablation resulted in 74.8% vertigo control and 24.8% incidence of hearing loss. Hence, although complete ablation was more effective in controlling vertigo, the incidence of hearing loss increased.

A recent meta-analysis of 14 prospective studies involving 599 patients including two RCTs further corroborates the success of vertigo control with IT-Gent. Successful (Class A/B) vertigo control can be achieved in 87.5% of patients. This study, however, showed no significant difference in vertigo control between fixed dose (87.5%) versus titration method (88.2%). In this review, 1.8% of patients experienced profound deafness. Mean changes in pure tone average (PTA) and WDS were not significantly different between the two methods, although greater tinnitus improvement was seen in the titration method.[71]

Comparison of vertigo outcomes across different treatment modalities has also been performed. Derebery et al. compared vertigo control rates for patients undergoing ESS versus a group of IT-Gent patients. In their series, 82% of patients in the ESS group had complete control of vertigo, whereas only 71% of their control group had such results. They concluded that ESS was better for vertigo control; however, the "control group" used in their comparison was a pooled sample taken from other literature sources.[72]

A recent double-blind randomized trial involving 60 patients assessed vertigo control between IT-steroids (methylprednisolone 62.5 mg/mL) and IT-Gent (40 mg/mL). There was a significant reduction in vertigo in both treatment arms (IT-steroids 90%; IT-Gent

87%) at 18–24 months posttreatment compared with 6 months before intervention. There was no significant difference in audiometric outcomes and functional levels between the two cohorts.[73] In contrast, another randomized trial assessing vertigo control between IT-Dex (4 mg/mL) and low-dose IT-Gent showed inferior 2-year vertigo control outcomes in the steroid group (Class A/B control of 61% vs. 93.5%).[74]

Thus, although there is evidence to support the use of IT-steroids and IT-gentamicin as a means for successful vertigo control in the majority of patients with MD, further large randomized trials are needed to study the long-term control compared with ablative therapies.

Vestibular nerve section and labyrinthectomy. Selective sectioning of the vestibular nerve can be performed via several approaches: translabyrinthine (TL) VNS, retrolabyrinthine (RL) VNS, retrosigmoid (RS) VNS, middle fossa (MF) VNS, and combined retrolabyrinthine-retrosigmoid (RR) VNS. A labyrinthectomy can be performed via the TML or transcanal labyrinthectomy (TCL) approach.

The TCL approach is typically performed under local anesthesia in medically frail individuals who cannot undergo a procedure under general anesthesia. However, care must be taken to sedate these patients enough during the procedure, as they will immediately develop severe vertigo and nausea after the saccule is punctured.

Rosenberg et al. demonstrated that vertigo control was achieved in 95%, 90%, and 92% of patients who had an RLVNS, RSVNS, and RRVNS, respectively. In the 47 patients who were studied, hearing levels improved in 34%, remained the same in 32%, and worsened in 34%.[75]

By reviewing their results in 143 patients who underwent a modified RLVNS (including a portion of the cochlear nerve to ablate the cochleovestibular fibers), Nguyen et al. showed that vertigo control (cured or better) was obtained in 92%, hearing remained unchanged or improved in two-thirds of patients, and the percentage of patients with severe disability dropped from 42% preoperatively to 7% following the RLVNS.[76] Of those patients who continued to have vertigo following VNS, some (9%) demonstrated evidence of residual ipsilateral vestibular function on postoperative testing (VNG, VEMP), and half of those went on to develop contralateral MD.[77]

What Influences the Surgeon's Decision in Selecting the Type of a Destructive Surgical Procedure?

A national survey of the preferred surgical approach showed that 77% of surgeons performed RSVNS, 14%

performed MFVNS, and 9% performed RLVNS.[12] When contemplating a nerve section, several factors should be considered in choosing the approach:

1. Position of the sigmoid sinus
   - Far-forward: RSVNS
   - Posterior or lateral: RLVNS
2. Status of residual hearing
   - PTA > 80 dB, WDS < 20%: TLVNS, TML, or TCL
3. Suspicion of cochleovestibular fibers
   - MFVNS
   - Retrosigmoid-internal auditory canal

Detailing the surgical technique is beyond the scope of this discussion, and the reader is encouraged to consult surgical otologic textbooks.

The most important factor in selecting the type of procedure is the status of the patient's residual hearing. If hearing is poor, a TML is offered. If hearing is serviceable, a selective VNS or chemical labyrinthectomy using IT-Gent is usually recommended.

Other factors may influence the type of approach. If the sigmoid is forward, an RS approach may provide better exposure. If a cleavage plane is not well visualized, the posterior lip of the internal auditory canal is typically drilled away. In patients with suspected active residual cochleovestibular fibers (Ort's cochleovestibular bundle of the inferior vestibular nerve) or vestibulofacial fibers (Rasmussen cochleofacial bundle of the superior vestibular nerve), a more laterally placed exposure of the fundus of the internal auditory canal via an MF approach can provide better surgical exposure.[78,79] These fibers leave the vestibular nerve shortly after the main trunk exits the lamina cribrosa. Failure to section these bridging fibers may result in residual vestibular function and symptoms after a vestibular nerve section (RL, RS, and RRVNS).

Vestibular nerve section versus labyrinthectomy

Teufert et al. reviewed the House Ear Clinic experience with 25 patients undergoing TML and 17 patients undergoing TLVNS.[80] In their series, 64% of TML patients and 64.7% of TLVNS had MD. Class A and B vertigo control was achieved in 86% of the TML group and 88% of the TLVNS group. Despite the comparable vertigo control, the resolution of the chronic imbalance and disequilibrium was seen in 82% of the TLVNS and 52% of the TML group, a significant difference. TLVNS was thus recommended.

Diaz et al., using a disease-specific outcome questionnaire in 44 patients with MD who underwent TML, showed that 98% of their patients reported an improvement in their overall quality of life.[81] The resultant hearing loss did not significantly affect their quality of life.

Vestibular nerve section versus intratympanic perfusion of gentamicin

Coletti et al. reviewed their results in 209 patients who underwent an RSVNS and 24 patients who received IT-Gent.[82] Gentamicin (80 mg/mL) was mixed with 8.4% buffer (26 mg per injection) and injected up to once per week for 6 weeks. Class A and B vertigo control was obtained in 95.8% and 75% of patients in the RSVNS and IT-Gent groups, respectively. In the IT-Gent group, hearing was significantly worse than in the RSVNS group. In the IT-Gent group, the average PTA decreased from 50.1 to 74.7 dB and the WDS changed from 87% to 65%.

Kaylie et al. compared their postsurgical vertigo control rate with IT-Gent.[83] Class A and B vertigo control at 18 and 24 months was obtained in 100%, 82.8%, and 72.3% of patients who underwent a TML, VNS, and ESS, respectively. Compared with IT-Gent, TML offered better vertigo control, VNS was comparable, and ESS was less effective. Postoperative PTA and WDS worsened (PTA > 15 dB and WDS worsened by > 20%) in 11% of their patients who underwent ESS or VNS. They felt that these results were slightly better than the hearing preservation rate following IT-Gent.

Two years following the TML, A.S. began complaining of a sensation of aural fullness, increasing subjective tinnitus, and decreased subjective hearing in the contralateral ear. An audiogram showed moderate SNHL. The WDS was 76%. A repeat MRI was normal. ECoG showed an elevated SP/AP ratio. An infectious and autoimmune workup was negative. She was diagnosed with BMD. Her vertigo spells resolved following a course of oral prednisone and IT-Dex; however, her hearing remained unchanged. She was fit with a hearing aid in the left ear. Approximately 4 months later, she had further decline in her left-sided hearing and an increase in subjective tinnitus on the left. An audiogram showed severe left-sided SNHL (Fig. 13.1G), with a WDS of 36%. Another course of steroids failed to improve her hearing. She continued to use a hearing aid on that side with some auditory benefit for sound awareness. After 4 months, she completed a cochlear implant evaluation and was deemed to be an appropriate candidate audiologically. She then received a cochlear implant in the side that had had the labyrinthectomy. On the other hand, she continued to be troubled by frequent vertigo spells and was offered an ELS decompression only without shunting on the left side. She underwent the ESS but unfortunately continued to complain of biweekly vertigo and constant disequilibrium. A VNG showed absent caloric responses in the labyrinthectomized side and markedly reduced vestibular responses on the nonlabyrinthectomized side. Rotary chair testing showed bilateral vestibular hypofunction with abnormally low vestibulo-ocular reflex gain and significant asymmetry. She underwent 4 months of vestibular rehabilitation, which helped with the chronic disequilibrium and overall quality of life but did not significantly affect her vertigo spells. After several discussions, she was offered intramuscular streptomycin at 1 g IM BID. After a cumulative dose of 25 g her vertigo spells ceased. On her last follow-up, she described rare episodes of oscillopsia and was free of vertigo spells.

What Are the Challenges in the Diagnosis and Treatment of Bilateral Meniere's Disease?

In this patient, the contralateral ear involvement was delayed in time and is consistent with BMD. The incidence in the literature of BMD ranges from 2% to 70%.[84] Although the incidence is likely lower than 70%, there is an increasing likelihood of contralateral ear involvement over time. Furthermore, there is a significant overlap with vestibular migraine and autoimmune disease in patients with bilateral symptoms. The Meniere's Disease Consortium recently provided a subgroup analysis of BMD patients. They found that the majority of patients have metachronous (43%) or simultaneous (17%) SNHL without migraine or a history of autoimmune disease. Several other BMD subgroups were identified, including a familial BMD pattern (13%), a comorbid migraine group (12%), and a group who also carried a diagnosis of rheumatoid arthritis (11%).[84]

Role of diagnostic tests

In patients who develop bilateral disease at a short interval, it is reasonable to consider entities that cause BMD-like symptoms.[5] These can be infectious (otosyphilis),[6,39] neoplastic (bilateral ELS tumors in a patient with von Hippel-Lindau disease),[85] or immune-mediated (Cogan's syndrome).[8]

Several years after the initial presentation, it is reasonable to repeat the MRI. In patients with BMD-like symptoms secondary to immune-mediated symptoms, gadolinium-MRI can evaluate for intralabyrinthine enhancement and is helpful in determining the stage of the inflammatory vestibulocochleitis. The initial enhancement seen at the acute labyrinthitis stage fades away during the subacute phase. The absence of fluid signal on T2-weighted images in the cochlea and labyrinth denotes a fibrous or sosseous obliteration of the cochlear lumen. Computed tomography scan assists in determining whether this is due to fibrous reaction or

neo-ossification. Cochlear obliteration can be seen in 50% of cases with autoimmune or immune-mediated inner ear diseases.[86]

Given the increased frequency of autoimmune disease in the BMD group, further serological studies for autoimmunity should be pursued. Antinuclear antibody screening with reflexive specific antibody titers should be obtained.

Migraine is common in this group also, and as such, symptoms for typical or atypical migraine should be sought. The International Headache Society has published extensive diagnostic criteria regarding the diagnosis and classification of the myriad headache syndromes, and the reader is directed to those publications for further reading (also see Chapter 11).[87]

Vertigo control in patients with bilateral Meniere's disease and failed medical therapy

The risk of deafness and oscillopsia following complete bilateral cochleovestibular ablation renders the management of BMD a challenging task. Although cochlear implantation provides acceptable hearing rehabilitation for deafened individuals, the quality of life is poor, and the degree of disability resulting from severe bilateral vestibular hypofunction is dreadful.

Most physicians agree that a destructive procedure is contraindicated in the management of the second ear in patients with bilateral disease. Nevertheless, some physicians may offer nondestructive procedures for the second ear in patients with BMD.

Shea et al. demonstrated good vertigo control in patients with BMD using intramuscular streptomycin. All 11 patients treated in this series had complete vertigo control. One patient developed oscillopsia, and hearing worsened in three patients after treatment.[88]

Hearing Rehabilitation in Meniere's Disease

For many patients, the hearing loss that accompanies MD has a significant negative impact on their quality of life, although it is not the most disabling symptom of the disorder. Consequently, patients should be offered options for auditory rehabilitation. The body of literature regarding treatment for single-sided deafness is significant. CROS/BiCROS and osseointegrated bone conduction devices have been used effectively for many years. However, as there is currently an interest in restoring ipsilateral auditory perception in single-sided deafness to improve the binaural hearing, we will focus on cochlear implantation in MD.

Recently there has been significant interest in cochlear implantation for MD patients, both for those with bilateral SNHL and those with single-sided deafness due to their MD. Numerous groups have demonstrated improved auditory performance following implantation.[89-92] Although the MD group of cochlear implant users receives benefit from the device, they do not perform as well as patients who are implanted for other causes of SNHL.[93] For those with intractable vertigo, TML is not a contraindication for cochlear implantation.[94] Using promontory stimulation testing in labyrinthectomized patients, investigators confirmed cochlear viability.[95] Thus, patients may have ablative surgery for vertigo but still receive a cochlear implant at a later date. MRI should be performed before cochlear implant surgery to confirm cochlear duct patency.[96,97] Several reports of cochlear implantation in a labyrinthectomized ear yielded good auditory performance.[98] Bilateral implantation may also be advisable for patients who are candidates.[99] Interestingly, patients undergoing cochlear implantation without vestibular ablation have reported variable hearing with their cochlear implant during episodes of vertigo.[93] Although the mechanism behind this has not been elucidated, it seems possible that the underlying pathophysiology affecting the membranous labyrinth may also affect neural function.

Management of Meniere's Disease in an Only Hearing Ear

MD in an only hearing ear is difficult to treat. A survey of 165 members of the American Neurotological Society showed that 99% of physicians recommended dietary modifications as a first-line therapy.[100] Only 39% of surveyed members offered oral corticosteroids as a first-line treatment, whereas 71% offered surgery for the only hearing ear when deemed appropriate. Patients may be somewhat comforted in the fact that cochlear implantation can restore some degree of hearing; nevertheless, the prospect of bilateral deafness is extremely upsetting to most patients. However, all efforts should be made to preserve native cochlear function as long as possible.

CONCLUSION

Diagnosis and treatment of MD continues to challenge many physicians. Current treatment strategies ranging from nondestructive, function-preserving interventions to destructive, function-ablative procedures are effective in controlling vertigo attacks. To date, no therapy has been shown to successfully prevent the progressive cochlear dysfunction seen in MD. Nevertheless, current hearing rehabilitative strategies using acoustic or electric auditory stimulation can help restore hearing to the affected ear. Unfortunately, many patients continue to be disabled by the severe tinnitus and chronic imbalance that accompanies progressive disease.

REFERENCES

1. Meniere P. Maladies de L'oreille interne offrant les symptomes de la congestion cerebrale apoplecaforme. *Gaz Med de Paris.* 1861;16:88.
2. Arenberg IK, Balkany TJ, Goldman G, Pilsbury 3rd RC. The incidence and prevalence of Meniere's disease – a statistical analysis of limits. *Otolaryngol Clin North Am.* 1980;13(4):597–601.
3. Stahle J, Stahle C, Arenberg IK. Incidence of Meniere's disease. *Arch Otolaryngol.* 1978;104(2):99–102.
4. Committe on Hearing and Equlibrium. Guidelines for the diagnosis and evaluation of therapy in Meniere's disease. *Otolaryngol Head Neck Surg.* 1995;113:181.
5. Lopez-Escamez JA, Carey JP, Chung WH, et al. Diagnostic criteria for Meniere's disease. *J Vestib Res.* 2015;25:1–7.
6. Pulec JL. Meniere's disease of syphilitic etiology. *Ear Nose Throat J.* 1997;76(8):508–510.
7. Lempert T, Olesen J, Furman J, et al. Vestibular migraine: diagnostic criteria. *J Vestib Res.* 2012;22:167–172.
8. Hughes GB, Barna BP, Kinney SE, Calabrese LH, Nalepa NJ. Clinical diagnosis of immune inner-ear disease. *Laryngoscope.* 1988;98(5):251–253.
9. Cmejrek RC, Megerian CA. Obstrucign lesions of the endolymphatic sac and duct mimicking Meniere's disease. *Ear Nose Throat J.* 2004;83(11):753–756.
10. Lui YF, Xu H. The intimate relationship between vestibular migraine and Meniere disease: a review of pathogenesis and presentation. *Behav Neurol.* 2016;2016. Epub ahead of print.
11. Cha YH, Brodsky J, Ishiyama G, Sabatti C, Baloh RW. The relevance of migraine in patients with Meniere's disease. *Acta Otolaryngol.* 2007;127(12):1241–1245.
12. Kim HH, Wiet RJ, Battista RA. Trends in the diagnosis and the managment of Meniere's disease: results of a survey. *Otolaryngol Head Neck Surg.* 2005;132(5):722–726.
13. Gatland DJ, Billings RJ, Youngs RP, Johnson NP. Investigation of the physiological basis of summating potential changes in endolymphatic hydrops. *Acta Otolaryngol.* 1988;105(3–4):218–222.
14. Ge X, Shea Jr JJ. Transtympanic electrocochleography: a 10-year experience. *Otol Neurotol.* 2002;23(5):799–805.
15. Al-Momani MO, Ferraro JA, Gajewski BJ, Ator G. Improved sensitivity of electrocochleography in the diagnosis of Meniere's disease. *Int J Audiol.* 2009;48(11):811–819.
16. Rauch SD, Zhou G, Kujawa SG, Guinan JJ, Hermann BS. Vestibular evoked myogenic potentials show altered tuning in patients with Meniere's disease. *Otol Neurotol.* 2004;25(3):333–338.

17. Timmer FC, Zhou G, Guinan JJ, Kujawa SG, Hermann BS, Rauch SD. Vestibular evoked myogenic potential (VEMP) in patients with Meniere's disease with drop attacks. *Laryngoscope*. 2006;116(5):776–779.

18. Lin MY, Timmer FC, Oriel BS, et al. Vestibular evoked myogenic potentials (VEMP) can detect asymptomatic saccular hydrops. *Laryngoscope*. 2006;116(6):987–992.

19. Johnson SA, O'Beirne GA, Lin E, Gourley J, Hornibrook J. oVEMPs and cVEMPs in patients with "clinically certain" Meniere's disease. *Acta Otolaryngol*. 2016;136(10):1029–1034.

20. Egami N, Ushio M, Yamasoba T, Yamaguchi T, Murofushi T, Iwasaki S. The diagnostic value of vestibular evoked myogenic potentials in patients with Meniere's disease. *J Vestib Res*. 2013;23(4–5):249–257.

21. Lamounier P, de Souza TS, Gobbo DA, Bahmad Jr F. Evaluation of vestibular evoked myogenic potentials (VEMP) and electrocochleography for the diagnosis of Meniere's disease. *Braz J Otorhinolaryngol*. 2017;83(4):394–403.

22. Van Tilberg MJ, Hermann BS, Guinan JJ, Rauch SD. Serial cVEMP testing is sensitive to disease progression in Meniere's patients. *Otol Neurotol*. 2016;37(10):1614–1619.

23. Chen L, Xu H, Wang WQ, Zhang QQ, Lv QY, Song XC. Evaluation of the otolith function using c/oVEMPs in patients with Meniere's disease. *J Otolaryngol Head Neck Surg*. 2016;45(1):39.

24. Park HJ, Migliaccio AA, Della Santina CC, Minor LB, Carey JP. Search-coil head-thrust and caloric tests in Meniere's disease. *Acta Otolaryngol*. 2005;125(8):852.

25. Palomar-Asenjo V, Boleas-Aguirre MS, Sanchez-Ferrandiz N, Perez Fernandez N. Caloric and rotatory chair test results in patients with Meniere's disease. *Otol Neurotol*. 2006;27(7):945–950.

26. House J, Doherty JK, Fisher LM, Derebery MJ, Berliner KI. Meniere's disease: prevalence of contralateral ear involvement. *Otol Neurotol*. 2006;27(3):355–361.

27. Dornhoffer JL. Diagnosis of cochlear Meniere's disease with electrocochleography. *ORL J Otorhinolaryngol Relat Spec*. 1998;60(6):301–305.

28. Ikeda M, Sando I. Paravestibular canaliculus in Meniere's disease: a histopathological study. *Ann Otol Rhinol Laryngol Suppl*. 1985;118:11–16.

29. Masutani H, Nakai Y, Kato A. Microvascular disorder of the stria vascularis in endolymphatic hydrops. *Acta Otolaryngol Suppl*. 1995;519:74–77.

30. Paparella MM. The cause (multifactorial inheritance) and pathogenesis (endolymphatic malabsorption) of Meniere's disease and its symptoms (mechanical and chemical). *Acta Otolaryngol*. 1985;99(3–4):445–451.

31. Xenellis J, Morrison AW, McClowskey D, Festenstein H. HLA antigens in the pathogenesis of Meniere's disease. *J Laryngol Otol*. 1986;100(1):21–24.

32. Yoo TJ, Yazawa Y, Tomoka K, Floyd R. Type II collagen-induced autoimmune endolymphatic hydrops in guinea pigs. *Science*. 1983;222(4619):65–67.

33. Clark SK, Rees TS. Posttraumatic endolymphatic hydrops. *Arch Otolaryngol*. 1977;103(12):725–726.

34. Derebery M. Allergic and immunologic aspects of Meniere's disease. *Otolaryngol Head Neck Surg*. 1996;114(3):360–365.

35. Shea JJ, Ge X, Orchik DJ. Traumatic endolymphatic hydrops. *Am J Otol*. 1995;16(2):235–240.

36. Agre P, Kozono D. Aquaporin water channels: molecular mechanisms for human disease. *FEBS Lett*. 2003;555:72–78.

37. McCall AA, Ishiyama G, Lopez IA, Bhuta S, Vetter S, Ishiyama A. Histopathological and ultrastructural analysis of vestibular endorgans in Meniere's disease reveals basement membrane pathology. *BMC Ear Nose Throat Disord*. 2009;9:4.

38. Lopes Kde C, Sartorato EL, da Silva-Costa SM, de Macedo Adamov NS, Gananca FF. Meniere's disease: molecular analysis of Aquaporins 2.3 and potassium channel KCNE1 genes in Brazilian patients. *Otol Neurotol*. 2016;37(8):1117–1121.

39. Paparella MM. Pathogenesis of Meniere's disease and Meniere's syndrome. *Acta Otolaryngol Suppl*. 1984;406:10–25.

40. Salt AN. Regulation of endolymphatic fluid volume. *Ann N Y Acad Sci*. 2001;942:306–312.

41. Merchant SN, Adams JC, Nadol Jr JB. Pathophysiology of Meniere's syndrome: are symptoms caused by endolymphatic hydrops? *Otol Neurotol*. 2005;26(1):74–81.

42. Nakashima T, Naganawa S, Sugiura M, et al. Visualization of endolymphatic hydrops in patients with Meniere's disease. *Laryngoscope*. 2007;117(3):415–420.

43. Naganawa S, Yamakazi M, Kawaii H, et al. MR imaging of Meniere's disease after combined intratympanic and intravenous injection of gadolinium using HYDROPS2. *Magn Reson Med Sci*. 2014;13(2):133–137.

44. Yoshida T, Sugimoto S, Teranishi M, et al. Imaging of the endolymphatic space in patients with Meniere's disease. *Auris Nasus Larynx*. 2017. Feb 27, Epub ahead of print.

45. Santos PM, Hall RA, Synder JM, Hughes LF, Dobie RA. Diuretic and diet effect on Meniere's disease evaluated by the 1985 Committee on Hearing and Equilibrium guidelines. *Otolaryngol Head Neck Surg*. 1993;109(4):680–689.

46. Silverstein H, Smouha E, Jones R. Natural history vs. surgery for Meniere's disease. *Otolaryngol Head Neck Surg*. 1989;100(1):6–16.

47. Furstenberg AC, Lashmet FH, Lathrop F. Meniere's symptom complex: medical treatment. *Ann Otol Rhinol Laryngol*. 1934;43:1035–1046.

48. Boles R, Rice DH, Hybels R, Work WP. Conservative management of Meniere's disease: Furstenberg regimen revisited. *Ann Otol Rhinol Laryngol*. 1975;84(4 pt 1):513–517.

49. Thirlwall AS, Kundu S. Diuretics for Meniere's disease or syndrome. *Cochrane Database Syst Rev*. 2006;3:CD003599.

50. James AL, Burton MJ. Betahistine for Meniere's disease or syndrome. *Cochrane Databse Syst Rev*. 2001:CD001873.

51. Adrion C, Fischer CS, Wagner J, et al. Efficacy and safety of betahistine treatment in patients with Meniere's disease: primary results of a long term, multicenter, double blind, randomized, placebo controlled, dose defining trial (BEMED trial). *BMJ.* 2016;352:h6816.

52. Lambert PR, Nguyen S, Maxwell KS, et al. A randomized, double-blind, placebo-controlled clinical study to assess safety and clinical activity of OTO-104 given as a single intratympanic injection in patients with unilateral Meniere's disease. *Otol Neurotol.* 2012;33(7):1257–1265.

53. Boleas-Aguirre MS, Lin FR, Della Santina CC, Minor LB, Carey JP. Longitudinal results with intratympanic dexamethasone in the treatment of Meniere's disease. *Otol Neurotol.* 2008;29(1):33–38.

54. Phillips JS, Westerberg B. Intratympanic steroids for Meniere's disease or syndrome. *Cochrane Database Syst Rev.* 2011;7:CD008514.

55. Clyde JW, Oberman BS, Isildak H. Current managment practices in Meniere's disease. *Otol Neurotol.* 2017;38. Epub ahead of print.

56. Gottshall KR, Hoffer ME, Moore RJ, Balough BJ. The role of vestibular rehabilitation in the treatment of Meniere's disease. *Otolaryngol Head Neck Surg.* 2005;133(3):326–328.

57. van Sonsbeek S, Pullens B, van Benthem PP. Positive pressure therapy for Meniere's disease or syndrome. *Cochrane Database Syst Rev.* 2015;10(3):CD008419.

58. Sood AJ, Lambert PR, Nguyen SA, Meyer TA. Endolymphatic sac surgery for Meniere's disease: a systematic review and meta-analysis. *Otol Neurotol.* 2014;35(6):1033–1045.

59. Lim MY, Zhang M, Yuen HW, Leong JL. Current evidence for endolymphatic sac surgery in the treatment of Meniere's disease: a systematic review. *Singapore Med J.* 2015;56(11):593–598.

60. Quaranta A, Marini F, Sallustio V. Long-term outcome of Meniere's disease: endolymphatic mastoid shunt versus natural history. *Audiol Neurootol.* 1998;3(1):54–60.

61. Telischi FF, Luxford WM. Long-term efficacy of endolymphatic sac surgery for vertigo in Meniere's disease. *Otolaryngol Head Neck Surg.* 1993;109(1):83–87.

62. Wick CC, Manzoor NF, McKenna C, Semaan MT, Megerian CA. Long-term outcomes of endolymphatic sac shunting with local steroids for Meniere's disease. *Am J Otolaryngol.* 2017;38. Epub ahead of print.

63. Kato BM, LaRouere MJ, Bojrab DI, Michaelides EM. Evaluating quality of life after endolymphatic sac surgery: the Meniere's disease outcomes questionnaire. *Otol Neurotol.* 2004;25(3):339–344.

64. Brinson GM, Chen DA, Arriaga MA. Endolymphatic mastoid shunt versus endolymphatic sac decompression for Meniere's disease. *Otolaryngol Head Neck Surg.* 2007;136(3):415–421.

65. Chung JW, Fayad J, Linthicum F, Ishiymama A, Merchant SN. Histopathology after endolymphatic sac surgery for Meniere's disease. *Otol Neurotol.* 2011;32(4):660–664.

66. Blakley BW. Clinical forum: a review of intratympanic therapy. *Am J Otol.* 1997;18(4):520–531.

67. Nedzelski JM, Chiong CM, Fradet G, Schessel DA, Bryce GE, Pflaiderer AG. Intratympanic gentamicin instillation as treatment of unilateral Meniere's disease: update of an ongoing study. *Am J Otol.* 1993;14(3):278–282.

68. Forge A, Li L. Apoptotic death of hair cells in mammalian vestibular sensory epithelia. *Hear Res.* 2000;139(1–2):97–115.

69. Nakagawa T, Yamane H, Shibata S, Nakai Y. Gentamicin ototoxicity induced apoptosis of the vestibular hair cells in guinea pigs. *Eur Arch Otorhinolaryngol.* 1997;254(1):9–14.

70. Chia SH, Gamst AC, Anderson JP, Harris JP. Intratympanic gentamicin therapy for Meniere's disease: a meta-analysis. *Otol Neurotol.* 2004;25(4):544–552.

71. Huon LK, Fang TY, Wang PC. Outcomes of intratympanic gentamicin injection to treat Meniere's disease. *Otol Neurotol.* 2012;5:706–714.

72. Derebery MJ, Fisher LM, Berliner KI, Chung J, Green K. *Otol Neurotol.* 2010;31(4):649–655.

73. Patel M, Agarwal K, Arshad Q, et al. Intratympanic methylprednisolone versus gentamicin in patients with unilateral Meniere's disease: a randomized, double-blind, comparative effectiveness trial. *Lancet.* 2016;10061:2753–2762.

74. Casani AP, Piaggi P, Cerchial N, Seccia V, Franceschini SS, Dallan I. Intratympanic treatment of intractable unilateral Meniere disease: gentamicin or dexamethasone? A randomized controlled trial. *Otolaryngol Head Neck Surg.* 2012;3:430–437.

75. Rosenberg SI, Silverstein H, Hoffer ME, Thaler E. Hearing results after posterior fossa vestibular neurectomy. *Otolaryngol Head Neck Surg.* 1996;114(1):32–37.

76. Nguyen CD, Brachmann DE, Crane RT, Linthicum Jr FH, Hitselberger WE. Retrolabyrinthine vestibular nerve section: evaluation of technical modification in 143 cases. *Am J Otol.* 1992;13(4):328–332.

77. Schlegel M, Vibert D, Ott SR, Hausler R, Caversaccio MD. Functional results and quality of life after retrosigmoid vestibular neurectomy in patients with Meniere's disease. *Otol Neurotol.* 2012;33(8):1380–1385.

78. Green JD, Shelton C, Brackmann DE. Middle fossa vestibular neurectomy in retrolabyrinthine neurectomy failures. *Arch Otolaryngol Head Neck Surg.* 1992;118(10):1058–1060.

79. Silverstein H, Jackson LE. Vestibular nerve section. *Otolaryngol Clin North Am.* 2002;35(3):655–673.

80. Teufert KB, Berliner KI, De la Cruz A. Persistent dizziness after surgical treatment of vertigo:an exploratory study of prognostic factors. *Otol Neurotol.* 2007;28(8):1056–1062.

81. Diaz RC, LaRouere MJ, Bojrab DI, Zappia JJ, Sargent EW, Shaia WT. Quality-of-life assessment of Meniere's disease patients after surgical labyrinthectomy. *Otol Neurotol.* 2007;28(1):74–86.

82. Colletti V, Carner M, Colletti L. Auditory results after vestibular nerve section and intratympanic gentamicin for Meniere's disease. *Otol Neurotol.* 2007;28(2):145–151.

83. Kaylie DM, Jackson GG, Gardner EK. Surgical management of Meniere's disease in the era of gentamicin. *Otolaryngol Head Neck Surg.* 2005;132(3):443–450.

84. Frejo L, Soto-Varela A, Santos-Perez S, et al. Clinical subgroups in bilateral Meniere disease. *Front Neurol.* 2016;7:182.

85. Megerian CA, Semaan MT. Evaluation and management of endolymphatic sac and duct tumors. *Otolaryngol Clin North Am.* 2007;40(3):463–478.

86. Aftab S, Semaan MT, Murray GS, Megerian CA. Cochlear implantation outcomes in patients with autoimmune and immune-mediated inner ear disease. *Otol Neurotol.* 2010;31(8):1337–1342.

87. Headache classification committee of the International Headache Society. The international classification of headache disorders, 3rd edition. *Cephalagia.* 2013;33(9):629–808.

88. Shea JJ, Ge X, Orchik DJ. Long-term results of low dose intramuscular streptomycin for Meniere's disease. *Am J Otol.* 1994;15(4):540–544.

89. McRackan TR, Gifford RH, Kahue CN, et al. Cochlear implantation in Meniere's disease patients. *Otol Neurotol.* 2014;3:421–425.

90. Hansen MR, Gantz BJ, Dunn D. Outcomes after cochlear implantation for patients with single-sided deafness, including those with recalcitrant Meniere's disease. *Otol Neurotol.* 2013;34(9):1681–1687.

91. Heywood RL, Atlas MD. Simultaneous cochlear implantation and labyrinthectomy for advanced Meniere's disease. *J Laryngol Otol.* 2016;130(2):204–206.

92. Lustig LR, Yeagle J, Niparko JK, Minor LB. Cochlear implantation in patients with bilateral Meniere's disease. *Otol Neurotol.* 2003;24(3):397–403.

93. Samy RN, Houston L, Scott M, Choo DL, Meinzen-Derr J. Cochlear implantation in patients with Meniere's disease. *Cochlear Implants Int.* 2015;16(4):208–212.

94. Doobe G, Ernst A, Ramalingam R, Mittmann P, Todt I. Simultaneous labyrinthectomy and cochlear implantation for patients with single-sided Meniere's disease and profound sensorineural hearing loss. *Biomed Res Int.* 2015;2015:457318.

95. Kartush JM, Linstrom CJ, Graham MD, Kulick KC, Bouchard KR. Promontory stimulation following labyrinthectomy: implications for cochlear implantation. *Laryngoscope.* 1990;100(1):5–9.

96. Sargent EW, Liao E, Gonda Jr RL. Cochlear patency after transmastoid labyrinthectomy for Meniere's syndrome. *Otol Neurotol.* 2016;37(7):937–939.

97. Charlett SD, Biggs N. The prevalence of cochlear obliteration after labyrinthectomy using magnetic resonance imaging and the implications for cochlear implantation. *Otol Neurotol.* 2015;36(8):1328–1330.

98. Zwolan TA, Shepard NT, Niparko JK. Labyrinthectomy with cochlear implantation. *Am J Otol.* 1993;14(3):220–223.

99. Holden LK, Neely G, Gotter BD, Mispagel KM, Firszt JB. Sequential bilateral cochlear implantation in a patient with bilateral Meniere's disease. *J Am Acad Audiol.* 2012;23(4):256–268.

100. Peterson WM, Issacson JE. Current managment of Meniere's disease in an only hearing ear. *Otol Neurotol.* 2007;28(5):696–699.

CHAPTER 14

Uncommon Causes of Disequilibrium in the Adult

MARCELLO CHERCHI, MD, PHD

UNCOMMON CAUSES OF CHRONIC DISEQUILIBRIUM IN THE ADULT

Bilateral Vestibular Loss

Epidemiology. Bilateral vestibular loss is uncommon.[1] In some patients the cause is known, whereas in other patients the condition seems to be idiopathic, and these patients tend to be older adults.

Pathophysiology. The percentage of patients with ideopathic bilateral vestibular loss varies from 21% to 51%.[2,3] In the remaining patients the most common cause is ototoxicity, accounting for 17%–66%,[2,4] with gentamicin being the most common ototoxin. Other causes include bilateral (usually sequential) vestibular neuritis and autoimmune inner ear disease. The underlying pathophysiology is either dysfunction of the peripheral vestibular receptors (as in gentamicin ototoxicity) or dysfunction of the vestibular nerve (as in vestibular neuritis).

Typical presentation. The common complaints are imbalance, disequilibrium, dizziness and oscillopsia ("jumpy vision" or the appearance that the world moves with each step or when riding in a car that goes over a bump). Patients will also be very dependent on their vision for maintaining balance; therefore, falls will often result when trying to walk in the dark, or when closing the eyes in the shower. Depending on the cause, the chronology of symptoms is variable. In idiopathic cases, the development of symptoms may be insidious. In gentamicin ototoxicity, the onset of symptoms usually occurs within several weeks of starting intravenous gentamicin and is unrelated to peak and trough levels. In addition, a mitochondrial genetic mutation on the MT-RNR1 gene confers particular susceptibility to aminoglycoside ototoxicity.[5]

Physical examination. Patients will be obviously unsteady on physical examination. They fail tandem Romberg stance with eyes closed. On dynamic visual acuity testing, they typically lose four or more lines when the head is oscillating in a sinusoidal pattern around the vertical axis compared with when the head is stationary. On fundoscopy, if the head is similarly oscillated, the retinae appear to move (rather than staying entirely steady).

Diagnostic testing. The gold standard test for bilateral vestibular loss is rotary chair testing, which shows the combination of low vestibulo-ocular reflex (VOR) gain and VOR phase lead (more so in the lower frequencies) during sinusoidal harmonic oscillation, and low VOR gain and short vestibular time constants on step velocity testing. Vestibular evoked myogenic potentials are absent. Caloric responses, including ice water calorics, are absent. Video head impulse testing shows low VOR gain bilaterally and overt saccades (if the bilateral loss is recent), or covert saccades (if the bilateral loss is more remote and is now compensated). Computerized dynamic posturography shows a "vestibular" pattern on sensory analysis, as well as an "ankle dominant" pattern (especially in conditions 5 and 6) on strategy analysis. Imaging of the brain and internal auditory canals is usually normal, although when the etiology involves vestibular neuritis, there may be enhancement of the vestibular nerve.

Treatment. Treatment is generally limited to physical therapy for vestibular rehabilitation and strategies for personal safety and fall prevention. These patients can improve but retain significant dependence on vision and proprioception for balance.

Progressive Supranuclear Palsy and Other Atypical Parkinsonisms

Parkinson's disease and the other parkinsonian disorders often involve disequilibrium at some point in the course of the disease. Idiopathic Parkinson's disease is by far the most common pathology in this family of diseases but will usually have come to the attention of a neurologist long before referral to a subspecialty clinic of balance disorders. The other diseases in this family include progressive supranuclear palsy (PSP; or the Steele-Richardson-Olszewski syndrome), multiple systems atrophy, corticobasal ganglionic degeneration, and dentatorubropallidoluysian atrophy. Of these, we have selected to focus on PSP because it often presents with disequilibrium early in the course of the disease and may elude diagnosis initially, or be initially misdiagnosed as idiopathic Parkinson's disease.

Epidemiology. The prevalence of PSP has been estimated variably at 1.39–6.4 per 100,000 and is more common in men. The age of onset is usually 40's to 60's.

Pathophysiology. PSP is a tauopathy, and histopathologic studies demonstrate accumulation of abnormal tau protein that is seen as globose neurofibrillary tangles in the prefrontal cortex, globus pallidus, substantia nigra, and subthalamic nucleus.

Typical presentation. By the time the diagnosis is made, symptoms have often been present for several years. Often the initial presentation will be a complaint of unsteadiness or falling, typically backward. Descending stairs sometimes poses a particular challenge. Patients have usually developed some degree of dysphagia by the time the diagnosis is confirmed. Patients with PSP frequently seem to be oblivious to their deficits and consequently exhibit poor judgment regarding their ability to ambulate and to negotiate stairways. As the disease advances, patients become progressively immobilized and are eventually confined to a wheelchair and then to a bed. The mean disease duration from the first onset of symptoms until death is 8.0 ± 4.1 years.[6] Patients usually die within about 5 years of being diagnosed,[7] with death typically resulting from the usual diseases affecting immobilized patients (e.g., aspiration, infections, thromboembolism).

Physical examination. There is usually axial hypertonia manifesting as truncal and neck stiffness (often with tonic hyperextension), although distracting maneuvers (such as having the patient open and close the hands) may be required to elicit this sign. The extremities usually have normal tone initially and lack the resting tremor of Parkinson's disease, although as the disease advances, symmetrical appendicular hypertonia may develop. Facies eventually become masked; although in contradistinction to Parkinson's disease, the tone of the periorbital musculature tends to produce the appearance of a "frightened stare." Oculomotor examination shows obvious slowing down of voluntary vertical saccades, although reflexive vertical saccades may initially be preserved. More subtle findings include convergence insufficiency and square wave jerks. Later in the disease, horizontal saccades are also affected. Cognitive evaluation reveals mild to moderate dementia with apathy and impaired executive function.

Diagnostic testing. Videonystagmography corroborates and quantifies the clinical oculomotor examination. Caloric testing is normal. Rotary chair testing sometimes exhibits "hang-up" of the eyes at the extremes of lateral gaze on optokinetic testing. Sometimes vestibular evoked myogenic potentials are reduced out of proportion to age. MRI sometimes demonstrates midbrain atrophy.

Treatment. Only symptomatic treatment is available. Sometimes a medication for idiopathic Parkinson's disease (such as levodopa-carbidopa) will bring about a modest, transient response that is never sustained.

Spinocerebellar Ataxias

Epidemiology. The spinocerebellar ataxias (SCAs) are rare and were originally referred to as autosomal dominant ataxias because of their mode of inheritance. They comprise a family of over 20 diseases whose number continues to grow as more forms are recognized.[8] Mutations for most of the SCAs involve trinucleotide repeat expansions, although some are point mutations.

Pathophysiology. Each of the SCAs produces different combinations of pathology in the cerebellum, pons, inferior olives, and spinal cord. The pathology in the cerebellum usually affects Purkinje cells, although SCA3 (Machado-Joseph disease) is an exception in this respect.

Typical presentation. Despite the distinct genetics of each of the SCAs, there is considerable overlap in the clinical presentations. The age of onset is in the 20s' to 40's, although SCA6 can present as late as the 60s. Most of the diseases involve gradually progressive ataxia.

Physical examination. Most SCAs exhibit a variety of cerebellar signs, such as dysmetria, dysdiadochokinesia, and dysarthria. Oculomotor signs include saccadic dysmetria (both hypometria and hypermetria), poor smooth pursuit, and spontaneous nystagmus. In some of the SCAs (types 1 and 7), saccades are slow; SCA2 in particular has markedly slow horizontal saccades. The "spinal" component of the "SCAs" often manifests as pyramidal tract signs, such as hyperreflexia and pathological reflexes (Babinski sign, Hoffman sign), although not all of the SCAs exhibit such findings.

Diagnostic testing. The various types of SCAs generally cannot be distinguished on clinical examination alone; genetic testing is available. Occasionally, one finds that a single patient has mutations of two or more SCAs. Imaging often demonstrates progressive cerebellar atrophy. There may also be atrophy of the pons, medulla, and cervical spinal cord.

Treatment. No treatment is available; personal safety and fall prevention are paramount.

Mal de Debarquement

Epidemiology. Mal de debarquement (MDD) is rare, although its incidence is unknown. 95% of patients are middle age females (mean 49.3 years).[9,10] Migraine is a frequent comorbidity.

Pathophysiology. The pathophysiology is unknown.

Typical presentation. Most cases of MDD seem to be triggered by exposure to motion that is quite prolonged, typically 4 h or more,[9] and consequently the history usually begins after a boat cruise or long train ride. The patient will usually say that the ride was uneventful in that it induced no motion sickness. Immediately after disembarking, the patient has the feeling of "still being on the boat" or train. While many normal people may have this sensation for several hours after such a ride, in patients with MDD the symptoms continue for 6 months to 10 years (mean 3.5 ± 2.5 years).[9] Patients will complain that they always feel as if they are in motion, typically with a rocking or swaying sensation, although a notable exception is that this sensation completely disappears when they ride in a car or other vehicle (including boats). This is an important clue, as virtually no other form of disequilibrium *improves* when the patient is subjected to additional vestibular stimulation. Occasionally, one sees patients who lack the initial prolonged exposure to motion; however, the history (including improvement with movement and response to benzodiazepines) is otherwise consistent with MDD. Such patients have migraine-associated vertigo as a differential diagnosis.

Physical examination. The physical examination is usually entirely normal.

Diagnostic testing. Diagnostic testing is normal. Occasionally, videonystagmography will show direction-changing positional nystagmus.[11]

Treatment. Because of the rarity of this disease, no systematic studies of its treatment have been conducted. Usually, patients have some response to benzodiazepines, such as clonazepam.[9,10] A recent study by Dai and colleagues[12] reports that a treatment protocol involving combined simultaneous visual stimuli and motion exposure may bring about "readaptation of the VOR" and thereby diminish the symptoms of MDD, although this finding needs to be replicated.[10]

UNCOMMON CAUSES OF EPISODIC DISEQUILIBRIUM IN THE ADULT

Psychogenic Disequilibrium

Epidemiology. Disequilibrium due exclusively to psychiatric factors is somewhat uncommon, although the epidemiology is difficult to assess because many patients with primary otologic and neurologic causes of disequilibrium may secondarily develop psychologic enhancement of that symptom. Cases of purely psychogenic disequilibrium usually involve anxiety and panic disorders.

Pathophysiology. The mechanism by which psychiatric pathology causes disequilibrium is unknown.

Typical presentation. Patients usually describe episodes of disequilibrium lasting several minutes, often accompanied by symptoms of nausea, shortness of breath, palpitations, and diaphoresis. They may or may not describe associated feelings of anxiety or panic.

Physical examination. The physical examination is normal.

Diagnostic testing. Purely psychogenic disequilibrium should be a diagnosis of exclusion. A screening otologic and neurologic workup should be undertaken to exclude nonpsychologic etiologies.

Treatment. Anxiolytics or antidepressants are reasonable to try.

Vestibular Paroxysmia

Epidemiology. Vestibular paroxysmia (VP) is uncommon, although its exact incidence is unknown.

Pathophysiology. VP is believed to result from episodic irritability of the vestibular nerve. Occasionally, this appears to be due to radiographically demonstrable microvascular compression (typically by the superior cerebellar artery or an aberrant loop of another small branch artery).[13,14] In some cases VP probably arises as a consequence of a lesion of the vestibular nerve by vestibular neuritis, or from a traction injury (as in head trauma). In the majority of cases the underlying pathophysiology is unknown.

Typical presentation. Usually, patients will experience a very disturbing first event consisting of extremely abrupt-onset disequilibrium (with no prodrome) that lasts a fraction of a second and then completely stops, with no residual symptoms. The disequilibrium itself may be perceived as a spin, as a "shove" in the lateral or anteroposterior axis, or as a drop. In some cases the disequilibrium lasts a few seconds, but rarely longer. The frequency of recurrence is variable; it can occur as frequently as multiple times per day, or as infrequently as only a few times per year. The episodes are dangerous insofar as they have no warning and are quite violent. Occasional cases present with episodic tinnitus that is simultaneous with the paroxysmal vestibular events.[15]

Physical examination. Usually physical examination is normal. On video oculography, there is sometimes a modest baseline nystagmus beating away from the lesion. In some cases, hyperventilation induces nystagmus (after a delay of 30–120 s) beating toward the lesion. This pattern is believed to be due to an increased rate of tonic firing of the lesioned vestibular nerve that in turn is triggered by the change in acid-base balance resulting from hyperventilation.[16]

Diagnostic testing. In some cases there is a reduced caloric response or reduced vestibular myogenic potential on the lesioned side. Sometimes microvascular compression can be demonstrated by good quality imaging (magnetic resonance imaging with and without contrast).

Treatment. Therapy with oxcarbazepine or other antiepileptic medications can reduce the frequency of the episodes. Some patients are fortunate enough to have the episodes completely stop after such therapy is initiated. For medically refractory cases in which microvascular compression can be confidently identified, surgical intervention is sometimes considered.[17]

Episodic Ataxia, Type 1

Epidemiology. Episodic ataxia type 1 (EA1) is rare. It is a dominantly inherited condition.

Pathophysiology. EA1 results from several different missense mutations on chromosome 12 affecting the gene that encodes the KCNA1 potassium channel.[18] This potassium channel is highly expressed in the cerebellum, and it is presumed that its episodic dysfunction is responsible for the clinical manifestations of the disease.

Typical presentation. Symptom onset may be during infancy, and symptoms typically resolve by young adulthood. Patients suffer from episodes of incoordination, abnormal movements, and slurred speech. Usually, the episodes occur spontaneously, but sometimes they appear to be triggered by a physiologic stressor or after being startled. The episodes typically last seconds to minutes, although their frequency is quite variable.

Physical examination. During episodes, patients exhibit appendicular cerebellar signs but do not usually have nystagmus. Between episodes, patients may exhibit myokymia in the hands and periorbital musculature.

Diagnostic testing. Genetic testing is available. Imaging is usually normal; specifically, there is no cerebellar atrophy.

Treatment. Patients sometimes have a modest response to acetazolamide. They may also respond to carbamazepine. For those patients whose episodes are reliably triggered by particular activities, avoidance of triggers is often adequate.

Episodic Ataxia, Type 2

Epidemiology. Episodic ataxia type 2 (EA2) is rare. It is a dominantly inherited condition. Half of patients with EA2 have migraines.

Pathophysiology. EA2 results from several different mutations on chromosome 19 affecting the gene that encodes the α1A subunit of the CACNA1A calcium channel.[18,19] This calcium channel is expressed in the cerebellar granular cells and Purkinje cells. A different mutation in this gene manifests as familial hemiplegic migraine.[20]

Typical presentation. Patients usually present in the teenage years with spontaneous episodes of truncal ataxia lasting for hours to days, often associated with vertigo, nausea, and vomiting.

Physical examination. During an episode, patients exhibit truncal ataxia and spontaneous nystagmus. Between episodes, patients may have gaze-evoked nystagmus and rebound nystagmus,[21] as well as impaired fixation suppression of the VOR.[22] Some patients also develop spontaneous downbeating nystagmus. As the disease progresses, patients begin to exhibit subtle cerebellar signs even between attacks, resulting in mild chronic ataxia.

Diagnostic testing. Genetic testing is available. Imaging may demonstrate atrophy of the cerebellar vermis.

Treatment. Patients often have a good response to acetazolamide. They may also respond to carbamazepine.

Vestibular Seizures

Epidemiology. Vestibular seizures (also referred to as epileptic vertigo) are rare. The exact incidence is unknown.

Pathophysiology. Vestibular seizures, by definition, involve abnormal electrical activity (seizure) affecting those parts of the cerebral cortex believed to mediate vestibular sensation (superoposterior temporal cortex and temporoparietal junction). The rarity of this phenomenon is due to the fact that seizure activity rarely remains restricted exclusively to the small area of vestibular cortex. Seizure activity will more commonly spread, and when it does, other sensory, motor, and cognitive symptoms will ensue, and the salience of these other symptoms tends to overshadow the vestibular symptoms.[23]

Typical presentation. Vestibular seizures typically start abruptly and last seconds to minutes.

Physical examination. The physical examination is normal.

Diagnostic testing. Electroencephalography may reveal abnormalities over the temporal or temporoparietal regions. Brain imaging should be performed to exclude focal anatomic lesions, such as tumors and cortical strokes.

Treatment. Antiepileptic medications are used for treatment.

Cervicogenic Vertigo

Epidemiology. Cervicogenic vertigo is uncommon but probably also underreported. This diagnosis is controversial. Clinicians are frequently confronted with patients who complain of neck symptoms and dizziness, and although a thorough workup usually reveals no abnormalities, logic suggests a relationship between neck pathology and imbalance. Cervicogenic vertigo is frequently suspected as a cause of imbalance in patients who have sustained a neck injury, but because such injuries frequently lead to medical-legal disputes (such as litigation regarding whiplash injury—see Chapter 7), symptom enhancement for secondary gain may cloud the picture, making this phenomenon difficult to study.

Pathophysiology. The pathophysiology of cervicogenic vertigo is poorly understood.[24,25] Although torquing of, or impingement on, a vertebral artery seems like an obvious mechanism, such impairment of circulation would typically result in a constellation of brainstem symptoms rather than simply isolated disequilibrium. Another proposed mechanism involves abnormalities of proprioception mediating head-on-body position, or other somatosensory inputs.[16]

Typical presentation. Often there is some inciting event, such as a neck injury, and patients are often in litigation with respect to that injury. After the inciting event, patients usually complain of disequilibrium that is episodic insofar as it is exacerbated by head-on-neck movements, although they may also complain of a component of milder chronic disequilibrium. They may describe the disequilibrium in different ways, typically using descriptors such as "floating," "drifting," or "rocking." In addition, patients usually have complaints such as neck pain, neck stiffness, or limited range of motion of the neck.

Physical examination. Physical examination may reveal tension of neck muscles. Rarely, video oculography will detect horizontal nystagmus when the head is maintained in a position rotated to one or the other side and the eyes are maintained in a neutral position (with respect to the orbits).

Diagnostic testing. Otologic, vestibular, and imaging studies are usually normal.

Treatment. Usually, physical therapy directed at the neck and vestibular rehabilitation are the only available therapies.

REFERENCES

1. Hain TC, Cherchi M, Yacovino DA. Bilateral vestibular loss. *Semin Neurol.* 2013;33(3):195–203.
2. Rinne T, Bronstein AM, Rudge P, Gresty MA, Luxon LM. Bilateral loss of vestibular function: clinical findings in 53 patients. *J Neurol.* 1998;245(6–7):314–321.
3. Zingler VC, Cnyrim C, Jahn K, et al. Causative factors and epidemiology of bilateral vestibulopathy in 255 patients. *Ann Neurol.* 2007;61(6):524–532.
4. Gillespie MB, Minor LB. Prognosis in bilateral vestibular hypofunction. *Laryngoscope.* 1999;109(1):35–41.
5. Prezant TR, Agapian JV, Bohlman MC, et al. Mitochondrial ribosomal RNA mutation associated with both antibiotic-induced and non-syndromic deafness. *Nat Genet.* 1993;4:289–294.
6. O'Sullivan SS, Massey LA, Williams DR, et al. Clinical outcomes of progressive supranuclear palsy and multiple system atrophy. *Brain.* 2008;131(Pt 5):1362–1372.
7. Bower JH, Maraganore DM, McDonnell SK, Rocca WA. Incidence of progressive supranuclear palsy and multiple system atrophy in Olmsted County, Minnesota, 1976 to 1990. *Neurology.* 1997;49(5):1284–1288.
8. Storey E. Genetic cerebellar ataxias. *Semin Neurol.* 2014; 34(3):280–292.
9. Hain TC, Hanna PA, Rheinberger MA. Mal de debarquement. *Arch Otolaryngol Head Neck Surg.* 1999;125(6):615–620.
10. Hain TC, Cherchi M. Mal de debarquement syndrome. *Handb Clin Neurol.* 2016;137:391–395.
11. Brown JJ, Baloh RW. Persistent mal de debarquement syndrome: a motion-induced subjective disorder of balance. *Am J Otolaryngol.* 1987;8(4):219–222.
12. Dai M, Cohen B, Smouha E, Cho C. Readaptation of the vestibulo-ocular reflex relieves the mal de debarquement syndrome. *Front Neurol.* 2014;5:124.
13. Hufner K, Barresi D, Glaser M, et al. Vestibular paroxysmia: diagnostic features and medical treatment. *Neurology.* 2008;71(13):1006–1014.
14. Brandt T, Strupp M, Dieterich M. Vestibular paroxysmia: a treatable neurovascular cross-compression syndrome. *J Neurol.* 2016;263(suppl 1):S90–S96.
15. Chang TP, Wu YC, Hsu YC. Vestibular paroxysmia associated with paroxysmal pulsatile tinnitus: a case report and review of the literature. *Acta Neurol Taiwan.* 2013; 22(2):72–75.
16. Cherchi M, Hain TC. Provocative maneuvers for nystagmus. In: Eggers S, Zee D, eds. *Vertigo and Imbalance: Clinical Neurophysiology of the Vestibular System.* Amsterdam: Elsevier; 2009:111–134.
17. Jannetta PJ, Moller MB, Moller AR. Disabling positional vertigo. *N Engl J Med.* 1984;310(26):1700–1705.
18. D'Adamo MC. Episodic ataxia type 1. In: Pagon RA, Adam MP, Ardinger HH, et al., eds. *GeneReviews(R).* Seattle, WA; 1993.
19. Spacey S. Episodic ataxia type 2. In: Pagon RA, Adam MP, Ardinger HH, et al., eds. *GeneReviews(R).* Seattle, WA; 1993.

20. Vahedi K, Taupin P, Djomby R, et al. Efficacy and tolerability of acetazolamide in migraine prophylaxis: a randomised placebo-controlled trial. *J Neurol.* 2002;249(2): 206–211.

21. Baloh RW. Episodic vertigo: central nervous system causes. *Curr Opin Neurol.* 2002;15(1):17–21.

22. Baloh RW, Yue Q, Furman JM, Nelson SF. Familial episodic ataxia: clinical heterogeneity in four families linked to chromosome 190. *Ann Nerol.* 1997;41:8–16.

23. Tarnutzer AA, Lee SH, Robinson KA, Kaplan PW, Newman-Toker DE. Clinical and electrographic findings in epileptic vertigo and dizziness: a systematic review. *Neurology.* 2015;84(15):1595–1604.

24. Yacovino DA, Hain TC. Clinical characteristics of cervicogenic-related dizziness and vertigo. *Semin Neurol.* 2013;33(3):244–255.

25. Hain TC. Cervicogenic causes of vertigo. *Curr Opin Neurol.* 2015;28(1):69–73.

CHAPTER 15

The Cardiovascular Dizziness Connection: Role of Vestibular Autonomic Interactions in Aging and Dizziness

JORGE M. SERRADOR, PHD

INTRODUCTION

Without a doubt, vestibular dysfunction can cause dizziness; however, other systems that interact with the vestibular system can also be involved. The goal of this chapter is to discuss the role of cardiovascular reflexes in contributing to dizziness.

A common symptom that often causes a patient to seek medical attention for the evaluation of dizziness is presyncope: the feeling of "lightheadedness" before fainting. Even young healthy individuals with intact vestibular systems commonly report dizziness and lightheadedness during tilt table testing. Participants generally report *dizziness* but not true vertigo. So why are these individuals reporting dizziness during an upright tilt?

Although the mechanism remains unclear, the assumption is that reductions in cerebral blood flow (CBF) result in symptoms associated with presyncope. In fact, recent evidence has found that both orthostatic hypotension (decreased blood pressure when standing)[1] and cerebral hypoperfusion (reduction in brain blood flow)[2] are related to incidents of dizziness. To understand why CBF would be reduced during upright posture requires an understanding of how blood pressure and CBF are regulated when we are standing or when we rise from a supine or seated position. To explore this connection, blood pressure regulation and regulation of brain blood flow are described in this chapter.

In addition, fascinating evolving evidence suggests that the vestibular system provides important signals that assist in the regulation of blood pressure[3] and brain blood flow.[4] This chapter also explores these

vestibular connections in the context of their impact on the development of dizziness and vertigo.

REGULATION OF BLOOD PRESSURE

Regulation of blood pressure is essential to health because blood flow through all organs is dependent on adequate driving pressure. To produce that pressure, the heart pumps approximately 86,000 times/day to maintain blood flow and pressure throughout the body. Pressure at the aorta, where blood is ejected from the left ventricle, is determined by the following equation:

$$MAP = CO \times TPR \qquad (15.1)$$

where MAP is the mean arterial pressure, CO is the cardiac output (total blood flow out of the heart each minute), and TPR is the total peripheral resistance of blood vessels throughout the body. Cardiac output is determined by the heart rate multiplied by the stroke volume, the amount of blood pumped in one contraction of the left ventricle. Thus to maintain adequate pressure we must maintain the stroke volume. Because the heart is a passive pump (i.e., it fills passively), the volume it ejects is based on how much blood is returned to the heart and how forcefully the heart contracts. The return of blood to the heart is determined by a number of properties, but because we are interested in the relationship to dizziness and vertigo, which are symptoms that normally occur when upright, we must consider the importance of the upright posture in cardiovascular regulation.

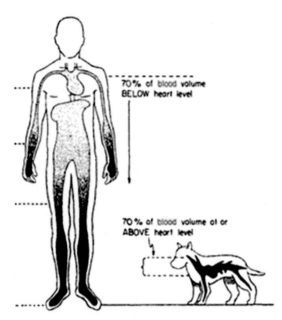

FIG. 15.1 Distribution of blood when upright in a human versus a quadruped. Note that a significant amount of blood volume is located below the heart in a standing human compared with the quadruped. (From Rowell. *Human Cardiovascular Control.* Oxford University Press; 1993; with permission.)

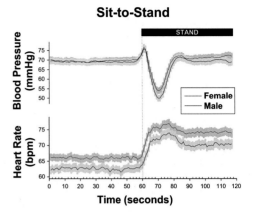

FIG. 15.2 Changes in heart rate and blood pressure in group of elderly individuals (308 females, 236 males) when moving from a sitting position to a standing position and remaining standing for 1 min. Note the significant decrease in blood pressure upon standing with a compensatory increase in heart rate to return blood pressure to baseline levels within 30 sec. (Data collected as part of MOBILIZE Boston study.)

Humans are bipedal and, unlike quadrupeds, during upright standing, there is a significant distance between the head and the feet. This unique posture results in substantial movement of blood from the upper torso to the legs (Fig. 15.1).

Sufficient cardiac output is required to maintain blood pressure (MAP; Eq. 15.1). Cardiac output is the product of heart rate and stroke volume, and stroke volume is determined by venous return (the amount of blood returning to the heart); therefore, assumption of the upright position results in considerable reduction in venous return. The result of this reduction in venous return is a drop in mean arterial blood pressure, which if uncompensated results in syncope (i.e., loss of consciousness). An example of this response was demonstrated in a group of elderly males and females who participated in the Maintenance of Balance, Independent Living, Intellect and Zest in the Elderly (MOBILIZE) Boston study (Fig. 15.2).

Note that within 10 seconds of initiating the stand, the participants had roughly a 20-mmHg drop in mean arterial pressure (MAP). The decrease in pressure was transient, and by 30 seconds the blood pressure had returned to baseline levels. This regulation of blood pressure is essential to maintaining consciousness. Returning to Eq. (15.1), some variables can be modified to maintain pressure. One of these variables is cardiac output, which is dependent on the stroke volume and heart rate. When humans stand upright, there is translocation of blood to the lower limbs and reduction in stroke volume. This results in a reduction in arterial pressure as seen in Fig. 15.2. To return blood pressure to normal levels, there is a need to modify (increase) the heart rate and/or resistance, which is accomplished by the baroreflex.

BAROREFLEX REGULATION OF BLOOD PRESSURE

The baroreflex is a mechanism that regulates blood pressure in response to sudden pressure changes. The baroreflex senses pressure changes through stretch receptors located in the aortic arch and carotid arteries at the bifurcation of the common carotid artery into the external and internal carotid arteries. Stretch of these arteries is interpreted as an increase in pressure and results in increased neural firing (Fig. 15.3). These neural signals result in the activation of cardiovascular control centers in the brainstem, which in turn results in changes in the heart rate and resistance. The detailed neural networks involved in the baroreflex response are well described but beyond the scope of this chapter.

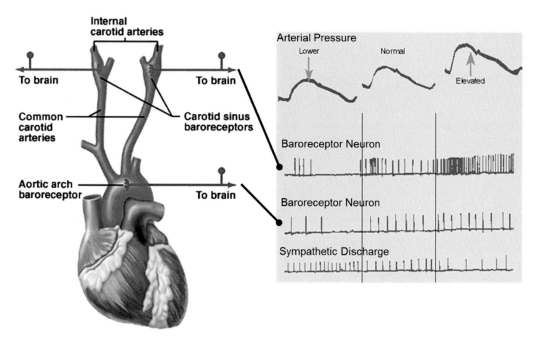

FIG. 15.3 Effects of increasing pressure on firing of single baroreceptor neurons and the resulting effect on sympathetic discharge. (Adapted from Heesch. Reflexes that control cardiovascular function. *Adv Physiol Educ.* 1999;22:S234–S243; with permission.)

Briefly, the baroreflex is able to modulate the heart rate by activating the autonomic nervous system, which directly controls the heart rate. By activating the parasympathetic system, the heart rate **slows**, and this effect can occur within one beat. Heart rate control under 100 beats per minute is primarily parasympathetic mediated, so the fastest response to a decrease in blood pressure is parasympathetic *withdrawal*, which allows the heart rate to increase immediately. The baroreflex can cause an increase not only in the heart rate by decreasing parasympathetic tone but also in the contractility of the heart by increasing sympathetic activity to the heart. However, this mechanism is more likely to predominate at higher heart rates, such as those achieved during exercise.

The other baroreflex-mediated response to blood pressure changes is to change peripheral vascular resistance. In humans, parasympathetic activity seems to have little effect on vascular resistance, unlike in many quadrupeds. In contrast, increases in sympathetic activity to the peripheral vessels result in vasoconstriction and an increase in peripheral vascular resistance.

To return to how humans respond to assuming the upright posture, Fig. 15.2 illustrates that there is a reduction in blood pressure. This is sensed by the stretch receptors, resulting in the baroreflex initiating an immediate increase in the heart rate to compensate for the decrease in stroke volume caused by blood moving into the lower limbs. As can be seen in Fig. 15.2, there is an immediate increase in the heart rate resulting from baroreflex-mediated parasympathetic withdrawal. Despite the increase in heart rate, blood pressure continues to fall. At the same time as the heart rate increases, to maintain mean arterial blood pressure, there is a baroreflex-mediated increase in sympathetic activity to peripheral blood vessels resulting in vasoconstriction. This increase in resistance, which takes approximately 10 seconds, results in increased total peripheral resistance and thus increased MAP (Eq. 15.1; $MAP = CO \times TPR$). As can be seen in Fig. 15.2, roughly 10 seconds after standing, blood pressure begins to rise and returns to baseline levels in approximately 25 seconds. One can also see that the heart rate begins to decrease within 20 seconds after standing, as resistance compensates for reduced stroke volume.

Returning to the discussion of what this has to do with dizziness and vertigo, without this baroreflex response to drops in pressure, humans would be unable to maintain adequate blood flow to the brain when standing, which would produce dizziness (presyncope) and even loss of consciousness. In fact, in a study of 11,429 patients, orthostatic hypotension (i.e., abnormally low blood pressure when upright) in the first minute of standing was strongly related to dizziness. Because that first minute is the period during which the baroreflex must adjust for the shift of blood into the lower limbs, these data highlight the importance of considering the baroreflex and blood pressure regulation in patients with dizziness, especially when dizziness occurs after standing.

It is well known that aging results in blunting of the baroreflex.[5] This is thought to be the result of stiffening of large vessels, which reduces stretch during changes in blood pressure. Thus, if the same pressure decrease results in an attenuated stretch because of vessel stiffening, an inappropriately low or diminished heart rate increase would be expected. Furthermore, aging processes appear to hinder the ability of increased sympathetic outflow to effect vasoconstriction and increased resistance.[6] Thus elderly individuals are at a greater risk for orthostatic hypotension, which produces dizziness. In addition, some blood pressure medications (e.g., alpha blockers, calcium channel blockers) dampen the ability of peripheral blood vessels to vasoconstrict, and other blood pressure medications (e.g., beta blockers) do not allow the heart to increase its rate to maintain blood pressure.

Thus far this chapter has focused on blood pressure regulation based on the assumption that orthostatic hypotension could be contributing to reductions in CBF and thus the development of dizziness. However, the picture is more complicated than this. It is necessary to understand how CBF is regulated to examine its possible role in dizziness.

REGULATION OF BRAIN BLOOD FLOW

Regulation of CBF is critical for proper neural function. Therefore alterations in CBF regulation caused by aging or age-related disease may have important clinical consequences, such as cognitive impairment, gait disorders, falls, and the development of symptoms such as dizziness. This section reviews mechanisms of CBF regulation and their changes with hypertension and aging, with particular attention to the possible etiologies of dizziness in some patients.

The regulation of CBF involves several interacting mechanisms.[7,8] Barcroft in 1914 proposed that the cerebral flow was matched to metabolic demands.[7] This has since been validated in both animal and human studies. Cognitive activation in humans increases both global and local blood flow to the brain.[9–11] The ability to augment flow is critical, for example, cognitive deficits with cerebral ischemia are reversed by increases in global CBF.[12] Despite the fact that vasodilation occurs locally around activated neurons because of neurovascular

coupling, this vasodilation may be insufficient if global cerebral flow is significantly reduced. To ensure sufficient CBF is available, cerebral vessels must dilate or constrict in response to the prevailing blood pressure. The ability to maintain brain blood flow over a wide range of pressures is termed cerebral autoregulation.[8] Thus, impairment of cerebral autoregulation could adversely affect global CBF during orthostatic hypotension.

AUTOREGULATION OF CEREBRAL BLOOD FLOW

Cerebral autoregulation maintains blood flow relatively constant across a wide range of cerebral perfusion pressures (CPPs). CBF is determined by CPP and cerebrovascular resistance (CVR), with CPP being a result of arterial pressure minus intracranial pressure. The relationship between these variables can be defined as:

$$CBF = \frac{CPP}{CVR} \qquad (15.2)$$

Thus, vascular resistance must be adjusted to maintain CBF constant in the face of changing perfusion pressure. This is accomplished by dilation of cerebral vessels.[8] Fig. 15.4 demonstrates that within a normal pressure range, CVR adjusts to the prevailing CPP to maintain flow relatively constant. When pressure becomes excessively low, resulting in maximal vasodilation, resistance can no longer adjust to decreasing perfusion pressures and CBF falls. In contrast, when pressures become too high, cerebral vessels are forced open by the driving pressure and thus resistance decreases, resulting in an increase in CBF. This condition is termed autoregulatory breakthrough.

Why is cerebral autoregulation important in the consideration of other mechanisms that may contribute to dizziness? Most people have had the experience of getting up quickly in the morning, becoming lightheaded, and needing to sit down again. The reason for this lies in the CBF response to the sudden pressure change associated with the change in posture from supine to upright. The cerebral flow velocity response has been examined by studying the response of individuals to a change in pressure during a "sit to stand" maneuver or induced by release of two thigh cuffs that were inflated above systolic blood pressure for 3 min.

Three important events preceding the baroreflex are highlighted in Fig. 15.5: the first is initiation of the blood pressure drop (marked by dotted lines at time point 0), the second is the nadir of the cerebral flow velocity response (dotted lines at approximately 4 seconds), and the third event is when cerebral flow

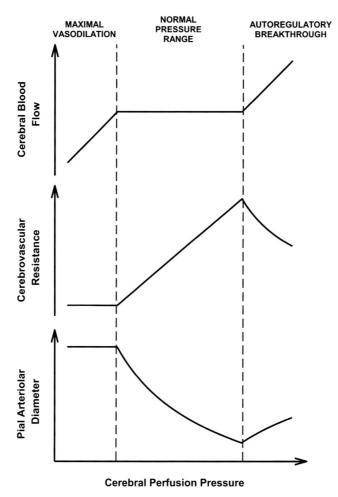

FIG. 15.4 Representation of cerebral autoregulation demonstrating that cerebral blood flow is kept relatively constant over a wide range of pressures (top panel) by adjusting cerebrovascular resistance.

velocity has returned to baseline levels (dotted lines at approximately 11 seconds). Fig. 15.5 demonstrates that blood pressure continues to drop after the flow velocity has hit its nadir. It is also important to note that CBF velocity returns to baseline before blood pressure returns to baseline. Recall that, according to Eq. (15.2), CBF is driven by the pressure unless resistance is changed. These data indicate that cerebral vessels must dilate to improve CBF before baroreflex return of CBF to baseline.[13] This is cerebral autoregulation in action. Thus, when cerebral autoregulation is impaired, CBF continues to decrease when blood pressure drops, likely producing symptoms of dizziness, as has been reported in a group of patients with Parkinson disease [14] and patients referred to an autonomic clinic.[2]

Although autoregulation is an important mechanism, previous research has found that autoregulation is fairly robust. It is well known that changing arterial carbon dioxide levels results in changes in CBF without affecting cerebral autoregulation.[8] Similarly, stimulation of the fastigial nucleus in primates has been found to result in vasodilation, which causes increases in CBF without affecting autoregulation.[15,16] This vasodilation may be mediated by parasympathetic pathways.[17] Autoregulation even seems to be maintained during hypotension in both chronic local cerebral hypoperfusion and orthostatic hypotension.[7,18–20]

An increased sympathetic outflow caused by the baroreflex is another possible mechanism by which cerebral autoregulation could be altered. There is some evidence of decreased ability to regulate CBF during

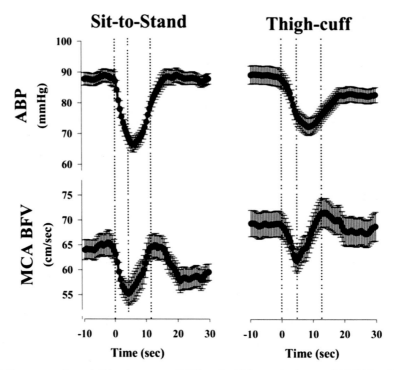

FIG. 15.5 Response of arterial blood pressure (ABP) and middle cerebral artery (MCA) blood flow velocity (BFV) during sit to stand maneuver (left panel, upright at time point 0) or thigh cuff release (right panel). (Adapted from Sorond FA, Serrador JM, Jones RN, Shaffer ML, Lipsitz LA. The sit-to-stand technique for the measurement of dynamic cerebral autoregulation. *Ultrasound Med Biol.* 2009;35(1):21–29; with permission.)

pressure fluctuations caused by lower body negative pressure[21] or upright tilt.[22] However, early studies of cats found no effect of acute sympathetic denervation on autoregulatory responses.[23] Consistent with this, animal studies have found no effect on autoregulation from chronic or acute sympathetic denervation or from electrical stimulation when blood pressure is kept stable.[24,25] In humans, sympathetic activation caused by upright tilt does not impair the ability to regulate against pressure fluctuations,[26,27] despite creating decreases in cerebral flow velocity similar to previous studies, all to suggest that sympathetic activation does not impair cerebral autoregulation.[21,22]

Thus, based on these data, it seems that the cerebral autoregulatory system is robust and that reduction in CBF caused by an inability of the cerebral autoregulatory system to handle pressure changes is unlikely, although no studies have examined the relationship between cerebral autoregulation and dizziness. However, other mechanisms related to aging may affect the baroreflex, resulting in cerebral hypoperfusion.

EFFECTS OF AGE ON CEREBRAL BLOOD FLOW

Aging is associated with a well-documented decrease in global CBF[28–34] and an increase in cerebral vascular resistance.[28] This raises the question of whether aging may impair cerebral autoregulation and thus contribute to cerebral hypoperfusion in the elderly. In fact, previous work has demonstrated that older rats are less able to tolerate hypotensive stimuli, have reduced cerebrovascular reactivity to CO_2 (often used as an indicator of intact autoregulation), and have an increased lower limit of autoregulation.[35–39] These findings suggest that autoregulation could be impaired as a result of aging.

Studies of CBF in elderly humans have produced conflicting results. Studies that examined the response to changes in arterial CO_2 levels have reported that aging either has no effect on cerebrovascular reactivity[40–42] or is associated with reduced reactivity.[43–47] Myogenic tone in isolated human pial arteries was found to be unaffected by age, suggesting intact autoregulatory capacity.[48] Furthermore, measures of cerebral autoregulation in elderly humans, based on the response of CBF to spontaneous fluctuations in blood pressure, have found that autoregulation remains intact.[42,44,49–54]

In fact, in the largest study of autoregulation in an elderly population, Deegan et al. found that cerebral autoregulation remained intact as shown in (Fig. 15.6).[42] It has been suggested in a smaller cross-sectional dataset that autoregulation may be impaired as individuals get older,[55] but this is in contrast to the many studies that have found intact autoregulation.

If impaired autoregulation is not involved in the reduction in CBF, could a direct, sympathetically mediated vasoconstriction be the cause? Sympathetic innervation of cerebral vessels has been found in animals originating in the superior cervical ganglion, stellate ganglion, and via several central pathways, including the locus coeruleus, fastigial nucleus, dorsal raphe nucleus, dorsal medullary reticular formation, and rostral ventrolateral medulla.[56] However, the role of sympathetic pathways in autoregulation in humans remains unclear. For example, blockade of sympathetic activity through the stellate ganglion has been found to increase CBF, as measured by single-photon emission computed tomography (SPECT), presumably through the blockade of a sympathetic vasoconstrictor signal.[57] However, MRI measures of CBF using the same blocking technique found no change in internal carotid artery flow but demonstrated an increase in common carotid flow, suggesting vasodilation in extracerebral beds.[58] Therefore, it is possible that the increase in CBF observed with SPECT was partly due to the increased scalp and facial blood flow. In contrast, direct stimulation of cervical ganglia (and presumably sympathetic pathways) during surgery has been shown to cause an increase in CBF and arterial pressure.[59] However, patients in this study were anesthetized with isoflurane, which has been shown to ablate autoregulation, as has nitrous oxide, which is a potent vasodilator, particularly when used in combination with isoflurane.[60,61] These considerations suggest that the elevated cerebral perfusion was the result of increased arterial pressure augmenting cerebral flow through vessels with pharmacologically impaired autoregulation.

In primates, cerebral vasoconstriction has been found with stimulation of the locus coeruleus.[62] This vasoconstriction was unaffected by sectioning of the vagus nerve or sympathetic trunk, suggesting an absence of peripheral sympathetic influence. In humans, direct measures of middle cerebral artery diameter using MRI during sympathetic activation induced by lower body negative pressure did not demonstrate vasoconstriction at the basal artery

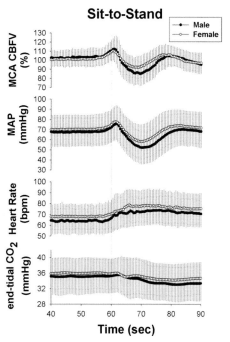

FIG. 15.6 Response of 308 females and 236 males over the age of 70 years in a sit to stand protocol. Notice that the middle cerebral artery cerebral blood flow velocity (MCA CBFV) begins to return to baseline levels before mean arterial pressure (MAP), indicating intact autoregulation. (From Deegan BM, Sorond FA, Galica A, Lipsitz LA, O'Laighin G, Serrador JM. Elderly women regulate brain blood flow better than men do. *Stroke*. 2011;42(7):1988–1993; with permission.)

level, even though flow decreased, suggesting that the constriction occurred at peripheral resistance arteries.[63] Direct intrathecal infusion of the locus coeruleus with clonidine, an α2-agonist that at low doses inhibits central sympathetic activity, resulted in a reduction in cerebral flow velocity in one patient, presumably through downstream vasoconstriction.[64] In healthy individuals, clonidine has been found to minimize the decrease in cerebral flow velocity during sympathetic activation by the cold pressor test, presumably by reducing sympathetic activation.[64,65] Furthermore, the use of β-blockers attenuated the decrease in CBF velocity of patients with orthostatic intolerance during head up tilt testing.[66] In these studies it was proposed that the observed changes in CBF were due to a decrease in CVR as a result of reduced cerebral sympathetic activity. However, low-dose clonidine also produced hypotension and caused a reduction in baseline cerebral flow velocity, suggesting cerebral vasoconstriction.[64] This reduction in flow was present even when the hypotension was eliminated with phenylephrine.[67]

In contrast, increasing peripheral sympathetic activity using cold face stimulation or skin surface cooling did not increase CVR.[68,69] Increasing muscle sympathetic nerve activity by approximately 50% using static hand grip did not cause a reduction in cerebral flow velocity, suggesting absence of sympathetically mediated cerebral vasoconstriction.[70] Similarly, ganglionic blockade and sympathoexcitation using lower body negative pressure did not change the response of subjects to CO_2 or improve their CBF response.[71–73] Interruption of the sympathetic pathway through stellate ganglion block causes a reduction in cerebral flow velocity without a change in pressure, suggesting cerebral vasoconstriction rather than vasodilation, as would be expected if sympathetic vasoconstriction were interrupted.[74] Similarly, patients with cervical spinal cord injuries who should have interrupted sympathetic pathways through the stellate ganglia demonstrate decreases in cerebral flow velocity similar to controls with intact pathways.[75,76] Finally, direct infusion of norepinephrine in both anesthetized and conscious patients[77–79] has not been shown to affect CBF or vascular resistance; therefore, the role of sympathetic activation on cerebrovascular tone is as yet unclear.

If not direct sympathetic vasoconstriction, other mechanisms may be involved in age-related decline in CBF. Infusion of adenosine, a vasodilator, has been found to produce attenuated vasodilatory responses in aged rats.[80] Similarly, endothelium-dependent vasodilation is attenuated in aged animals.[81–83] In addition, cholinergic vasodilator systems are impaired in older rats.[84,85] In contrast, application of a high dose of intravascular serotonin, a dose-dependent vasoconstrictor, produced augmented vasoconstriction in aged rats.[86] These data suggest that, in older animals, vasoconstrictor stimuli may dominate. Extrapolating these mechanisms to elderly humans may prove difficult, because there appear to be inherent differences in the cerebrovascular systems of older animals compared with humans. For example, myogenic tone remains intact with age in isolated human pial arteries but is reduced in older rat cerebral arteries, which reduces their ability to dilate or constrict in response to pressure changes.[48,81]

Finally, aging is associated with general cerebral atrophy that includes the loss of gray matter.[32] Thus, reductions in CBF may simply be the result of reduced metabolic demand resulting from reduced volume of neural tissue. Yoshii et al.[87] found that age-related reductions in global cerebral metabolic rate were eliminated when metabolic rate was normalized to brain volume. However, use of advanced imaging techniques over the last decade suggests that reductions in cerebral metabolic rate with aging, especially in the frontal lobes, are independent of brain atrophy.[32]

Although current data do not provide a clear mechanism for the reduction in CBF with aging, it appears that older individuals are still able to regulate fluctuations in pressure (i.e., cerebral autoregulation is intact). Regardless of the mechanism, it is possible that reductions in CBF that occur with aging may make individuals more susceptible to additional decreases in CBF. For example, older adults have a high prevalence of orthostatic and postprandial hypotension, which not only are risk factors for falls and syncope but also are related to dizziness.[1] Thus one could argue that, if older individuals have reductions in global CBF, transient drops in flow when assuming the upright posture could result in significant hypoperfusion, which would cause dizziness and increase their risk of falling (Fig. 15.6).

Because humans spend most of their time in the upright posture, these data raise concerns regarding the effects repeated bouts of transient cerebral hypoperfusion in the setting of reductions in global CBF may have on global cerebral function.

UNIQUE CHARACTERISTICS OF THE UPRIGHT POSTURE IN HUMANS

Thus far this chapter has presented information concerning MAP, pressure at the heart, and CPP. This section highlights an additional unique factor: the hydrostatic gradient. The concept of the hydrostatic gradient is that the pressure in a column of fluid increases toward the bottom of the column because of the weight of the fluid within the column. This is why pressure increases with diving under water. Similarly, pressure in the atmosphere decreases at higher altitudes because there is a reduction in the amount of air above.

When humans are supine, pressure is similar across the body, such that if MAP at the heart is 90 mmHg, it is also 90 mmHg at the head (Fig. 15.7). Because humans are bipedal, and the cardiovascular system is essentially a fluid-filled column, pressure at the feet increases during upright stance. Based on normal blood viscosity, this pressure increase is roughly 0.7788 mmHg/cm of vertical distance. This means that pressure at the feet increases to approximately 180 mmHg, whereas pressure at the head decreases to near 70 mmHg.

Recalling that Eq. (15.2) predicts that CBF is proportional to driving pressure, a reduction in driving pressure would cause a reduction in CBF. Thus, maintaining CBF when upright requires dilation of the vessels in the

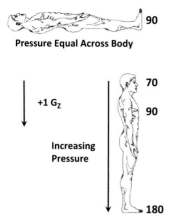

FIG. 15.7 Representation of effects of the hydrostatic gradient on cerebral perfusion pressure (CPP). When supine, pressure is equal at the heart and head. The effect of gravity during upright posture causes pressure at the feet to be higher and pressure at the head to be lower, resulting in a decrease in CPP from 90 to 70 mmHg.

brain. For example, getting out of bed and standing up in the morning demands that the brain deal with roughly a 20 mmHg transient drop in pressure associated with the translocation of blood from the thorax to the legs, and the brain also must handle the 20 mmHg hydrostatic gradient that develops in the process. Thus, it is not surprising that people get dizzy and lightheaded getting out of bed in the morning. A common suggestion for avoiding this is to sit on the bed for a minute or so before getting up, to allow the cerebral vasculature to dilate in response to the hydrostatic gradient before throwing the transient drop in pressure at it.

In addition, assuming an upright posture results in a reduction in end tidal and arterial CO_2 of approximately 2 mmHg (Fig. 15.6).[88,89] Arterial CO_2 is a very potent cerebral vasodilator that results in nearly a 3%/mmHg change in CBF,[42] so that, in addition to effects from the hydrostatic gradient, CBF decreases by another 6% because of decreases in arterial CO_2. This of course assumes that the individual does not hyperventilate (perhaps because of anxiety from feeling dizzy), which drives the end tidal CO_2 down even further, resulting in even greater drops in CBF and subsequently increasing dizziness.

To add to the complexity of the situation, there is increasing evidence that even if blood pressure is maintained, CBF may decrease. In fact, Serrador, Shoemaker et al. found that, in a group of healthy individuals immediately following exposure to the National Aeronautics and Space Administration parabolic flight program, those

who developed presyncopal symptoms (e.g., lightheadedness and dizziness) when upright had significantly greater drops in CBF velocity than those who did not experience symptoms, even though both groups had similar levels of end tidal CO_2 and higher blood pressures.[26] These data illustrate that individuals can demonstrate reductions in CBF *even without orthostatic hypotension*.

This finding is further supported by the work of Novak. In this study, 1279 patients who had been referred to an autonomic clinic were retrospectively examined and 102 patients were found to have orthostatic dizziness. In the patients with orthostatic dizziness, there was no difference in orthostatic blood pressure or end tidal CO_2, although CBF decreased $24.1 \pm 8.2\%$ compared with only $4.2 \pm 5.6\%$ decrease in patients without dizziness.[2] None of the patients in this study had a vestibular evaluation, so it is unclear whether or how vestibular dysfunction may have been a contributing factor.

Thus, humans have a number of challenges when assuming the upright posture. Not only does this require that balance be maintained but brain blood flow also must be maintained. This raises questions regarding how human adaptions to the upright posture may be integrated. Could the vestibular system assist with maintaining brain blood flow?

VESTIBULAR EFFECTS ON BLOOD PRESSURE AND CEREBRAL BLOOD FLOW

As discussed earlier in this chapter, humans have several adaptive systems that help maintain blood pressure (baroreflex) and CBF (cerebral autoregulation) during the transition from the supine to the upright position. Of course, both baroreflex and cerebral autoregulation are feedback systems, meaning that pressure drops must occur before the systems adjust to return the blood pressure or CBF to baseline levels.

In contrast, the vestibular system can notify the brain of a change in posture in milliseconds, well before blood pressure or CBF begins to drop. There is emerging evidence that the vestibular system contributes to autonomic responses to help maintain blood pressure.[3] Earlier work in animals has demonstrated that sectioning the vestibular nerve to remove information regarding head position relative to gravity results in a dramatic increase in postural hypotension.[90–94] Evidence from patients also demonstrates a role for vestibular inputs in cardiovascular regulation.[95]

Although contributions of the vestibular system in autonomic responses to the upright position have been documented, there has been little work examining how

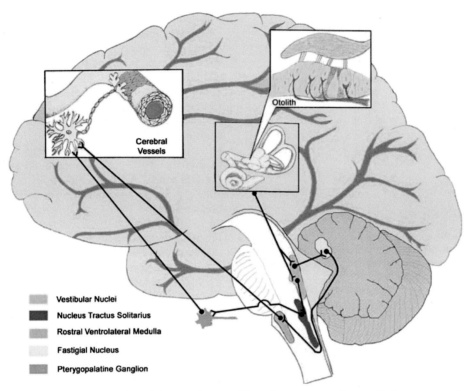

Vestibular Nuclei

Nucleus Tractus Solitarius

Rostral Ventrolateral Medulla

Fastigial Nucleus

Pterygopalatine Ganglion

FIG. 15.8 Anatomic connections demonstrating possible pathways connecting vestibular organs and cerebral vessels. (From Serrador J, Schlegel T, Black FO, Wood S. Vestibular effects on cerebral blood flow. *BMC Neurosci.* 2009;10(1):119; with permission.)

vestibular inputs may affect CBF directly. Anatomic evidence in animals demonstrates that neural connections are present between vestibular nuclei and cerebral vessels through two possible pathways (Fig. 15.8). Connections have been identified between vestibular nuclei and the fastigial nucleus,[96] then to the rostral ventrolateral medulla,[97] followed by vasodilatory connections to cerebral vessels.[98] Similarly, neurons travelling from vestibular nuclei to the nucleus tractus solitarius[99] and then to the pterygopalatine ganglion[100] can produce cerebral vasodilation[17,101,102]; however, the role these connections play in humans is as yet unclear.

To examine how vestibular signals may affect CBF in humans, studies have examined caloric vestibular stimulation of horizontal semicircular canals. Caloric stimulation results in an increased blood flow in the basilar and middle cerebral arteries,[103,104] as well as the parietal lobe,[105] while decreasing blood flow in the posterior cerebral artery.[104] However, it is unclear whether changes in CBF are due to semicircular canal activation or increases in neural activity in areas such as the sensory cortex in response to the increased input.

Because perception of change in position relative to gravity is mediated by otolith organs (utricle and saccule), it seems more likely that otolith activation would be involved in some kind of dilation of cerebral vessels.

Our laboratory has found that subjects exposed to 30 minutes of hypergravity demonstrate impaired CBF regulation that returns to normal upon assumption of the upright posture.[106] Furthermore, this impairment has been found to correlate with noninvasive measures of otolith sensitivity, providing indirect evidence of a contribution from otolith activation. Similarly, using head down neck flexion, we have found modulation of CVR that may be due to otolith activation.[107] Finally, in subjects who develop nausea during centrifugation, CBF is reduced almost 2 minutes before actual nausea.[108] We also found that we could cause changes in CBF that matched the frequency of vestibular stimulation during both pitch tilt and centrifugation.[4] Because centrifugation was performed in the dark with no visual cues, these data support the hypothesis that input from vestibular organs can affect CBF.

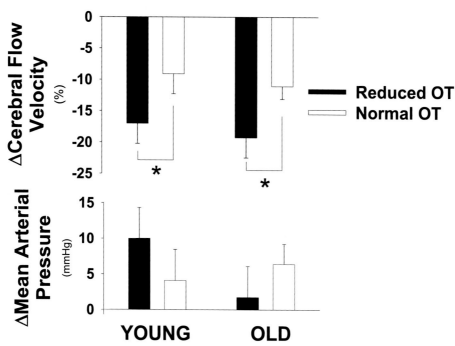

FIG. 15.9 Decrease in steady cerebral flow velocity during upright tilt in young and older subjects with either normal ocular torsion (OT) or reduced OT, as an indicator of otolith function.

In one study, we recruited 155 subjects across a wide age range who had previously participated in a study that measured ocular torsion.[109] Both young and old subjects with either normal ocular torsion (>0.2 degrees of ocular torsion per degree of tilt) or reduced ocular torsion (<0.16 degrees) participated in the study. Tilt table testing was performed with the subjects blindfolded to minimize visual inputs. Interestingly, regardless of age, reduced ocular torsion was associated with a significantly greater decrease in cerebral flow velocity when upright (Fig. 15.9). Surprisingly, this did not affect the MAP response. This demonstrated another situation in which individuals showed significant drops in CBF even when MAP was maintained. Although none of these healthy subjects developed symptoms, these data support a role for otolith input in maintaining CBF when upright.

One possible explanation for these findings is that the otolith effect on blood pressure was not seen because the baroreflex was effective and was able to maintain blood pressure despite otolith activation. Recall that one function of otolith organs is to assist in the maintenance of CBF when upright by compensating for the hydrostatic gradient. Therefore, when otolith organs detect a change in posture relative to gravity, a dilatory signal is provided to cerebral vessels to help maintain flow, notwithstanding the hydrostatic gradient. If otolith function is impaired, this dilation does not occur, and CBF decreases, resulting in cerebral hypoperfusion and dizziness.

SUMMARY

Dizziness is an extremely common symptom that is seen across all ages. Although it is clear that dizziness can be the result of vestibular dysfunction, the possible role of cardiovascular and cerebrovascular function must be considered. Patients who demonstrate orthostatic hypotension may be suffering from cerebral hypoperfusion that produces presyncopal symptoms, such as dizziness, lightheadedness, and vertigo. There is a growing body of evidence revealing that hypotension does not need to be present for cerebral hypoperfusion to occur during upright stance. Thus, reduced CBF could be a contributing factor for many patients who experience dizziness when standing.

In addition, emerging evidence highlighting the importance of vestibular system involvement in cardiovascular adaptations to the upright posture suggests that patients with vestibular dysfunction, particularly older patients, may be especially vulnerable to orthostatic hypotension or orthostatic cerebral hypoperfusion. These comingling health issues increase patients' risks of presyncope, falls, and fall-related injury. Consideration of both the vestibular and cardiovascular systems and their interactions is essential to evaluation and management of patients with dizziness.

REFERENCES

1. Juraschek SP, Daya N, Rawlings AM, et al. Association of history of dizziness and long-term adverse outcomes with early vs later orthostatic hypotension assessment times in middle-aged adults. *JAMA Intern Med.* 2017;177(9).
2. Novak P. Orthostatic cerebral hypoperfusion syndrome. *Front Aging Neurosci.* 2016;8(22).
3. McCall AA, Miller DM, Yates BJ. Descending influences on vestibulospinal and vestibulosympathetic reflexes. *Front Neurol.* 2017;8(112).
4. Serrador J, Schlegel T, Black FO, Wood S. Vestibular effects on cerebral blood flow. *BMC Neurosci.* 2009;10(1):119.
5. Monahan KD. Effect of aging on baroreflex function in humans. *Am J Physiol Regul Integr Comp Physiol.* 2007;293(1):R3–R12.
6. Joyner MJ, Charkoudian N, Wallin BG. The sympathetic nervous system and blood pressure in humans: individualized patterns of regulation and their implications. *Hypertension.* 2010;56(1):10–16.
7. Lassen NA. Cerebral blood flow and oxygen consumption in man. *Physiol Rev.* 1959;39(2):183–238.
8. Paulson OB, Strandgaard S, Edvinsson L. Cerebral autoregulation. *Cerebrovasc Brain Metab Rev.* 1990;2(2):161–192.
9. Gur RC, Jaggi JL, Ragland JD, et al. Effects of memory processing on regional brain activation: cerebral blood flow in normal subjects. *Int J Neurosci.* 1993;72(1–2):31–44.
10. Perani D, Gilardi MC, Cappa SF, Fazio F. PET studies of cognitive functions: a review. *J Nucl Biol Med.* 1992;36(4):324–336.
11. Ramsay SC, Adams L, Murphy K, et al. Regional cerebral blood flow during volitional expiration in man: a comparison with volitional inspiration. *J Physiol.* 1993;461:101.
12. Nunn J, Hodges H. Cognitive deficits induced by global cerebral ischaemia: relationship to brain damage and reversal by transplants. *Behav Brain Res.* 1994;65(1):1–31.
13. Sorond FA, Serrador JM, Jones RN, Shaffer ML, Lipsitz LA. The sit-to-stand technique for the measurement of dynamic cerebral autoregulation. *Ultrasound Med Biol.* 2009;35(1):21–29.
14. Park J, Kim HT, Park KM, et al. Orthostatic dizziness in Parkinson's disease is attributed to cerebral hypoperfusion: a transcranial doppler study. *J Clin Ultrasound.* 2017;45(6):337–342.
15. Goadsby PJ, Lambert GA. Electrical stimulation of the fastigial nucleus increases total cerebral blood flow in the monkey. *Neurosci Lett.* 1989;107(1–3):141–144.
16. McKee JC, Denn MJ, Stone HL. Neurogenic cerebral vasodilation from electrical stimulation of the cerebellum in the monkey. *Stroke.* 1976;7(2):179–186.
17. Toda N, Tanaka T, Ayajiki K, Okamura T. Cerebral vasodilatation induced by stimulation of the pterygopalatine ganglion and greater petrosal nerve in anesthetized monkeys. *Neuroscience.* 2000;96(2):393–398.
18. Keunen RW, Eikelboom BC, Stegeman DF, Ackerstaff RG. Chronic cerebral hypotension induces a downward shift of the cerebral autoregulation: a hypothesis based on TCD and OPG-GEE studies in ambulatory patients with occlusive cerebrovascular disease. *Neurol Res.* 1994;16(6):413–416.
19. Novak V, Novak P, Spies JM, Low PA. Autoregulation of cerebral blood flow in orthostatic hypotension. *Stroke.* 1998;29(1):104–111.
20. Nanda RN, Wyper DJ, Harper AM, Johnson RH. Cerebral blood flow in paraplegia. *Paraplegia.* 1974;12(3):212–218.
21. Zhang R, Zuckerman JH, Giller CA, Levine BD. Transfer function analysis of dynamic cerebral autoregulation in humans. *Am J Physiol.* 1998;274(1 Pt 2):H233–H241.
22. Carey BJ, Manktelow BN, Panerai RB, Potter JF. Cerebral autoregulatory responses to head-up tilt in normal subjects and patients with recurrent vasovagal syncope. *Circulation.* 2001;104(8):898–902.
23. Fog M. Cerebral circulation. I. Reaction of pial arteries to epinephrine by direct application and intravenous injection. *Arch Neurol Psychiatr Chic.* 1939;41:109–118.
24. Eklof B, Ingvar DH, Kagstrom E, Olin T. Persistence of cerebral blood flow autoregulation following chronic bilateral cervical sympathectomy in the monkey. *Acta Physiol Scand.* 1971;82(2):172–176.
25. Waltz AG, Yamaguchi T, Regli F. Regulatory responses of cerebral vasculature after sympathetic denervation. *Am J Physiol.* 1971;221(1):298–302.
26. Serrador JM, Shoemaker JK, Brown TE, Kassam MS, Bondar RL, Schlegel TT. Cerebral vasoconstriction precedes orthostatic intolerance after parabolic flight. *Brain Res Bull.* 2000;53(1):113–120.
27. Diehl RR, Linden D, Chalkiadaki A, Diehl A. Cerebrovascular mechanisms in neurocardiogenic syncope with and without postural tachycardia syndrome. *J Auton Nerv Syst.* 1999;76(2–3):159–166.

28. Krejza J, Mariak Z, Walecki J, Szydlik P, Lewko J, Usty-mowicz A. Transcranial color Doppler sonography of basal cerebral arteries in 182 healthy subjects: age and sex variability and normal reference values for blood flow parameters. *AJR Am J Roentgenol.* 1999;172(1):213–218.

29. Marchal G, Rioux P, Petit-Taboue MC, et al. Regional cerebral oxygen consumption, blood flow, and blood volume in healthy human aging. *Arch Neurol.* 1992;49(10):1013–1020.

30. Catafau AM, Lomena FJ, Pavia J, et al. Regional cerebral blood flow pattern in normal young and aged volunteers: a 99mTc-HMPAO SPET study. *Eur J Nucl Med.* 1996;23(10):1329–1337.

31. Krausz Y, Bonne O, Gorfine M, Karger H, Lerer B, Chisin R. Age-related changes in brain perfusion of normal subjects detected by 99mTc-HMPAO SPECT. *Neuroradiology.* 1998;40(7):428–434.

32. Nobler MS, Mann JJ, Sackeim HA. Serotonin, cerebral blood flow, and cerebral metabolic rate in geriatric major depression and normal aging. *Brain Res Brain Res Rev.* 1999;30(3):250–263.

33. Schultz SK, O'Leary DS, Boles Ponto LL, Watkins GL, Hichwa RD, Andreasen NC. Age-related changes in regional cerebral blood flow among young to mid-life adults. *Neuroreport.* 1999;10(12):2493–2496.

34. Stoquart-ElSankari S, Baledent O, Gondry-Jouet C, Makki M, Godefroy O, Meyer ME. Aging effects on cerebral blood and cerebrospinal fluid flows. *J Cereb Blood Flow Metab.* 2007;27(9):1563–1572.

35. Larsen FS, Olsen KS, Hansen BA, Paulson OB, Knudsen GM. Transcranial Doppler is valid for determination of the lower limit of cerebral blood flow autoregulation. *Stroke.* 1994;25(10):1985–1988.

36. Hoffman WE, Miletich DJ, Albrecht RF. The influence of antihypertensive therapy on cerebral autoregulation in aged hypertensive rats. *Stroke.* 1982;13(5):701–704.

37. Hoffman WE, Albrecht RF, Miletich DJ. The influence of aging and hypertension on cerebral autoregulation. *Brain Res.* 1981;214(1):196–199.

38. Fujishima M, Sadoshima S, Ogata J, et al. Autoregulation of cerebral blood flow in young and aged spontaneously hypertensive rats (SHR). *Gerontology.* 1984;30(1):30–36.

39. Toyoda K, Fujii K, Takata Y, Ibayashi S, Fujikawa M, Fujishima M. Effect of aging on regulation of brain stem circulation during hypotension. *J Cereb Blood Flow Metab.* 1997;17(6):680–685.

40. Kastrup A, Dichgans J, Niemeier M, Schabet M. Changes of cerebrovascular CO_2 reactivity during normal aging. *Stroke.* 1998;29(7):1311–1314.

41. Ito H, Kanno I, Ibaraki M, Hatazawa J. Effect of aging on cerebral vascular response to PaCO2 changes in humans as measured by positron emission tomography. *J Cereb Blood Flow Metab.* 2002;22(8):997–1003.

42. Deegan BM, Sorond FA, Galica A, Lipsitz LA, O'Laighin G, Serrador JM. Elderly women regulate brain blood flow better than men do. *Stroke.* 2011;42(7):1988–1993.

43. Lartaud I, Bray-des-Boscs L, Chillon JM, Atkinson J, Capdeville-Atkinson C. In vivo cerebrovascular reactivity in Wistar and Fischer 344 rat strains during aging. *Am J Physiol.* 1993;264(3 Pt 2):H851–H858.

44. Lipsitz LA, Mukai S, Hamner J, Gagnon M, Babikian V. Dynamic regulation of middle cerebral artery blood flow velocity in aging and hypertension. *Stroke.* 2000;31(8):1897–1903.

45. Matteis M, Troisi E, Monaldo BC, Caltagirone C, Silvestrini M. Age and sex differences in cerebral hemodynamics: a transcranial Doppler study. *Stroke.* 1998;29(5):963–967.

46. Oblak JP, Zaletel M, Zvan B, Kiauta T, Pogacnik T. The effect of age on cerebrovascular reactivity to cold pressor test and head-up tilt. *Acta Neurol Scand.* 2002;106(1):30–33.

47. Bakker SL, de Leeuw FE, den Heijer T, Koudstaal PJ, Hofman A, Breteler MM. Cerebral haemodynamics in the elderly: the rotterdam study. *Neuroepidemiology.* 2004;23(4):178–184.

48. Thorin-Trescases N, Bartolotta T, Hyman N, et al. Diameter dependence of myogenic tone of human pial arteries. Possible relation to distensibility. *Stroke.* 1997;28(12):2486–2492.

49. Carey BJ, Eames PJ, Blake MJ, Panerai RB, Potter JF. Dynamic cerebral autoregulation is unaffected by aging. *Stroke.* 2000;31(12):2895–2900.

50. Fisher JP, Ogoh S, Young CN, Raven PB, Fadel PJ. Regulation of middle cerebral artery blood velocity during dynamic exercise in humans: influence of aging. *J Appl Physiol.* 2008;105(1):266–273.

51. Lewis PM, Smielewski P, Pickard JD, Czosnyka M. Slow oscillations in middle cerebral artery cerebral blood flow velocity and aging. *Neurol Res.* 2007;29(3):260–263.

52. Yam AT, Lang EW, Lagopoulos J, et al. Cerebral autoregulation and ageing. *J Clin Neurosci.* 2005;12(6):643–646.

53. Serrador JM, Sorond FA, Vyas M, Gagnon M, Iloputaife ID, Lipsitz LA. Cerebral pressure-flow relations in hypertensive elderly humans: transfer gain in different frequency domains. *J Appl Physiol.* 2005;98(1):151–159.

54. Carey BJ, Panerai RB, Potter JF. Effect of aging on dynamic cerebral autoregulation during head-up tilt. *Stroke.* 2003;34(8):1871–1875.

55. Xing CY, Tarumi T, Meijers RL, et al. Arterial pressure, heart rate, and cerebral hemodynamics across the adult life span. *Hypertension.* 2017;69(4):712–720.

56. Sandor P. Nervous control of the cerebrovascular system: doubts and facts. *Neurochem Int.* 1999;35(3):237–259.

57. Umeyama T, Kugimiya T, Ogawa T, Kandori Y, Ishizuka A, Hanaoka K. Changes in cerebral blood flow estimated after stellate ganglion block by single photon emission computed tomography. *J Auton Nerv Syst.* 1995;50(3):339–346.

58. Nitahara K, Dan K. Blood flow velocity changes in carotid and vertebral arteries with stellate ganglion block: measurement by magnetic resonance imaging using a direct bolus tracking method. *Reg Anesth Pain Med.* 1998;23(6):600–604.

59. Wahlgren NG, Hellstrom G, Lindquist C, Rudehill A. Sympathetic nerve stimulation in humans increases middle cerebral artery blood flow velocity. *Cerebrovasc Dis.* 1992;2(6):359–364.

60. Strebel S, Lam AM, Matta B, Mayberg TS, Aaslid R, Newell DW. Dynamic and static cerebral autoregulation during isoflurane, desflurane, and propofol anesthesia. *Anesthesiology.* 1995;83(1):66–76.

61. Strebel S, Kaufmann M, Anselmi L, Schaefer HG. Nitrous oxide is a potent cerebrovasodilator in humans when added to isoflurane. A transcranial Doppler study. *Acta Anaesthesiol Scand.* 1995;39(5):653–658.

62. Goadsby PJ, Duckworth JW. Low frequency stimulation of the locus coeruleus reduces regional cerebral blood flow in the spinalized cat. *Brain Res.* 1989;476(1):71–77.

63. Serrador JM, Picot PA, Rutt BK, Shoemaker JK, Bondar RL. MRI measures of middle cerebral artery diameter in conscious humans during simulated orthostasis. *Stroke.* 2000;31(7):1672–1678.

64. Bramanti P, Mariani CA, D'Aleo G, Malara A. The first in vivo experience of the effects of the continuous intrathecal infusion of clonidine on the locus coeruleus in the regulation of cerebral blood flow: a TCD study. *Ital J Neurol Sci.* 1997;18(3):139–144.

65. Micieli G, Tassorelli C, Bosone D, Cavallini A, Viotti E, Nappi G. Intracerebral vascular changes induced by cold pressor test: a model of sympathetic activation. *Neurol Res.* 1994;16(3):163–167.

66. Jordan J, Shannon JR, Black BK, Paranjape SY, Barwise J, Robertson D. Raised cerebrovascular resistance in idiopathic orthostatic intolerance: evidence for sympathetic vasoconstriction. *Hypertension.* 1998;32(4):699–704.

67. Lee HW, Caldwell JE, Dodson B, Talke P, Howley J. The effect of clonidine on cerebral blood flow velocity, carbon dioxide cerebral vasoreactivity, and response to increased arterial pressure in human volunteers. *Anesthesiology.* 1997;87(3):553–558.

68. Brown CM, Sanya EO, Hilz MJ. Effect of cold face stimulation on cerebral blood flow in humans. *Brain Res Bull.* 2003;61(1):81–86.

69. Durand S, Cui J, Williams KD, Crandall CG. Skin surface cooling improves orthostatic tolerance in normothermic individuals. *Am J Physiol Regul Integr Comp Physiol.* 2004;286(1):R199–R205.

70. Ainslie PN, Ashmead JC, Ide K, Morgan BJ, Poulin MJ. Differential responses to CO_2 and sympathetic stimulation in the cerebral and femoral circulations in humans. *J Physiol.* 2005;566(Pt 2):613–624.

71. Przybylowski T, Bangash MF, Reichmuth K, Morgan BJ, Skatrud JB, Dempsey JA. Mechanisms of the cerebrovascular response to apnoea in humans. *J Physiol.* 2003;548(Pt 1):323–332.

72. Zhang R, Levine BD. Autonomic ganglionic blockade does not prevent reduction in cerebral blood flow velocity during orthostasis in humans. *Stroke.* 2007;38(4):1238–1244.

73. LeMarbre G, Stauber S, Khayat RN, Puleo DS, Skatrud JB, Morgan BJ. Baroreflex-induced sympathetic activation does not alter cerebrovascular CO_2 responsiveness in humans. *J Physiol.* 2003;551(Pt 2):609–616.

74. Gupta MM, Bithal PK, Dash HH, Chaturvedi A, Mahajan RP. Effects of stellate ganglion block on cerebral haemodynamics as assessed by transcranial Doppler ultrasonography. *Br J Anaesth.* 2005;95(5):669–673.

75. Handrakis JP, DeMeersman RE, Rosado-Rivera D, et al. Effect of hypotensive challenge on systemic hemodynamics and cerebral blood flow in persons with tetraplegia. *Clin Auton Res.* 2009;19(1):39–45.

76. Houtman S, Serrador JM, Colier WN, Strijbos DW, Shoemaker K, Hopman MT. Changes in cerebral oxygenation and blood flow during LBNP in spinal cord-injured individuals. *J Appl Physiol.* 2001;91(5):2199–2204.

77. Strebel SP, Kindler C, Bissonnette B, Tschaler G, Deanovic D. The impact of systemic vasoconstrictors on the cerebral circulation of anesthetized patients. *Anesthesiology.* 1998;89(1):67–72.

78. Olesen J. The effect of intracarotid epinephrine, norepinephrine, and angiotensin on the regional cerebral blood flow in man. *Neurology.* 1972;22(9):978–987.

79. Kimmerly DS, Tutungi E, Wilson TD, et al. Circulating norepinephrine and cerebrovascular control in conscious humans. *Clin Physiol Funct Imaging.* 2003;23(6):314–319.

80. Jiang HX, Chen PC, Sobin SS, Giannotta SL. Age related alterations in the response of the pial arterioles to adenosine in the rat. *Mech Ageing Dev.* 1992;65(2–3):257–276.

81. Geary GG, Buchholz JN. Selected contribution: effects of aging on cerebrovascular tone and $[Ca^{2+}]i$. *J Appl Physiol.* 2003;95(4):1746–1754.

82. Geary GG, Buchholz JN, Pearce WJ. Maturation depresses mouse cerebrovascular tone through endothelium-dependent mechanisms. *Am J Physiol Regul Integr Comp Physiol.* 2003;284(3):R734–R741.

83. Mayhan WG, Arrick DM, Sharpe GM, Sun H. Age-related alterations in reactivity of cerebral arterioles: role of oxidative stress. *Microcirculation.* 2008;15(3):225–236.

84. Sato A, Sato Y, Uchida S. Regulation of cerebral cortical blood flow by the basal forebrain cholinergic fibers and aging. *Auton Neurosci.* 2002;96(1):13–19.

85. Uchida S, Suzuki A, Kagitani F, Hotta H. Effects of age on cholinergic vasodilation of cortical cerebral blood vessels in rats. *Neurosci Lett.* 2000;294(2):109–112.

86. Hajdu MA, McElmurry RT, Heistad DD, Baumbach GL. Effects of aging on cerebral vascular responses to serotonin in rats. *Am J Physiol.* 1993;264(6 Pt 2):H2136–H2140.

87. Yoshii F, Barker WW, Chang JY, et al. Sensitivity of cerebral glucose metabolism to age, gender, brain volume, brain atrophy, and cerebrovascular risk factors. *J Cereb Blood Flow Metab.* 1988;8(5):654–661.

88. Serrador JM, Bondar RL, Hughson RL. Ventilatory response to passive head up tilt. In: Hughson RL, Cunningham DA, Duffin J, eds. *Advances in Modeling and Control of Ventilation.* New York: Plenum Press; 1998:133–139.

89. Serrador JM, Hughson RL, Kowalchuk JM, Bondar RL, Gelb AW. Cerebral blood flow during orthostasis: role of arterial CO_2. *Am J Physiol Regul Integr Comp Physiol.* 2006;290(4):R1087–R1093.

90. Yates BJ, Miller AD. Physiological evidence that the vestibular system participates in autonomic and respiratory control. *J Vestib Res.* 1998;8(1):17–25.

91. Yates BJ, Holmes MJ, Jian BJ. Adaptive plasticity in vestibular influences on cardiovascular control. *Brain Res Bull.* 2000;53(1):3–9.

92. Wilson TD, Cotter LA, Draper JA, et al. Vestibular inputs elicit patterned changes in limb blood flow in conscious cats. *J Physiol.* 2006;575(Pt 2):671–684.

93. Wilson TD, Cotter LA, Draper JA, et al. Effects of postural changes and removal of vestibular inputs on blood flow to the head of conscious felines. *J Appl Physiol.* 2006;100(5):1475–1482.

94. Yates BJ, Jian BJ, Cotter LA, Cass SP. Responses of vestibular nucleus neurons to tilt following chronic bilateral removal of vestibular inputs. *Exp Brain Res.* 2000;130(2):151–158.

95. Yates BJ, Bronstein AM. The effects of vestibular system lesions on autonomic regulation: observations, mechanisms, and clinical implications. *J Vestib Res.* 2005;15(3):119–129.

96. Shaikh AG, Ghasia FF, Dickman JD, Angelaki DE. Properties of cerebellar fastigial neurons during translation, rotation, and eye movements. *J Neurophysiol.* 2005;93(2):853–863.

97. Yates BJ, Goto T, Bolton PS. Responses of neurons in the rostral ventrolateral medulla of the cat to natural vestibular stimulation. *Brain Res.* 1993;601(1–2):255–264.

98. Golanov EV, Christensen JRC, Reis DJ. The medullary cerebrovascular vasodilator area mediates cerebrovascular vasodilation and electroencephalogram synchronization elicited from cerebellar fastigial nucleus in Sprague–Dawley rats. *Neurosci Lett.* 2000;288(3):183–186.

99. Yates BJ, Grelot L, Kerman IA, Balaban CD, Jakus J, Miller AD. Organization of vestibular inputs to nucleus tractus solitarius and adjacent structures in cat brain stem. *Am J Physiol.* 1994;267(4 Pt 2):R974–R983.

100. Agassandian K, Fazan VP, Margaryan N, Dragon DN, Riley J, Talman WT. A novel central pathway links arterial baroreceptors and pontine parasympathetic neurons in cerebrovascular control. *Cell Mol Neurobiol.* 2003;23(4–5):463–478.

101. Talman WT, Corr J, Nitschke Dragon D, Wang D. Parasympathetic stimulation elicits cerebral vasodilatation in rat. *Auton Neurosci.* 2007;133(2):153–157.

102. Toda N, Ayajiki K, Tanaka T, Okamura T. Preganglionic and postganglionic neurons responsible for cerebral vasodilation mediated by nitric oxide in anesthetized dogs. *J Cereb Blood Flow Metab.* 2000;20(4):700–708.

103. Heckmann JG, Leis S, Muck-Weymann M, Hilz MJ, Neundorfer B. Vestibular evoked blood flow response in the basilar artery. *Acta Neurol Scand.* 1999;100(1):12–17.

104. Tiecks FP, Planck J, Haberl RL, Brandt T. Reduction in posterior cerebral artery blood flow velocity during caloric vestibular stimulation. *J Cereb Blood Flow Metab.* 1996;16(6):1379–1382.

105. Takeda N, Hashikawa K, Moriwaki H, et al. Effects of caloric vestibular stimulation on parietal and temporal blood flow in human brain: a consecutive technetium-99m-HMPAO spect study. *J Vestib Res.* 1996;6(2):127–134.

106. Serrador JM, Wood SJ, Picot PA, et al. Effect of acute exposure to hypergravity (GX vs. GZ) on dynamic cerebral autoregulation. *J Appl Physiol.* 2001;91(5):1986–1994.

107. Wilson TD, Serrador JM, Shoemaker JK. Head position modifies cerebrovascular response to orthostatic stress. *Brain Res.* 2003;961(2):261–268.

108. Serrador JM, Schlegel TT, Black FO, Wood JS. Cerebral hypoperfusion precedes nausea during centrifugation. *Aviat Space Environ Med.* 2005;76(2):91–96.

109. Serrador JM, Lipsitz LA, Gopalakrishnan GS, Black FO, Wood SJ. Loss of otolith function with age is associated with increased postural sway measures. *Neurosci Lett.* 2009;465:10–15.

CHAPTER 16

Vertebrobasilar Infarcts and Ischemia

GAIL ISHIYAMA, MD • DAVID S. LIEBESKIND, MD • AKIRA ISHIYAMA, MD

Clinical Vignette

A 68-year-old male with a history of myocardial infarction 5 years ago, hypertension, hypercholesterolemia, and diabetes presents with the acute onset of rotational vertigo with nausea and vomiting and hearing loss in the right ear. Left-beating nystagmus is present in center gaze and increases velocity in left gaze. The head impulse test, originally known as the Halmagyi-Curthoys test, demonstrates catch-up saccades with head impulses to the right. There is no skew deviation and no other abnormal eye movements. No other focal neurologic symptoms or signs are noted except a mild peripheral neuropathy. When asked, he recalls having some episodes of leg numbness lasting 5 or 10 minutes recently, and 2 months ago he had a drop attack in which his legs gave out and buckled without loss of consciousness.

INTRODUCTION

The history and presentation of the patient described in the vignette should alert the clinician to the possibility of a posterior circulation stroke. The next sequence of events for this patient may be gradual onset of increasing lethargy, bilateral leg spasms and hyper-reflexia, and ultimately the recognition of an impending basilar artery stroke. It is important to note that vascular supply for the inner ear labyrinth is usually the same as for the anterior cerebellum: the anterior inferior cerebellar artery (AICA), which is a small branch of the larger basilar artery. Thus an AICA infarct presenting with acute vertigo and hearing loss can be the first sign of an impending basilar artery stroke resulting from a small embolic piece of the growing basilar artery atherosclerotic clot dislodging and traveling into the AICA, in an artery-to-artery embolic stroke. Occlusion of the basilar artery is often fatal and portends a poor prognosis if not treated quickly. Reasons for heightened suspicion of infarct include (1) sudden onset of symptoms; (2) combined vertigo and unilateral hearing loss; (3) vascular risk factors of age, diabetes, myocardial atherosclerotic disease, and hypercholesterolemia; and (4) past history of transient ischemic attacks (TIAs) in the posterior circulation.

In this review, we first present "state of the science" information regarding interventions and outcome studies demonstrating the superiority of treating large cerebral vessel occlusions with endovascular thrombectomy and intravenous tissue plasminogen activator (tPA). In addition, we review the most recent studies analyzing typical presentation of patients with posterior circulation strokes: clinical presentation, magnetic resonance imaging (MRI) and computed tomography (CT) findings, stroke etiologies, as well as important considerations for managing patients with these conditions.

The second section addresses the anatomy and vascular supply of the posterior cerebral circulation and inner ear, with particular attention to major branches and the labyrinthine circulation. The third section describes common presentations of stroke syndromes in the posterior circulation related to symptoms of vertigo and dizziness, with particular stroke syndromes and their presentation described in detail. We elaborate on critical components and key questions of the clinical examination and on the relationship of stroke with migraine.

EXCITING NEW HORIZONS IN STROKE TREATMENT

Vertebrobasilar Ischemia and Infarcts

Historically, ischemic strokes were treated supportively, and a delay in diagnosis did not have significant consequences. With the development of proven treatments, it is now widely acknowledged that "time is brain" and that each minute of untreated stroke in the frontal lobes allows an estimated 1.9 million neurons to be destroyed.[2] More recently, there has been rapid development of effective interventions for the treatment of stroke, with outcome measures demonstrating that early intervention results in better patient recovery and also extends the post-stroke time interval for additional potentially brain-saving interventions. The presentation of the patient described earlier should result in hospitalization and expedited referral to specialists in cerebrovascular disease, preferably within a leading stroke center. TIAs within the last 72 hours and recent increase in the frequency of TIAs also merit rapid assessment and management.

Acute Ischemic Stroke

Several landmark trials have rapidly transformed the standard of care for acute ischemic stroke treatment, with the most dramatic results demonstrating unequivocal benefit of acute endovascular intervention for a select group of patients with large vessel occlusions in the anterior circulation.[3,4] These dramatic changes in the treatment of acute stroke make it even more imperative that the clinician who first sees a patient with a potential stroke recognizes the key signs and initiates immediate evaluation. Technological advances and workflow efficiencies have facilitated an even more rapid delivery of acute stroke interventions, and the world of stroke medicine has become exquisitely dynamic, ever evolving, and rapidly advancing.

During a ground-breaking investigational multicenter randomized trial involving 39 centers in the United States and Europe, entitled Solitaire With the Intention For Thrombectomy as Primary Endovascular Treatment (SWIFT-PRIME), investigators stopped the study early because of clear demonstration of superior patient outcomes with thrombectomy with a stent retriever plus intravenous tPA. This protocol was reported to reduce disability at 90 days following anterior circulation stroke, with 60% of patients demonstrating functional independence compared with only 35% of patients who received conventional intravenous treatment demonstrating functional independence at 90 days.[3] Data from multiple studies (e.g., SWIFT PRIME, Endovascular Treatment for Small Core and Anterior Circulation Proximal Occlusion with Emphasis on Minimizing CT to Recanalization Times [ESCAPE trial], Extending the Time for Thrombolysis in Emergency Neurological Deficits—Intra-Arterial [EXTEND-IA trial], Randomized Trial of Revascularization With the Solitaire FR Device Versus Best Medical Therapy in the Treatment of Acute Stroke Due to Anterior Circulation Large Vessel Occlusion Presenting Within Eight Hours of Symptom Onset [REVASCAT trial]) were pooled to investigate the efficacy and safety of stent thrombectomy in anterior circulation ischemic stroke with the primary analysis including 787 patients, demonstrating that thrombectomy was highly effective and significantly reduced disability. This has led to the highest level of recommended guidelines in the United States, Europe, and Canada supporting mechanical stent thrombectomy within 6 hours of ischemic stroke for patients with large vessel stroke caused by internal carotid and middle cerebral artery occlusions.[4] The meta-analysis of studies conducted in participating countries demonstrated that

modern thrombectomy devices achieve faster and more complete reperfusion, with a common odds ratio for improvement in the modified Rankin score at 2.4 and a P value of 10^{-10}. Quality-of-life scores at 24 months follow-up remain high for patients with stroke using this protocol, with no significant difference for patients who received intravenous thrombolysis plus thrombectomy versus thrombectomy alone.[5,6] A review of pooled data from five separate trials also demonstrates the efficacy of this treatment in important subsets of patients: patients 80 years and older, patients in whom thrombectomy was performed more than 5 hours after stroke onset, and patients not eligible for intravenous alteplase.[7] Taken together, these data illustrate that endovascular thrombectomy is a highly effective treatment for large vessel occlusive stroke in the anterior circulation, and rapid multimodal imaging to identify these patients is crucial.

As mentioned, imaging has an important role in the selection of patients who are likely to benefit from endovascular reperfusion therapy following anterior circulation stroke. In a retrospective study of patients who had undergone endovascular reperfusion, perfusion imaging-selected patients were more likely to have positive outcomes compared with noncontrast CT-selected patients, whereas CT-selected patients and MR-selected patients had roughly similar outcomes.[8] One study using CT perfusion demonstrated superiority of endovascular therapy initiated within 18 hours of symptom onset.[9] Imaging is absolutely essential in the analysis of the acute presentation of a potential cerebrovascular event: evaluating for cerebrovascular stenosis, atherosclerotic burden, silent cerebrovascular cortical infarcts, and perfusion deficits, as well as evaluating for vascular anomalies, tumors, metastatic disease, or other diseases such as multiple sclerosis, cerebellar atrophy syndromes, and Chiari malformation.

Endovascular Therapy in the Posterior Circulation

Vertigo as a presenting symptom in a patient with an evolving or impending stroke localizes to the posterior circulation, and as with the patient with anterior circulation stroke, it may be wise to consider the patient presenting with an acute vestibular syndrome as having a posterior circulation stroke until proven otherwise. This is particularly true for patients who have risk factors for stroke.

Large vessel atherosclerotic disease of the vertebral or basilar arteries accounts for approximately one-third of ischemic events in the posterior circulation.[10,11] The question has been raised regarding whether the patient with vertebrobasilar TIAs secondary to atherosclerosis or large vessel disease is likely to suffer a recurrence and if so, should vertebrobasilar stenosis be investigated in patients with potential TIAs localized to the posterior circulation. A pooled analysis of prospective studies demonstrated that the 90-day risk of stroke from the first event (TIA or stroke) in patients with vertebrobasilar stenosis was 24.6% compared with 7.2% in patients without stenosis.[12] Identification of stenosis in the posterior circulation in the acute setting of a TIA or stroke should prompt the managing healthcare provider to initiate preventative measures and to educate the patient regarding warning signs of stroke, which some studies suggest occur in one of four patients within 90 days. Therefore, imaging studies, including MRI/magnetic resonance angiography (MRA; see later discussion), in this group of patients with potential posterior circulation events would likely be high yield and may warrant active medical therapeutic preventatives or preemptive interventions.

Basilar artery occlusion, a subset of posterior circulation strokes, is potentially amenable to thrombectomy similar to large vessel occlusions in the anterior circulation. Basilar artery occlusion often mimics other nonstroke entities and can be misdiagnosed as meningitis, vestibular neuritis, or seizures because of the nonspecific clinical manifestations and the common stuttering symptom course. It is important for the clinician to know that dizziness and vertigo are common early prodromal symptoms of basilar artery occlusion.

Not surprisingly, posterior circulation strokes are associated with a delayed time to intervention compared with anterior circulation strokes.[13] In a large systematic review of 71,010 patients with ischemic stroke in the Austrian Stroke Unit Registry, the onset-to-door times (ODTs) and door-to-needle times (DNTs) were compared for anterior and posterior circulation strokes. Overall, the ODT for posterior circulation stroke was 170 minutes compared with 110 minutes for anterior circulation stroke. Furthermore, posterior circulation strokes were associated with a delay in DNT.[14] The **FAST** algorithm (Face, Arm, Speech, Time) is designed to help identify strokes for patients and their families, ambulance personnel, and persons in the field. However, in an analysis of 736 strokes, 14.1% of patients did not have any FAST symptoms at presentation, and of these, 42% had gait imbalance or leg weakness and 40% had visual symptoms, symptoms not included in the FAST mnemonic. With the addition of balance disturbance and eye movement abnormalities, a significantly higher proportion of patients with stroke would be correctly identified.[15] The authors propose **BE-FAST** as an acronym to reduce the proportion of missed strokes: Balance, Eyes, Face, Arm, Speech, Time. Missed strokes often are posterior circulation strokes, which commonly present with dizziness or nystagmus and diplopia. In summary, posterior circulation strokes are associated with delays

in OTD and DNT and are also more likely to be missed by current emergency examination protocols. Therefore, it is essential to educate healthcare providers and the public that "time is brain" and "time is brainstem."

Imaging in identification and management of posterior circulation stroke

In an editorial, Liebeskind recognized the importance of addressing patients with the most complex conditions and the role that advanced multimodal imaging has played in the rapid advancement of stroke interventions, as well as the need for precision medicine. As such, precision medicine in acute stroke depends largely on the phenotypic characterization provided by diagnostic neuroimaging.[16,17] A study using imaging-based scores for the prediction of early stroke risk after TIA demonstrated an increased sensitivity in the identification of these high-risk patients. Traditional parameters used to predict stroke include the following: age, blood pressure, clinical symptoms, duration, and diabetes (ABCD2), useful for nonspecialists in the community who may not have access to diagnostic neuroimaging. A proposed ABCD3-I model (age, blood pressure, clinical symptoms, duration, diabetes, dual events, and imaging) uses additional prognostic utility of detailed MRI variables, which include vascular imaging information.[18] An example of MRI data for potential risk stratification is the high incidental cerebellar cortical infarcts (35%) seen on the initial MRI of patients presenting with vertebrobasilar stroke or TIA and vertebral artery stenosis.[19] If validated, the presence of cerebellar cortical infarcts and vertebral artery stenosis on an MRI may be indicative of an impending vertebrobasilar stroke. The gathering of high-resolution MRI findings in patients presenting with cerebrovascular ischemia needs to be recognized as an important subset of precision medicine.

BRIEF SUMMARY OF THE ANATOMY OF THE POSTERIOR CIRCULATION

The vertebrobasilar vascular system provides blood supply to the posterior region of the brain, which includes the brainstem, cerebellum, and inner ear. The vertebrobasilar system represents about 20% of cerebral blood flow.[20] When vertigo is the presenting symptom of a TIA or stroke, the cerebrovascular region involved is the vertebrobasilar system. Ischemic attacks in the anterior circulation, that is, carotid system, may present with lightheadedness but will not present with rotational vertigo. Vertigo can result from ischemia of the inner ear, brainstem, or cerebellar structures perfused by the posterior circulation. Posterior circulation TIAs and strokes represent about 20% of all TIAs and strokes.[21]

The vertebral arteries originate from the subclavian arteries, which in turn originate from the thoracic aorta. The two vertebral arteries are only rarely the same size, and in 72% of participants in an anatomic study, one vertebral artery was at least double the size of the other.[22] The vertebral artery is designated into four sections: V1, which includes the origin and the extracranial prevertebral portion; V2, which is the extracranial foraminal or cervical artery; V3, which is the extracranial postforaminal artery at the atlantic region; and V4, which is the intracranial artery and includes the junction with the basilar artery. The most common sites of stenosis are at V1 and V4, particularly at the origin of the vertebral artery as it comes off of the subclavian artery and at the vertebrobasilar junction. There is a predilection for development of atherosclerotic plaques at sites with turbulent flow such as bifurcation points and at the origin of arteries.[23]

The two vertebral arteries converge to form the midline basilar artery, which courses along the ventral surface of the pons. The basilar artery gives off penetrating median, paramedian, and short circumferential branches. The posteroinferior cerebellar artery (PICA) is the largest branch of the vertebral artery. It generally originates 1–2 cm below the basilar artery but in angiograms has been shown to sometimes originate below the level of the foramen magnum.[24] The PICAs supply the lateral medulla, including the vestibular nuclei and the posteroinferior cerebellum. The largest circumferential branches are the AICAs, which arise from the proximal third of the basilar artery. In addition to supplying the labyrinth, the AICAs supply the lateral pontine tegmentum, the brachium pontis, the flocculus, and part of the anterior cerebellum. An AICA infarct typically involves the middle cerebellar peduncle.[25,26] There is often a close relationship between the PICA and ipsilateral AICA; if one PICA is hypoplastic, the ipsilateral AICA may be large and the contralateral PICA small.[27]

The vascular anatomy of the inner ear has been studied in many species.[28] The inner ear consists of the auditory and vestibular end organs, for hearing and balance, respectively. The vestibular labyrinth is composed of three semicircular canals (SCCs) and two otolith organs, the saccule and utricle. The vestibular end organs are involved in sensing head movement and position, more precisely, angular acceleration and linear acceleration. Vascular supply for the inner ear is provided by the internal auditory artery (also known as the labyrinthine artery), which arises most commonly as a branch of the ipsilateral AICA and may also be a branch of PICA or the basilar artery. Within the internal auditory canal, the internal auditory artery branches into two arteries: (1) the common cochlear artery, which feeds most of the cochlea, and the posterior vestibular artery, which feeds the inferior saccule and posterior SCC, and (2) the anterior vestibular branch, which feeds the horizontal and anterior SCC, the utricle, and a small portion of the saccule. The labyrinthine arteries are end arteries—they do not anastomose with other major arterial branches; therefore, if blood flow is interrupted for 15 seconds or more, the auditory nerve fibers become inexcitable.[29] In contrast, there are abundant anastomoses in the brainstem and overlying territories in the cerebellum, and thus the inner ear appears to be more vulnerable to interruption of blood flow than the brainstem or cerebellum.

Before dividing into the two posterior cerebral arteries (PCAs), the basilar artery gives off the superior cerebellar arteries (SCAs). The cerebellum is fed by the AICAs, PICAs, and SCAs with prominent anastomoses provided by these arteries on the cerebellar surface. These arteries feed areas of the brainstem related to wakefulness and consciousness, and there is a high degree of collateralization in this critical area. In contrast, there is little collateralization within the inner ear. This fact may explain why vertebrobasilar insufficiency can present with isolated labyrinthine infarctions[30] and cochlear hearing loss.[26]

The cause of vertebrobasilar insufficiency or ischemia (VBI) is usually atherosclerotic disease of the subclavian, vertebral, or basilar arteries. However, clinicians should realize that it has been estimated that one in five posterior circulation infarcts is cardioembolic and another one in five infarcts occurs from intra-arterial emboli originating in the extracranial and intracranial vertebral arteries.[31] Emboli travel to the distal arterial branches, often causing an isolated cerebellar infarction in the distribution of the SCA, AICA, or PICA. Therefore patients with isolated cerebellar infarctions should be evaluated carefully for an embolic source. The evaluation should include a search for a cardiac source of embolism and visualization of the intracranial and extracranial vertebrobasilar arteries, including the origin of the vertebral artery. There may be a tendency for cardiac catheterization embolic events to involve the posterior vertebrobasilar system.[32]

Another potential cause of VBI results from the fact that the extracranial vertebral arteries are susceptible to dissection, which refers to a tear in an artery, usually involving the middle layer, referred to as the medial coat. Sudden neck movements, such as neck manipulation, or even trivial motions such as extending the neck to take medications, can be an inciting event.

Dissections usually occur in portions of the extracranial arteries that are mobile rather than at the origins of arteries (e.g., at the distal extracranial vertebral artery V3). The extracranial and intracranial vertebrobasilar system is well visualized using present-day noninvasive imaging modalities. There are heritable disorders of connective tissue disease such as Ehlers-Danlos type IV, which are associated with arterial dissection, and can occur at multiple sites.[33] However, transient emboli are often not visualized and very small infarcts in communicating areas may not be seen on MRI. Therefore, the diagnosis of posterior circulation TIA or stroke is sometimes made on a clinical basis. Dissection in the vertebral artery, in addition to neurologic signs and symptoms, also causes severe neck pain, a clinical hallmark of vertebral artery dissection.

Microvascular ischemia may also be the cause of age-related atrophy of inner ear structures, a well-studied phenomenon in human temporal bones.[34,35] There is significant loss of spiral ligament volume of approximately 12% and a 32% loss of stria vascularis volume in humans older than 60 years compared with those younger than 40 years.[36] In the Fisher rat, there is an age-related decrease in blood flow of 75% in capillaries of the posterior crista ampullares.[37] Cells in the inner ear, especially those such as the strial marginal cells and the auditory and vestibular hair cells may be exceptionally vulnerable to ischemia because of the high volume density of mitochondria, which is associated with high energy demand.

The Posterior Circulation: Mechanisms of Stroke and Transient Ischemic Attacks

A large study of 407 consecutive patients with posterior circulation events, of whom 59% had strokes without TIA, 24% had TIAs followed by strokes, and 16% had only TIAs, demonstrated that embolism was the most common stroke mechanism, of which 24% were cardiac, 14% were intra-arterial, and 2% were combined cardiac and intra-arterial. In 32%, large artery atherosclerotic occlusive disease caused hemodynamic vertebrobasilar ischemia.[11] Distal infarcts, meaning those within the PCA, SCA, and top of the basilar artery territory, had a high likelihood of cardiac or artery-to-artery embolism. Areas that commonly demonstrated stenosis (>50%) included the origin of the vertebral artery in 131 patients (32.2%), intracranial vertebral artery in 132 patients (32.4%), basilar artery in 109 patients (26.8%), and PCA in 38 patients (9.3%). Fourteen percent of patients had penetrating and branch artery disease, meaning disease of the branch artery without disease of the parent artery. Most PCA infarcts were embolic. Patients with cardiac emboli had a poorer prognosis than patients with other stroke mechanisms. Consistent with prior studies, lateral medullary strokes were most often caused by atherosclerotic vertebral artery disease (see section on PICA territory infarcts).

DIZZINESS, VERTIGO, AND VERTEBROBASILAR ISCHEMIA

The clinician must distinguish a few salient symptom characteristics when a patient complains of dizziness. Global cerebral hypoperfusion, such as that caused by orthostatic hypotension, is likely to present with a sense of lightheadedness and an impending fainting sensation. Presyncopal lightheadedness is rather nonspecific and may arise from cardiac arrhythmias, cardiac valvular disease, orthostatic hypotension, and vasovagal reactions. In contrast, vertigo, the sensation of movement of the environment or of oneself, often in a rotational manner, is a common presentation of vertebrobasilar insufficiency, that is, diminished blood flow to the posterior circulation of the brain. Likewise, vertebrobasilar ischemia is a common cause of vertigo in the aging population; therefore, it is critical to distinguish whether the dizziness is vertigo or lightheadedness. Important questions to ask the patient include:

- *"Do you feel as though you are about to pass out?"* This would be consistent with global hypoperfusion.
- *"Do you feel as though the world is moving even when you are sitting still?"* This would be consistent with true vertigo.
- *"How long is the actual vertigo spell, and is the onset abrupt or gradual?"*
- *"How often do the spells occur, and is the frequency of the spells increasing?"*
- *"Are the spells provoked by positional changes of the head?"* This may indicate benign paroxysmal positional vertigo (BPPV), but vertigo from any cause can be associated with sensitivity to head movement. Moving the head or neck may also further compromise blood flow through a stenotic portion of the extracranial vertebral artery, so motion-provoked vertigo may be a sign of, or consistent with, vertebrobasilar ischemia.
- *"Are there any otological accompanying signs with the spells of vertigo: aural fullness, hearing loss, tinnitus?"* These may be indicative of Meniere's disease, and can also be seen in basilar migraine as well as TIAs in the AICA distribution.
- *"Are there any accompanying focal neurologic signs with the spells of vertigo, or in isolation?"* (see Table 16.1). These would be indicative of vertebrobasilar TIAs.

TABLE 16.1
Neurologic Review of Systems

Have you experienced any of the following symptoms? Please check yes or no and indicate if constant or in episodes.
1. Double vision, blurred vision, or blindness
2. Numbness of the face or extremities
3. Weakness in arms or legs
4. Clumsiness in arms or legs
5. Confusion or loss of consciousness
6. Difficulty with speech
7. Difficulty swallowing
8. Pain in neck or shoulder

- *"Is the episode followed by a headache?"* Note that this does not necessarily indicate migraine-associated vertigo: strokes, TIAs, arterial dissections, and seizures are often accompanied by headache.
- *"Is there a personal history of hypertension, hyperlipidemia, diabetes mellitus, cancer, coronary artery disease, peripheral vascular disease, migraine with aura or complicated migraine, strokes, or TIAs in the past?"*
- *"Is there a family history of the above risk factors, hearing loss, dizziness, connective tissue diseases, or migraine?"*

True vertigo is not present with presyncopal lightheadedness. In the case of posterior circulation ischemia, the onset of vertigo is usually abrupt and spontaneous rather than position induced, and there may be a flurry of spells within a few weeks' time.

The Importance of the Neurologic Examination and of Imaging the Vertebrobasilar Arteries

Any patient presenting with vertigo or hearing loss should be evaluated for focal neurologic signs that localize to the brainstem. We typically include in the questionnaire a neurologic review of systems that localizes to the posterior circulation[38] (see Table 16.1).

On examination, the patient presenting with vertigo, with or without hearing loss, should be evaluated for:
1. Facial weakness, which can be peripheral or central in AICA and PICA infarcts;
2. Facial sensory loss, which can be tested using a cold tuning fork or pinprick or by testing the corneal reflex with a cotton tip;
3. Eye movement abnormalities, including skew deviation, diplopia, and nystagmus. Gaze-evoked nystagmus or down-beat nystagmus is typical of a cerebellar infarct;
4. The visual fields; most PCA infarcts exhibit a visual field cut;

5. Crossed sensory loss, which is an important clue for brainstem involvement. This can manifest as ipsilateral loss of facial sensation and contralateral loss of extremities sensation;
6. Horner syndrome, tested in darkness for an ipsilateral smaller pupil because the anisocoria or asymmetry is accentuated in darkness. This occurs because of the loss of sympathetic outflow, which results in pupillary dilation, ptosis, miosis, and anhydrosis.
7. Limb ataxia; tests include finger to nose, finger to finger, and heel to shin;
8. Gait ataxia, which is generally exhibited by a wide-based gait or inability to walk;
9. Truncal ataxia, tested by asking the patient to sit up without back support and with arms crossed;
10. Head impulse test, which can reveal catch-up saccades in purely peripheral disorders, such as vestibular neuritis or gentamicin ototoxicity. However, it is important to note that the head impulse test demonstrates catch-up saccades in up to 70% of patients with an AICA infarct.[39]

Symptoms that may localize to a PICA infarct should be queried, including hiccoughs, inability to swallow, facial sensory and motor loss, and limb ataxia. In a patient with vertigo, hearing should always be tested at the bedside.

It is important to note that most vertebrobasilar ischemic attacks are due to large artery atherosclerosis. Large artery atherosclerosis as an etiologic mechanism of TIA is prone to recurrence or early progression to stroke.[40] In a large study of all consecutive cerebrovascular events (strokes and TIAs), events in the posterior (vertebrobasilar) circulation were more likely to be associated with significant stenosis (26.2%) than those in the anterior (carotid) circulation (11.5%).[41] Therefore imaging studies in this group of patients with posterior circulation events would be high yield. Furthermore, patients with vertebrobasilar TIAs secondary to atherosclerosis are even more likely to suffer early recurrence of a vascular event or progress to a stroke than patients with symptomatic carotid stenosis.[42] For these reasons, the possibility of vertebrobasilar TIA should be assessed with a stroke protocol MRI that includes assessment of the intracranial and extracranial anterior and posterior cerebral vasculature.

In the past, the only way to assess the posterior circulation accurately was to undertake a cerebral angiogram, an invasive procedure with risks. Fortunately, there are now noninvasive means of imaging the posterior circulation using contrast-enhanced MRA (CE-MRA) and CT angiography. CE-MRA has good sensitivity and specificity for the detection of 50%–99% vertebral or basilar stenosis, better than CT angiography, ultrasonography, or time-of-flight MRA.[43] The CE-MRA should image the great vessels from the aortic arch to the circle of Willis. In a large study of patients presenting with posterior circulation events, 39 patients had both CE-MRA and CTA, with corroborating results in 35 patients. In only 4 of 186 patients was it necessary to conduct intra-arterial subtraction angiography.[44] Previously, it was necessary to conduct traditional angiography to evaluate the V1 segment, in particular the origin or take-off of the vertebral artery, as it is not possible to visualize the origin of the vertebral artery well with noncontrast MRA. With the advent of CE-MRA and CTA, noninvasive means of visualizing this area is possible. The V1 and V4 areas were found to be the most common sites of stenosis (42.9% and 34.7%, respectively). Of those with stenosis in the V1 area, 12 of 39 (31%) were at the origin of the vertebral artery, making this the most common single site of stenosis of the vertebral artery.[44]

In patients presenting with symptoms attributable to the posterior circulation, a vertebral artery dissection may also be the cause. In a study by Gulli and colleagues of 216 consecutive posterior circulation strokes, 8 of these were secondary to vertebral artery dissection.[44] With current modern techniques, vertebral dissections can be evaluated using noninvasive imaging, CE-MRA, or CTA. Clinical suspicion for vertebral artery dissection should be high in the middle-aged patient with new-onset posterior circulation neurologic symptoms and severe, lancinating neck pain, usually after a strain or injury.

BEDSIDE EVALUATION OF THE PATIENT WITH ACUTE VESTIBULAR SYNDROME

The next relevant question is how to identify the patient at risk of vertebrobasilar stroke among patients presenting with vertigo. The term *acute vestibular syndrome* refers to a constellation of symptoms that includes vertigo, nystagmus, nausea, vomiting, ataxia, and intolerance of head movement that persists for at least 24 hours. Most of these patients have a peripheral vestibular disturbance, such as vestibular neuritis (see Chapter 10) as the cause of their symptoms; however, approximately 25% of patients with acute vestibular syndrome are found to have a brainstem or cerebellar stroke. In a retrospective, population-based study of patients who had been discharged from the emergency room with a diagnosis of peripheral vertigo, 0.18% of the patients had a stroke within 30 days. The relative risk of stroke within 30 days

was 9.3. To establish a context, qualifying patients were compared with patients diagnosed with renal colic, and it was noted that there was a 50-fold higher risk of stroke in the 7 days after discharge in patients presenting with vertigo than in patients with renal colic.[45] These findings are good reminders that early signs of stroke may mimic peripheral vestibular disorders. In a study of emergency room patients discharged with diagnosis of dizziness in Taiwan, 4.7% later suffered vascular events over a 3-year follow-up period, which was twice that of patients without the diagnosis of dizziness.[46] Newman-Toker argues that the emergency room physician should *not* feel reassured even if the risk of missing a sentinel stroke sign is extremely low.[47] He succinctly summarizes: "This translates to roughly 2600 to 10,500 patients each year in the United States who are told that they have a benign cause [of vertigo] and then suffer serious harms within 1 month."

The HINTS Plus algorithm (**H**ead **I**mpulse test, **N**ystagmus in different fields of gaze, and **T**est for **S**kew, **plus** new onset of hearing loss) has been proposed to distinguish peripheral from central etiologies in patients presenting with acute vestibular syndrome.[48] It is extremely important to note that the current literature reflects performance of HINTS testing by neurotologists and specifically trained neurologists or ophthalmologists. In a cross-sectional survey of emergency room physicians in the Kaiser Permanente Northern California system in 2013, respondents indicated the lowest use of and confidence in applying HINTS and the Epley maneuver as compared with other bedside tests, including gait and Romberg test, cranial nerve testing, limb testing, and application of ABCD2.[49] In a study of HINTS applied to acute vestibular syndrome, hearing loss was present in only 4 of 10 patients with an AICA infarct and the head impulse test was positive (i.e., catch-up saccades present with brief, rapid lateral head impulses) in 30% of patients with an AICA infarct. Skew deviation was present in 4 of 72 patients with vestibular neuritis and was absent in about half of the patients with a PICA infarct and 40% of the patients with an AICA infarct.[39] In these cases, the HINTS protocol demonstrated excellent sensitivity and specificity but required specific training in the correct performance of the HINTS components.

A subset of patients with acute vestibular syndrome demonstrate transient signs and symptoms, with nystagmus and vertigo lasting less than 24 hours. It may not be possible to use the HINTS protocol for these patients. It has been reported that 27% of patients with transient acute vestibular syndrome had ischemia, defined by a deficit on perfusion MRI, often in the cerebellum.[50] The addition of advanced MRI perfusion imaging in this study of transient vestibular syndromes captured posterior circulation ischemia, even when diffusion-weighted imaging (DWI) was negative. Lastly, the authors reported that acute vertigo lasting up to several hours was perfusion positive and often associated with vertebral stenosis, representing a new addition to currently recognized classic presentations of vertebrobasilar TIAs. Traditionally, it has been proposed that vertebrobasilar TIAs last 3–4 minutes and are abrupt in onset. This study demonstrates that acute-onset vertigo lasting up to 10 hours can be a vertebrobasilar TIA. The proposed use of multimodal imaging, which captures perfusion or flow parameters, is an excellent addition to identify the patient at risk of vertebrobasilar stroke.

Acute Vertebrobasilar Occlusion: Intervention Is Possible

Acute vertebrobasilar occlusion occurs when there is an occlusion or complete blockage of the basilar artery. This entity carries an extremely high morbidity and mortality. In young patients, the etiology can be from cardiac emboli or progression from a vertebral artery dissection. Dissections may occur with neck trauma, such as car accidents with whiplash, cervical neck manipulations, or spontaneously with a higher incidence in patients with a personal history of migraine. Local atherothrombosis is more common in elderly patients and in patients with metabolic syndrome. Early percutaneous treatment is associated with improved patient outcomes, and best results are achieved when intervention occurs within 4–6 hours. Even with successful and timely recanalization, the mortality rate is between 35% and 75%. Without intervention, mortality rates are as high as 80%–90%.[51]

Percutaneous interventions for vertebral artery stenosis are now possible. Noninvasive testing that includes Doppler studies can identify vertebral artery stenosis and reversed vertebral artery blood flow. Successful endovascular treatments have been reported in patients with vertebrobasilar stenosis.[52]

Advances in Intervention in Vertebrobasilar Ischemia and Infarcts

An important issue with regard to relying on bedside testing to replace multimodal imaging is that of time: if time is brain then the amount of time needed to perform further bedside testing to determine whether to conduct an MRI can result in a critical time delay in initiating immediate interventions. In the anterior circulation, this has been quantified: 1 minute earlier of endovascular thrombectomy DNT gains an average of more than 7 days of disability-free life in a patient under age 55 years.[53] Eligible patients must receive intravenous tPA and endovascular thrombectomy as quickly as possible because every minute saved results in quantifiably improved quality of life. This may also apply to basilar artery occlusion; clinical trials are under way.[54] In a retrospective single-center study, shorter delays in initiating intra-arterial therapy were associated with recanalization success and good neurologic outcomes in patients with acute basilar artery thrombosis.[55] Another single-center retrospective study demonstrated a favorable functional outcome following intra-arterial therapy in 50% of patients with basilar artery occlusion.[56a] Historically, basilar artery thrombosis managed with antiplatelet and/or anticoagulant therapy alone results in poor outcomes. Data from the Basilar Artery International Cooperation Study (BASICS), a prospective multicenter registry of patients with radiologically confirmed basilar artery occlusion has demonstrated that patients had a significantly increased likelihood of good functional outcome, as time to recanalization therapy is shorter with 35% of those treated within 6 hours having a good outcome compared with only 23% of those treated between 6 and 9 hours having a good outcome; beyond 9 hours, the prognosis was dismal.[56b] Of note, basilar artery occlusion strokes in 204 of 409 patients were preceded by prodromal symptoms, often recurrent vertigo spells, in 50% of these patients. Clinicians who see patients with vertigo must be alerted to refer patients to vascular neurologists promptly if vertebrobasilar ischemia is suspected.[56b] In a comparison of endovascular treatment with conservative intravenous or medical treatment for basilar artery occlusion, 45% of the endovascular-treated patients and none of the conservative treatment group had a favorable functional outcome.[57] These studies universally demonstrate that time is brainstem, and rapid endovascular treatment is the key to a good clinical outcome.

Peripheral Versus Central Causes of Vertigo in Vertebrobasilar Insufficiency

Common peripheral causes of vertigo include well-known otologic entities such as BPPV, vestibular neuritis, and Meniere's disease. Dizziness and imbalance are common problems among the elderly, with a population-based study reporting a prevalence of 24% of persons over age 72 years.[58] BPPV accounted for 39% of all cases of vertigo in the older population presenting to neurotology clinics.[59] Older individuals are also a well-known higher-risk group for cerebrovascular disease and stroke. Thus the presentation of an older patient with vertigo must address the issue of a cerebrovascular etiology, in particular vertebrobasilar ischemia.

A labyrinthine infarct is a peripheral cause of vertigo, and vestibular testing is typically read as "peripheral vestibular pathology with no signs of central involvement." However, a labyrinthine infarct can be a warning of an impending AICA infarct, which may be secondary to basilar artery thrombosis.[30] When dizziness is accompanied by other neurologic symptoms and signs, such as ataxia, sensory loss, visual loss, or a unilateral Horner sign, the diagnosis of a brainstem infarct is easily made. However, a TIA in the vertebrobasilar system may present with isolated vertigo or hearing loss, and clinicians need to consider that impending stroke is part of the differential diagnoses until ruled out conclusively. This is true even in BPPV, as estimates are that nearly 5% are secondary to vertebrobasilar insufficiency.[60] In fact, animal studies have demonstrated instability of otoconia after an ischemic attack of the labyrinthine artery.

Vertigo as a Presentation of Vertebrobasilar Insufficiency

Dizziness is likely the most common presenting complaint among patients 75 years and older in outpatient clinics, and dizziness accounted for 2.5% of all US Emergency Department presentations during the 10-year period from 1995 to 2004.[61,62] It was noted that the rate of visits for vertigo and dizziness increased each year, increasing by 37% over the decade with a disproportionate increase in the older population. The study reported a 67% increase in emergency room visits in patients over age 65 years compared with a 15% increase for those aged 45–64 years. This may be due in part to increasing public awareness that vertigo can be a sign of TIA, stroke, or impending stroke.

Studies have demonstrated that isolated vertigo can be the presentation of vertebrobasilar ischemia, and in fact, vertigo is the most common initial isolated symptom and sign of ischemia in the posterior circulation (see Table 16.1). It is critical that clinicians and emergency room physicians understand that transient vertebrobasilar ischemia, especially of the labyrinth, may not be evident on imaging studies. In a study of 42 patients with vertigo caused by vertebrobasilar insufficiency, there was a high incidence of isolated episodes of vertigo: 62% had at least one isolated episode of vertigo, and in 19% of these patients, the TIAs began with an isolated episode of vertigo.[63] Some patients with isolated vertigo attacks secondary to vertebrobasilar insufficiency also report transient focal neurologic symptoms such as visual loss or motor weakness, suggesting transient vertebrobasilar ischemia. In the classic synopsis on vertebrobasilar insufficiency, Williams and

TABLE 16.2
Initial Symptoms of Vertebrobasilar Insufficiency in 65 Patients

Symptoms	Number of Patients (Percentage)
Vertigo	32 (48)
Visual hallucinations	7 (10)
Drop attacks or weakness	7 (10)
Visceral sensations	5 (8)
Visual field defects	4 (6)
Diplopia	3 (5)
Headaches	2 (3)
Other	5 (8)

From Williams D, Wilson TG. The diagnosis of the major and minor syndromes of basilar insufficiency. *Brain*. 1962;85:741–774; with permission.

Wilson noted that vertigo was the initial symptom in 48% of the patients[38] (Table 16.2).

In addition to vertigo, visual symptoms such as diplopia, field defects, or illusions were the most common, noted in 69% of patients; other common symptoms noted in vertebrobasilar insufficiency were drop attacks in 33%, unsteadiness in 21%, confusion in 17%, headache in 14%, hearing loss in 14%, loss of consciousness in 10%, extremity numbness in 10%, dysarthria in 10%, and perioral numbness in 5%. Typically, the vertigo in vertebrobasilar TIAs is abrupt in onset and usually lasts several minutes; however, studies report vertigo spells lasting up to 10 hours, which may be accompanied by visual symptoms, dysarthria, extremity numbness, or drop attacks. Patients describe vertebrobasilar ischemic drop attacks as a buckling of the knees and bilateral lower extremity weakness, with or without a loss of consciousness.[38] This was first described by Kremer as being caused by a brainstem dysfunction, as a clinical entity, without imaging or angiographic evidence.[64] The clinical description remains accurate: "folding up at the knees." In contrast, drop attacks associated with Meniere's disease (i.e., otolithic crisis of Tumarkin) are characterized by a feeling of being pushed as if by an external force, and there is no loss of consciousness.[65]

Patients with vertebrobasilar ischemia have a very high prevalence of stroke risk factors

In a study of consecutive patients presenting to a large stroke center, the New England Medical Center Posterior Circulation Registry, the group of patients with extensive atherosclerotic disease involving the basilar artery had a very high prevalence of stroke risk factors. Hypertension was present in 70% and coronary artery disease in 60%. All patients with extensive atherosclerotic disease had one or more stroke risk factors. In all patients with posterior circulation disease, stroke risk factors with high incidence included hypertension (58%), smoking (42%), diabetes mellitus (24.7%), and hyperlipidemia (19%). Comorbidity of coronary artery disease (42%) and peripheral vascular disease (11%) was common. Other important modifiable lifestyle factors associated with stroke include alcohol abuse (13%), obesity (11%), and oral contraceptive pill use (2%).[66]

It is generally accepted that medical therapies in atherosclerotic disease should include lipid-lowering therapy. Regression of the stenosis has been demonstrated after 6 months of a statin lipid-lowering therapy in patients with intracranial arterial stenosis. Notably, there was a higher success rate with middle cerebral artery stenosis (59% of the 41 patients had regression) compared with basilar artery stenosis (38% of the 13 patients had regression).[67] Observational studies have reported rates of between 8% and 29% of regression and as high as 9%–33% progression in symptomatic intracranial stenosis.[68,69] However, the degree of regression of stenosis was not correlated with the degree of lipid lowering, as there were no differences in lipid profiles among patients.[67] This study was characterized by a relatively small number of participating patients, and there was no clear evidence for an improvement in clinical parameters associated with the regression of intracranial stenosis, and thus future, longitudinal studies are warranted.

Benign paroxysmal positional vertigo is associated with vertebrobasilar insufficiency

BPPV is likely the most common cause of vestibular vertigo, and there is a markedly increased incidence of BPPV in older subjects (see Chapter 9). In a large cross-sectional neurotologic survey, the 1-year prevalence of BPPV in subjects older than 60 years was nearly seven times higher than that of subjects 18–39 years old and the cumulative incidence of BPPV reached almost 10% by the age of 80 years.[70] However, although BPPV is a peripheral cause of vertigo spells, in a study of 240 consecutive patients with BPPV, 11 patients had typical symptoms of vertebrobasilar insufficiency.[60] The association between BPPV and vertebrobasilar ischemia may be caused by transient ischemia to the vestibular end organs resulting in otolith degradation or loosening of otoconia from the otolithic membrane. Inner ear

microvascular ischemia is believed to also mediate the association between migraine and BPPV.[71] Therefore, in the evaluation of a patient presenting with BPPV, the clinician should ask about symptoms related to vertebrobasilar insufficiency. Particular attention should be paid to these symptoms in the older patient with vascular risk factors noted previously.

The natural course of vertebral or basilar artery stenosis: a high risk of early recurrent stroke

It is critical for the clinician to recognize the first vertebrobasilar TIAs. Contrary to traditional beliefs, there seems to be a higher risk of stroke after vertebrobasilar TIAs than after carotid TIAs.[72,73] Furthermore, a meta-analysis has suggested that the risk of recurrent stroke is as high or higher for vertebrobasilar stroke as that for carotid stroke.[72] Using CE-MRA, and CT angiography when MRA could not be conducted (pacemaker or claustrophobia), Marquardt et al. evaluated consecutively presenting patients with vertebrobasilar ischemia and large artery stenosis. About 26% of patients (37 of 141) presenting with vertebrobasilar TIAs or stroke had significant vertebral or basilar stenosis.[41] Of these, there was a very high risk of 90-day recurrence of stroke (22%) and TIA or stroke (46%), despite medical management, which included aspirin, a statin, and antihypertensive treatment. Even in patients without large vessel stenosis, 21% had a posterior circulation event within 90 days of the initial symptoms. Vertebrobasilar events were associated with multiple TIAs shortly before first seeking medical attention, especially among patients with vertebrobasilar stenosis. Of interest, patients presenting with posterior circulation events with stenosis did not differ from those without stenosis with regard to treatable vascular risk factors, such as hypertension and hyperlipidemia.[41] Therefore, one cannot predict which patients are at higher risk for vertebrobasilar stenosis simply based on the presence and number of risk factors.

A study by Gulli and colleagues reported similar findings and added that visual disturbances, motor weakness, sensory disturbance, unsteadiness, ataxia, and vertigo were common transient precursors to posterior circulation stroke or TIA within 30–90 days. These reports highlight the recognition that the presence of stenosis in the vertebrobasilar distribution is a strong independent predictor of future stroke.

Another significant predictor of stroke after TIA is the presence of any lesions on DWI on MRI. In a study of 343 consecutive patients with TIA, DWI was positive in 40%. A total of 15 patients had strokes within 3 months, and in all but 1 patient, early strokes occurred in patients with DWI findings. The absolute risk of stroke after TIA was 1.5% at 7 days and 2.9% at 3 months. Patients with TIA with a positive DWI study result are approximately 10 times more likely to have a TIA or stroke than those with a negative DWI study.[74]

The bottom line is that vertebrobasilar insufficiency and posterior circulation events are highly likely to recur in patients with vertebrobasilar stenosis, apparently despite medical management. There are no apparent risk factors to predict which patients have large artery atherosclerotic stenosis; therefore, all patients need to be evaluated promptly for stenosis to identify which patients are at an increased risk for stroke recurrence. Patients with significant vertebrobasilar stenosis may be candidates for interventional procedures to prevent recurrences, and thus assessment by a stroke or interventional neuroradiologist should be timely. Vertebral angioplasty or stenting may be indicated, and initial studies show low complication rates.[75,76]

Anterior Inferior Cerebellar Artery Territory Infarcts and Audiovestibular Symptoms

Several studies have noted the association of hearing loss and prolonged vertigo associated with an AICA territory infarct.[25,77] A temporal bone histopathology study of a patient who had an AICA territory infarct showed complete loss of the sensory epithelium of the cochlea and vestibular labyrinth, indicative of labyrinthine infarct.[78] In a series of patients with AICA infarcts, five patients experienced abrupt onset of sensorineural hearing loss.[25] It is important for clinicians to realize that sudden deafness, tinnitus, or vertigo spells can occur as a TIA or infarct in the AICA distribution. Typically, audiovestibular TIAs occur with an abrupt onset, last a minute to a few minutes, and may precede the stroke by a few days to a few months.

Lee et al. conducted the largest and most complete study including complete auditory and vestibular testing of 82 consecutive patients with documented AICA infarcts.[79] The most common and dominant symptom was acute spontaneous prolonged (>24 hours) vertigo, with nausea and vomiting occurring in 80 of 82 patients (98%). The most common presentation of inner ear dysfunction was combined prolonged vertigo and hearing loss in 49 of 82 patients (60%). Of those with combined auditory and vestibular infarct, 13 had brief transient spells of vertigo or hearing loss lasting a few minutes within the month before the infarct. Isolated vestibular infarction without cochlear involvement was rare (5%), as was isolated cochlear infarction without vestibular involvement (3%). Electronystagmography

(ENG) testing revealed caloric paresis in 53 of 82 patients (65%), and nearly all had abnormal optokinetic or smooth pursuit eye movement findings or vestibulo-ocular reflex deficits (96%).

The Lee et al. study noted that patients with prodromal audiovestibular disturbances had a five times higher prevalence of severe basilar artery occlusive disease than those without prodromal audiovestibular disturbance (62% vs. 13%, $P<.001$). Given the low incidence of pure auditory or pure vestibular loss, the authors speculated that internal auditory artery ischemia seldom results in selective involvement of the anterior vestibular artery or main cochlear artery. Conversely, there is strong support for vascular ischemia or infarct in patients presenting with acute onset of combined auditory and vestibular loss.

In a study that followed up 12 consecutive patients with AICA infarcts, sensorineural hearing loss was identified in 11 (92%). Four of the patients had brief spells of hearing loss and/or tinnitus lasting a few minutes or isolated vertigo spells occurring from 1 day to 2 months before the AICA infarct. Audiologic testing in six patients revealed cochlear site of hearing loss. One patient had normal hearing, one had retrocochlear hearing loss, and four had hearing loss too profound to determine the site. In seven patients, there was variable recovery of hearing. On vestibular testing, the ENG showed unilaterally absent caloric response in 10 patients and a diminished caloric response in the other two patients, indicative of a labyrinthine infarct in the vestibular horizontal SCC. Optokinetic and smooth pursuit abnormalities were present in 11 patients.[26] These patients may present to neurologists, neurotologists, or general otolaryngologists. The key characteristics of the prodromal hearing loss or vertigo spells are the abrupt onset and duration of one to a few minutes. Of course, if there are accompanying neurologic complaints (e.g., facial palsy, ataxia, diminished sensation), the suspicion for a cerebrovascular event is raised. However, the vertigo or hearing loss/tinnitus may occur as isolated symptoms.

Because the labyrinthine artery has little or no collateralization with other arterial sources, the hearing loss in an AICA infarct would be predicted to be cochlear in etiology. In animal studies, the stria vascularis, spiral ligament, the organ of Corti, and spiral ganglion are strikingly vulnerable to occlusion of the AICA.[80] Furthermore, the retrocochlear cochlear nerve has abundant collateralization; therefore it is likely that in most cases, hearing loss in an AICA TIA or infarct stems from cochlear damage.[81] The vertigo may derive from the labyrinth (given caloric abnormalities) or the cerebellum and pons (given oculomotor abnormalities); however, given that the cerebellum and pons have more collateralization, the labyrinth is more likely the source of early brief spells of spontaneous vertigo.

The most common etiology for an AICA infarct is thrombosis or atheromatous formation of the basilar artery, blocking the origin of the AICA as noted in conventional angiography.[82] More recently, in a study of 23 consecutive patients with AICA infarcts, large artery atherosclerotic disease in the vertebrobasilar system was the main cause of stroke in 12 patients (52%), with coexisting large artery disease and cardiac embolic source in 4 patients (17%).[83] The most common MRA abnormality in a report by Lee and colleagues was diffuse or focal stenosis near the AICA origin of the basilar artery (20%). They also found that areas of infarct demonstrated on MRI were commonly the middle cerebellar peduncle (83%), anterior inferior cerebellum (46%), and lateral inferior pons (44%), with complete AICA infarction in 16%. Also, patients with basilar stenosis tended to have AICA infarcts as well as multiple posterior circulation infarcts. Lastly, it was previously reported that AICA infarcts have a high incidence of neurologic deficits localizing to the pons, whereas these brainstem deficits were relatively less frequent than expected: facial weakness (21%), facial sensory loss (28%), and body sensory loss (only 6%). Only 2 of the 82 patients had the complete syndrome as described by Adams.[84]

AICA infarcts may also occur in the setting of vertebrobasilar dolichoectasia, which is an elongation, tortuosity, and distension of the vertebrobasilar arteries. The basilar artery is most often affected, but the intracranial vertebral arteries can also be involved. Hypertensive and diabetic older subjects are more likely to develop dolichoectasia.[85] Thrombus can form in areas of turbulent flow and then embolize distally. Episodic symptoms may indicate that ischemia is caused by a thrombus blocking the origin of smaller branches such as the AICA, *or may be caused by* artery-to-artery embolic phenomenon. Episodic symptoms may indicate that ischemia is caused by thrombus blocking the origin of smaller branches such as AICA or by an artery-to-artery embolic phenomenon. On the other hand, progressive neurologic symptoms are more likely secondary to direct compression.[86] Both etiologies would be well visualized using noninvasive studies, such as CE-MRA or CT angiography.

Posterior inferior cerebellar artery syndrome or lateral medullary infarction

The classical syndrome associated with an infarct in the PICA distribution or dorsolateral medullary infarct has been termed "Wallenberg syndrome". Major symptoms include vertigo with nausea and vomiting secondary to vestibular nuclei or posteroinferior cerebellar infarct, severe imbalance likely related to damage to the cerebellum or cerebellar tracts, ipsilateral facial numbness (cranial nerve V and its nucleus), ipsilateral facial palsy (peripheral or central), crossed hemisensory loss (involvement of the sensory dorsal column tracts), dysphagia and dysphonia (due to involvement of the nucleus ambiguus). In a large study of 33 consecutive patients presenting with PICA infarcts, the most common symptom was vertigo (91%), followed by gait ataxia (88%), nausea/ vomiting (73%), nystagmus (67%), Horner's sign (73%), dysphagia (61%), hoarseness (55%), facial sensory change (85%) and hemibody sensory change (94%), mild central facial paresis (36%), mild hemiparesis (12%). Important to note is the very high proportion of symptoms in common with acute vestibular syndrome: vertigo, ataxia, nausea and vomiting, and nystagmus.[87] The authors identified what they termed "rostral" and "caudal" patient groups, based on MRI findings, which correlated with symptom clustering. The rostral group often had severe dysphagia, but only one had nystagmus in the primary gaze position. In the caudal group, none of the patients had dysphagia, whereas vertigo and gait ataxia were severe, and nystagmus was prominent in the primary gaze position. Kim conducted the largest study of pure lateral medullary infarction without cerebellar involvement in 130 consecutive patients (see Table 16.3).[88] The symptom clustering was similar, with patients who had rostral lesions exhibiting severe dysphagia, facial paresis, and dysarthria more often than patients with caudal lesions, and severe gait ataxia and headache less often than patients with caudal lesions.

Studies using both MRA and conventional angiograms demonstrate a high prevalence of vertebral artery disease, confirming findings of older studies of postmortem histopathology.[89] Large vessel infarction is common in lateral medullary syndrome, whereas arterial dissection, small vessel infarction, and cardiac embolism are less common.[88] Caudal lesions appear to be associated with dissection. In addition, isolated PICA pathology without vertebral artery pathology was more often secondary to cardioembolism.

Although most patients with lateral medullary stroke exhibit other neurologic deficits localizing to the brainstem, there are case reports of patients who presented with only vertigo and gait ataxia, without limb ataxia on examination. In these patients, there is strong lateropulsion toward the ipsilateral side causing inability to walk.[90] Clinicians may mistakenly diagnose this presentation as an inner ear disorder, as the lesion

TABLE 16.3

Frequency of Symptoms in 130 Consecutive Lateral Medullary Infarcts Without Cerebellar Involvement

Sensory symptoms and signs	125 (96%)
Gait ataxia	120 (92%)[a]
Horner sign	114 (88%)
Dysphagia	84 (65%)[b]
Dysarthria	28 (22%)[b]
Vertigo	74 (57%)
Nystagmus	73 (56%)
Limb ataxia	72 (55%)
Nausea and vomiting	67 (52%)
Headache	67 (52%)[a]
Skew deviation of eyes	53 (41%)
Diplopia	41 (32%)
Hiccoughs	33 (25%)
Facial palsy	27 (21%)[b]

[a]More common or severe in caudal group.
[b]More common or severe in rostral group.
From Kim JS. Pure lateral medullary infarction: clinical-radiological correlation of 130 acute, consecutive patients. *Brain*. 2003;126: 1864–1872; with permission.

may be small and missed on MRI. A key clinical difference in patients with lateral medullary stroke is the very strong lateropulsion, a prominent motor disturbance that causes a deviation toward the side of the lesion resulting in severe postural dyscontrol.[91] In contrast, with peripheral vestibular lesions, patients may fall or veer toward the affected side, but they are usually able to walk. Patients with stroke may also have a concomitant skew deviation, an ocular tilt reaction, and a head tilt.[92] The HINTS protocol may be particularly useful in identifying these patients.

Superior cerebellar artery infarcts are mainly embolic

The dominant features of SCA infarcts are ipsilateral limb ataxia, vertigo, nystagmus, and cerebellar signs, including dysarthria and gait ataxia. A study of 60 patients with SCA infarcts demonstrated that embolism was the predominant stroke mechanism, with artery-to-artery embolism from atherosclerotic vertebrobasilar artery disease in 20 of 60 (33%). Fourteen patients had a cardioembolic source (23%), and 10 patients had multiple lesions in the SCA and other vertebrobasilar

territories.[93] Previous studies also demonstrated the predominance of cardiac embolism as a source in SCA infarcts, with one study reporting 12 of 30[94] and another reporting 11 of 30.[95]

Basilar migraine and migraine-associated vertebrobasilar strokes

In 1961, Bickerstaff described a variant of migraine exhibiting symptoms localized to the posterior circulation.[96] In describing the alteration of consciousness that occurs in basilar migraine, Bickerstaff noted that it was "curiously slow in onset" and that patients seemed to be in a deep sleep. It has been proposed that this occurs secondary to dysfunction of the brainstem tegmentum. Hallmark symptoms associated with basilar migraine include the following:

- Visual symptoms in both temporal and nasal fields of both eyes
- Dysarthria
- Vertigo
- Tinnitus
- Decreased hearing
- Diplopia
- Ataxia
- Bilateral paresthesias
- Bilateral pareses
- Decreased level of consciousness

Olsson conducted a prospective study of 50 patients with basilar migraine and documented low-frequency sensorineural hearing loss in more than half of these patients.[97] Cutrer and Baloh described the spells of migraine-associated vertigo and reported 30% having spells lasting a few minutes to 2 hours and 49% having spells lasting more than 24 hours.[98] It is evident that the symptoms in basilar migraine are similar to those of vertebrobasilar insufficiency. Furthermore, although the original report described young adolescent girls with basilar migraine, there is evidence that basilar migraine can occur in middle-aged or elderly patients. The role of vasoconstriction and microvascular ischemia in migraine and migrainous aura is complex. Patients with migraine are reported to be sensitive to angiography, which can precipitate a migrainous attack. Migrainous aura may sometimes become permanent, and on evaluation it may be recognized that a stroke has occurred. The International Headache Society criteria for migrainous cerebral infarction include the following: (1) that the patient exhibits one or more migrainous aura symptoms not fully reversible within 7 days; (2) neuroimaging confirmation of ischemic infarction; (3) the present attack is typical of prior attacks, but neurologic deficits are not reversible within 7 days; and/or (4) neuroimaging shows an infarct in the relevant area in a patient who meets criteria for migraine with neurologic aura.[99]

To complicate matters for determining etiology, there are many disorders associated with strokes and migraine headaches, including antiphospholipid syndrome; mitochondrial myopathy, encephalopathy, lactic acidosis, and stroke (MELAS); and cerebral autosomal dominant arteriopathy with subcortical infarcts and leukoencephalopathy (CADACIL). There is likely a predominance of vertebrobasilar strokes associated with migrainous stroke. Bogousslavsky et al. reported nine PCA infarcts and two brainstem and cerebellar strokes among 22 patients with migrainous stroke.[100]

Patients who have migraine with aura seem to have a higher frequency of infarcts than those with common migraine, and the use of tryptans is considered contraindicated in basilar migraine. In patients with migraine who have transient unilateral hearing loss and tinnitus, we recommend the use of verapamil as the first-line agent, and we agree that tryptans would be relatively contraindicated.[101] In a longitudinal study of 18,725 patients (9044 men and 968 women) conducted in Iceland with a median follow-up period of 25.9 years, current, active migraine with aura was associated with an increased risk for cardiovascular disease mortality (hazard ratio 1.27) and greater risk of mortality from stroke (hazard ratio 1.40). There was no increased risk for persons with migraine without aura or non-migraine headache. In the Atherosclerosis Risk in Community study of 12,758 participants, migraine with visual aura in the late middle age was associated with an increased risk of cardioembolic stroke.[102] However, the added risk is likely to be modifiable with smoking cessation and effective management of hyperlipidemia and hypertension. Data from the Women's Health Study (n = 27,860 women 45 years or older) noted that women who had active migraine with aura had twice the risk for hemorrhagic stroke (hazard ratio 2.25).[103] Further studies are needed to evaluate whether this is related to medication treatment for the migrainous aura or some other comorbidity. In a study of patients with migraine, there was no correlation with excess atherosclerosis in large vessels in patients who had acute ischemic stroke.[104]

Modifiable risk factors and noninvasive medical interventions aimed at preventing vertebrobasilar stroke progression and recurrence

In a prospective study of 794 patients following first-time ischemic strokes of multiple types, the use of statins (fluvastatin, pravastatin, simvastatin, and atorvastatin) was associated with a significantly lower rate of secondary stroke (16% of those not receiving statins vs. 7.6% of those receiving statins had a recurrent stroke).[105] Those receiving statins also had an overall improved survival rate. The mechanism is likely not merely lowering of cholesterol but also other proposed mechanisms, including antithrombotic, antioxidative, antiinflammatory, vasodilatory, or plaque-stabilizing properties of statins. The evidence-based guidelines for the management of risk factors to prevent the first stroke have been published and updated.[106,107] The new American College of Cardiology and American Heart Association 2017 recommendations include treatment of hypertension to <130/80 in nondiabetic patients, who have a history of cardiac disease or stroke, abstention from tobacco, and tightly controlled hypertension for diabetic patients (<130/80 mm Hg) as primary or secondary cardiovascular and stroke prevention. Most recently, the American College of Cardiology and the American Heart Association Task Force published new guidelines for targeting a blood pressure of less than 130 mm Hg in elderly patients with hypertension, and guidelines for high-risk vascular patients may also change. The treatment of adults with diabetes with a statin to lower the risk of a first stroke is recommended. Other recommendations include screening for diabetes with HbA1C, screening for obesity with body mass index assessment, Mediterranean diet (class IIa, level of evidence C), sleep study/management of sleep apnea (class IIb, level of evidence B), and increased physical exercise.

In summary, vertigo may be the presenting symptom of a patient with vertebrobasilar ischemia. In fact, dizziness and vertigo are the most common symptoms of vertebrobasilar ischemia. Additionally, greater than 50% of patients with vertebrobasilar strokes due to basilar artery occlusion have prodromal vertigo spells before the strokes. These patients have a high risk of stroke recurrence or progression following a TIA, and prompt and accurate assessment and early intervention are critical for positive patient outcomes. The 90-day risk of stroke after a first event of TIA or stroke in patients with vertebrobasilar stenosis was nearly three times higher than in patients without stenosis. This demonstrates the predictive power of neuroimaging; patients with vertebrobasilar stenosis and potential TIAs (vertigo) should be referred for intensive medical treatment or other interventions. Multimodal imaging should include evaluation of the vasculature, and sensitivity is increased by perfusion imaging.

Cerebellar infarctions may mimic acute vestibular syndromes, and AICA infarction can present with catch-up saccades in the head impulse test, making the use of HINTS to diagnose AICA infarcts more challenging. It is important to note that the HINTS protocol cannot be used if the patient no longer has vertigo/nystagmus. For these reasons, the authors advocate the use of multimodal imaging to evaluate the vasculature and identify these high-risk patients. Just as in symptomatic and asymptomatic significant carotid stenosis, symptomatic vertebrobasilar stenosis is now recognized as a high-risk factor for stroke recurrence or progression, and prospective studies demonstrate that patients had an increased likelihood of good outcome if early treatment is initiated.

REFERENCES

1. Halmagyi GM, Curthoys IS. A clinical sign of canal paresis. *Arch Neurol.* 1988;45:737–739.
2. Saver JL. Time is brain-quantified. *Stroke.* 2006;37:263–266.
3. Saver JL, Goyal M, Bonafe A, et al. Stent-retriever thrombectomy after intravenous t-PA vs. t-PA alone in stroke. *N Engl J Med.* 2015;372(24):2285–2295.
4. Campbell BCV, Hill MD, Rubiera M, et al. Safety and efficacy of Solitaire stent thrombectomy: individual patient data meta-analysis of randomized trials. *Stroke.* 2016;47:798–806.
5. Van den Berg LA, Dijkgraaf MG, Berkhemer OA, et al. Two-year outcome after endovascular treatment for acute ischemic stroke. *N Engl J Med.* 2017;376(14):1341–1349.
6. Coutinho JM, Liebeskind DS, Slater LA, et al. Combined intravenous thrombolysis and thrombectomy vs. thrombectomy alone for acute ischemic stroke: a pooled analysis of the SWIFT and STAR studies. *JAMA Neurol.* 2017;74(3):268–274.
7. Goyal M, Menon BK, van Zwam WH, et al. Endovascular thrombectomy after large-vessel ischaemic stroke: a meta-analysis of individual patient data from five randomized trials. *Lancet.* 2016;387:1723–1731.
8. Prabhakaran S, Soltanolkotabi M, Honarmand AR, et al. Perfusion-based selection for endovascular reperfusion therapy in anterior circulation acute ischemic stroke. *Am J Neuroradiol.* 2014;35(7):1303–1308.
9. Lansberg MG, Christensen S, Kemp S, et al. Albers GW for CRISP investigators. CT perfusion to predict response to recanalization in ischemic stroke. *Ann Neurol.* 2017. https://doi.org/10.1002/ana.24953.
10. Caplan LR. Vertebrobasilar disease. *Adv Neurol.* 2003;92:131–140.
11. Caplan LR, Wityk RJ, Glass TA, et al. New England Medical Center posterior circulation registry. *Ann Neurol.* 2004;56:389–398.
12. Gulli G, Marquardt L, Rothwell PM, Markus HS. Stroke risk after posterior circulation stroke/transient ischemic attack and its relationship to site of vertebrobasilar stenosis: pooled data analysis from prospective studies. *Stroke.* 2013;44:598–604.
13. Sarraj A, Medrek S, Albright K, et al. Posterior circulation stroke is associated with prolonged door-to-needle time. *Int J Stroke.* 2015;10(5):672–678.
14. Sommer P, Seyfang L, Posekany A, et al. Prehospital and intra-hospital time delays in posterior circulation stroke: results from the Austrian stroke unit registry. *J Neurol.* 2017;264:131–138.
15. Aroor S, Singh R, Goldstein LB. BE-FAST (balance, eyes, face, arm, speech, time) reducing the proportion of strokes missed using the FAST mnemonic. *Stroke.* 2017;48:479–481.
16. Liebeskind DS. Editorial commentary: beyond the guidelines to expertise in precision stroke medicine. *Trends Cardiovasc Med.* 2017;27:67–68.
17. Hinman JD, Rost NS, Leung TW, et al. Principles of precision medicine in stroke. *J Neurol Neurosurg Psychiatry.* 2017;88:54–61.
18. Kelly PJ, Albers GW, Chatzikonstantinou A, et al. Validation and comparison of imaging-based scores for prediction of early stroke risk after transient ischaemic attack: a pooled analysis of individual-patient data from cohort studies. *Lancet Neurol.* 2016;15:1238–1247.
19. De Cocker LJ, Compter A, Kappelle LJ, Luijten PR, Hendrikse J, Van der Worp HB. Cerebellar cortical infarct cavities and vertebral artery disease. *Neuroradiology.* 2016;58(9):853–857.
20. Boyajian RA, Schwend RB, Wolfe MM, Bickerton RE, Otis SM. Measurement of anterior and posterior circulation flow contributions to cerebral blood flow contributions to cerebral blood flow. An ultrasound-derived volumetric flow analysis. *J Neuroimag.* 1995;5:1–3.
21. Cloud GC, Markus HS. Diagnosis and management of vertebral artery stenosis. *Q J Med.* 2003;96:27–54.
22. Stopford JSB. The arteries of the pons and medulla oblongata. *J Anat Physiol.* 1916;50:130–164.
23. Schmid-Schonbein H, Perktold K. Physical factors in the pathogenesis of atheroma formation. In: Caplan LR, ed. *Brain Ischemia: from Basic Science to Treatment.* London: Springer-Verlag Press; 1995.
24. Margolis MT, Newton TH. The posterior inferior cerebellar artery. In: Newton TH, Potts DG, eds. *Radiology of the Skull and Brain.* vol. 2. St. Louis: CV Mosby; 1974.
25. Matsushita K, Naritomi H, Kazui S, et al. Infarction in the anterior inferior cerebellar artery territory: magnetic resonance imaging and auditory brain stem responses. *Cerebrovasc Dis.* 1993;3:206–212.
26. Lee H, Sohn SI, Jung DK, et al. Sudden deafness and anterior inferior cerebellar artery infarction. *Stroke.* 2002;33(12):2807–2812.
27. Stevens RB, Stillwell DL. *Arteries and Veins of the Human Brain.* Springfield, Ill: CC Thomas; 1969.
28. Nakashima T, Naganawa S, Sone M, et al. Disorders of cochlear blood flow. *Brain Res Rev.* 2003;43:17–28.
29. Konishi T, Butler RA, Fernandez C. Effect of anoxia on cochlear potentials. *J Acoust Soc Am.* 1961;33:349–355.
30. Kim JS, Lee H. Inner ear dysfunction due to vertebrobasilar ischemic stroke. *Semin Neurol.* 2009;29:534–540.

31. Caplan LR. Brain embolism, revisited. *Neurology*. 1993;43: 1281–1287.

32. Keilson GR, Schwartz WJ, Recht LD. The preponderance of posterior circulation circulatory events is independent of the route of cardiac catheterization. *Stroke*. 1992;23:1358–1359.

33. Schievink WI, Michels W, Piepgras DG. Neurovascular complications of heritable connective tissue disorders. *Stroke*. 1994;25:889–903.

34. Johnsson LF, Hawkins JE. Vascular changes in the human ear associated with aging. *Ann Otol Rhinol Laryngol*. 1972;81:364–376.

35. Wright CG, Schuknecht HF. Atrophy of the spiral ligament. *Arch Otolaryngol*. 1972;96:16–21.

36. Ishiyama G, Tokita J, Lopez I, Ishiyama A. Unbiased stereological estimation of the spiral ligament and stria vascularis volumes in aging and Meniere's disease using archival human temporal bones. *J Assoc Res Otolaryngol*. 2007;8(1):8–17.

37. Lyon MF, Wanamaker HH. Blood flow and assessment of capillaries in the aging rat posterior canal crista. *Hear Res*. 1993;67(1-2):157–165.

38. Williams D, Wilson TG. The diagnosis of the major and minor syndromes of basilar insufficiency. *Brain*. 1962;85:741–774.

39. Carmona S, Martinez C, Zalazar G, et al. The diagnostic accuracy of truncal ataxia and HINTS as cardinal signs for acute vestibular syndrome. *Front Neurol*. 2016;7:125.

40. Purroy F, Montaner J, Molina CA, Delgado P, Ribo M, Alvarez-Sabin J. Patterns and predictors of early risk of recurrence after transient ischemic attack with respect to etiologic subtypes. *Stroke*. 2007;38:3225–3229.

41. Marquardt L, Kuker W, Chandratheva A, Geraghty O, Rothwell PM. Incidence and prognosis of ≥50% symptomatic vertebral or basilar artery stenosis: prospective population-based study. *Brain*. 2009;132:982–988.

42. Flossmann E, Touze E, Giles MF, Lovelock CE, Rothwell M. The early risk of stroke after vertebrobasilar TIA is higher than after carotid TIA (abstract). *Cerebrovasc Dis*. 2006;219(suppl 4):6.

43. Khan S, Cloud G, Kerry S, Markus HS. Imaging of vertebral artery stenosis: a systematic review. *J Neurol Neurosurg Psychiatry*. 2007;78:1218–1225.

44. Gulli G, Khan S, Markus HS. Vertebrobasilar stenosis predicts high early recurrent stroke risk in posterior circulation stroke and TIA. *Stroke*. 2009;40:2732–2737.

45. Atzema CL, Grewal K, Lu H, Kapral MK, Kulkarni G, Austin PC. Outcomes among patients discharged from the emergency department with a diagnosis of peripheral vertigo. *Ann Neurol*. 2016;79:32–41.

46. Lee DD, Ho HC, Su YC, et al. Increased risk of vascular events in emergency room patients discharged home with diagnosis of dizziness or vertigo: a 3 year follow up study. *PLoS One*. 2012;7(4).

47. Newman-Toker DE. Missed stroke in acute vertigo and dizziness: it is time for action, not debate. *Ann Neurol*. 2016;79:27–31.

48. Newman-Toker DE, Kerer KA, Hsieh YH. HINTS outperforms ABCD2 to screen for stroke in acute continuous vertigo and dizziness. *Acad Emerg Med*. 2013;20(10):986–996.

49. Kene MV, Ballard DW, Vinson DR, Rauchwerger AS, Iskin HR, Kim AS. CREST Network Investigators. Emergency physician attitudes, preferences, and risk tolerance for stroke as a potential cause of dizziness symptoms. *West J Emerg Med*. 2015;16(5):768–776.

50. Choi JH, Park MG, Choi SY, et al. Acute transient vestibular syndrome: prevalence of stroke and efficacy of bedside evaluation. *Stroke*. 2017;48:556–562.

51. Kamper L, Rybacki K, Mansour M, Winkler WV, Kempkes U, Haage P. Time management in acute vertebrobasilar occlusion. *Cardiovasc Interv Radiol*. 2009;32: 226–232.

52. Zavala-Alarcon E, Emmans L, Little R, Bant A. Percutaneous intervention for posterior fossa ischemia. A single center experience and review of the literature. *Int J Cardiol*. 2008;127(1):70–77.

53. Meretoja A, Keshrkaran M, Tatlisumak T, Donnan GA, Churilov L. Endovascular therapy for ischemic stroke: save a minute—save a week. *Neurology*. 2017;88:2123–2127.

54. Liu X, Xu G, Liu Y, et al. Acute basilar artery occlusion: Endovascular interventions versus standard medical treatment (BEST) trial-design and protocol for a randomized, controlled, multicenter study. *Int J Stroke*. 2017;12(7). [Epub Jan 1].

55. Tan ML, Mitchell P, Dowling R, Tacey M, Yan B. Shorter time to intervention improves recanalization success and clinical outcome post intra-arterial intervention for basilar artery thrombosis. *J Clin Neurosci*. 2012;19: 1397–1400.

56a. Van Houwelingen RC, Luijckx GJ, Mazuri A, BoKkkers RP, Eshghi OS, Uyttenboogaart M. Safety and outcome of intra-arterial treatment for basilar artery occlusion. *JAMA Neurol*. 2016;73(10):1225–1230.

56b. Vergouwen MDI, Algra A, Pfefferkorn T, et al. Time is brain(stem) in basilar artery occlusion. *Stroke*. 2012;43: 3003–3006.

57. Broussalis E, Hitzl W, McCoy M, Trinka E, Killer M. Comparison of endovascular treatment versus conservative medical treatment in patients with acute basilar artery occlusion. *Vasc Endovasc Surg*. 2013;47(6):429–437.

58. Tinetti ME, Williams CS, Gill TM. Dizziness among older adults: a possible geriatric syndrome. *Ann Intern Med*. 2000;132(5):337–344.

59. Katsarkas A. Dizziness in aging: a retrospective study of 1194 cases. *Otolaryngol Head Neck Surg*. 1994;110:296–301.

60. Baloh RW, Honrubia V, Jacobson K. Benign positional vertigo-clinical and oculographic features in 240 cases. *Neurology*. 1987;37:371–378.

61. Lalwani AK. Vertigo, disequilibrium, and imbalance with aging. In: Jackler RK, Brackmann DE, eds. *Neurotology*. 2nd ed. ; 2005:533–539.

62. Kerber KA, Meurer WJ, West BT, Fendrick AM. Dizziness presentations in U.S. emergency departments, 1995-2004. *Acad Emerg Med.* 2008;15:744–750.

63. Grad A, Baloh RW. Vertigo of vascular origin: clinical and ENG features in 84 cases. *Arch Neurol.* 1989;46:281–284.

64. Kremer M. Sitting, standing and walking. *Br Med J.* 1958;2:63–68.

65. Ishiyama G, Ishiyama A, Jacobson K, Baloh RW. Drop attacks in older patients secondary to an otologic cause. *Neurology.* 2001;57:1103–1106.

66. Caplan LR. *Posterior Circulation Disease: Clinical Findings, Diagnosis and Management.* Cambridge, Massachusetts, USA: Blackwell Science; 1996 [chapter 7].

67. Tan T-Y, Kuo Y-L, Lin W-C, Chen T-Y. Effect of lipid-lowering therapy on the progression of intracranial arterial stenosis. *J Neurol.* 2009;256:187–193.

68. Akins PT, Pilgrim TK, Cross III DT, Moran DJ. Natural history of stenosis from intracranial atherosclerosis by serial angiography. *Stroke.* 1998;29:433–438.

69. Mazighi M, Tanasescu R, Ducrocq X, et al. Prospective study of symptomatic atherothrombotic intracranial stenoses: the GESICA study. *Neurology.* 2006;66:1187–1191.

70. Von Brevern M, Radtke A, Lezius F, et al. Epidemiology of benign paroxysmal positional vertigo: a population-based study. *J Neurol Neurosurg Psychiatry.* 2007;78:710–715.

71. Ishiyama A, Jacobson KM, Baloh RW. Migraine and benign positional vertigo. *Ann Otol Rhinol Laryngol.* 2000;109:377–380.

72. Flossmann E, Rothwell PM. Prognosis of vertebrobasilar transient ischemic attack and minor stroke. *Brain.* 2003;126:1940–1954.

73. Flossmann E, Rothwell PM. Family history of stroke does not predict risk of stroke after transient ischemic attack. *Stroke.* 2006 Feb;37(2):544–546. Epub 2005 Dec 29.

74. Calvet D, Touze E, Oppenheim C, Turc G, Meder J-F, Mas J-L. DWI lesions and TIA etiology improve the prediction of stroke after TIA. *Stroke.* 2009;40:187–192.

75. Cloud GC, Crawley F, Clifton A, McCabe DJ, Brown MM, Markus HS. Vertebral artery origin angioplasty and primary stenting: safety and restenosis rates in a prospective series. *J Neurol Neurosurg Psychiatry.* 2003;74:586–590.

76. Hatano T, Tsukahara T, Ogino E, Aoyama T, Nakakuki T, Murakami M. Stenting for vertebrobasilar artery stenosis. *Acta Neurochir Suppl.* 2005;94:137–141.

77. Oas JG, Baloh RW. Vertigo and the anterior inferior cerebellar artery syndrome. *Neurology.* 1992;42:2274–2279.

78. Hinojosa R, Kohut RI. Clinical diagnosis of anterior inferior cerebellar artery thrombosis: autopsy and temporal bone histopathology study. *Ann Otol Rhinol Laryngol.* 1990;99:261–271.

79. Lee H, Kim JS, Chung E-J, et al. Infarction in the territory of anterior inferior cerebellar artery: spectrum of audiovestibular loss. *Stroke.* 2009;40:3745–3751.

80. Kimura R, Perlman HB. Arterial obstruction of the labyrinth. Part I. Cochlear changes. *Ann Otol Rhinol Laryngol.* 1958;67:5–24.

81. Mazzoni A. Internal auditory artery supply to the petrous bone. *Ann Otol Rhinol Laryngol.* 1972;81:13–21.

82. Caplan LR. Intracranial branch atheromatous disease. *Neurology.* 1989;39:1246–1250.

83. Kumral E, Kisabay A, Atac C. Lesion patterns and etiology of ischemia in the anterior inferior cerebellar artery territory involvement: a clinical-diffusion weighted-MRI study. *Eur J Neurol.* 2006;13(4):395–401.

84. Adams RD. Occlusion of the anterior inferior cerebellar artery. *Arch Neurol Psychiatry.* 1943;49:765–770.

85. Schwartz A, Rauenberg W, Hennerici M. Dolichoectatic intracranial arteries: review of selected aspects. *Cerebrovasc Dis.* 1993;3:273–279.

86. Smoker WR, Corbett JL, Gentry LR, Keyes MD, Price MJ, McKusker S. High resolution computed tomography of the basilar artery: vertebrobasilar dolichoectasia: clinical-pathologic correlation and review. *Am J Neuroradiol.* 1986;7:61–72.

87. Kim JS, Lee JH, Suh DC, Lee MC. Spectrum of lateral medullary syndrome: correlation between clinical findings and magnetic resonance imaging in 33 subjects. *Stroke.* 1994;25(7):1405–1410.

88. Kim JS. Pure lateral medullary infarction: clinical-radiological correlation of 130 acute, consecutive patients. *Brain.* 2003;126:1864–1872.

89. Fisher CM, Karnes WE, Kubik CS. Lateral medullary infarction: the pattern of vascular occlusion. *J Neuropathol Exp Neurol.* 1961;20:323–379.

90. Kim JS. Vertigo and gait ataxia without usual signs of lateral medullary infarction: a clinical variant related to rostral-dorsolateral lesions. *Cerebrovasc Dis.* 2000;10:471–474.

91. Bjerner K, Silfverskold BP. Lateropulsion and imbalance in Wallenberg's syndrome. *Acta Neurol Scand.* 1968;44:91–100.

92. Brandt T, Dieterich M. Skew deviation with ocular torsion: a vestibular brainstem sign of topographic diagnostic value. *Ann Neurol.* 1993;33:528–534.

93. Kumral E, Kisabay A, Atac C. Lesion patterns and etiology of ischemia in superior cerebellar artery territory infarcts. *Cerebrovasc Dis.* 2005;19(5):283–290.

94. Amarenco P, Levy C, Cohen A. Causes and mechanisms of territorial and non-territorial cerebellar infarcts in 115 consecutive patients. *Stroke.* 1994;25:105–112.

95. Kase C, Norrving B, Levine S. Cerebellar infarction: clinical and anatomic observations in 66 cases. *Stroke.* 1993;24:76–83.

96. Bickerstaff ER. Basilar artery migraine. *Lancet.* 1961;1:15–17.

97. Olsson JE. Neurotologic findings in basilar migraine. *Laryngoscope.* 1991;101:1–41.

98. Cutrer FM, Baloh RW. Migraine associated dizziness. *Headache.* 1992;32:300–304.

99. International Headache Society. Classification and diagnostic criteria for headache disorders, cranial neuralgias, and facial pain. *Cephalagia.* 1988;8:27.

100. Bogousslavsky J, Regli F, Van Melle G. Migraine stroke. *Neurology.* 1988;38:223–227.

101. Evans RW, Ishiyama G. Migraine with transient unilateral hearing loss and tinnitus. *Headache*. 2009;49(5):756–758.

102. Androulakis XM, Kodumuri N, Giamberardino LD, et al. Ischemic stroke subtypes and migraine with visual aura in the ARIC (atherosclerosis risk in communities) study. *Neurology*. 2016;87(24):2527–2532.

103. Kurth T, Kase CS, Schurks M, Tzourio C, Buring JE. Migraine and risk of haemorrhagic stroke in women: prospective cohort study. *BMJ*. 2010:341. PMID: 20736268.

104. Van Os HJA, Mulder IA, Broersen A, et al. *Stroke*. 2017. May 19 epub ahead of print.

105. Milionis HJ, Giannopoulos S, Kosmidou M, et al. Statin therapy after first stroke reduces 10-year stroke recurrence and improves survival. *Neurology*. 2009;72:1816–1822.

106. Goldstein LB, Adams R, Alberts MJ, et al. Primary prevention of ischemic stroke: a guideline from the American Heart Association/American Stroke Association Stroke Council: cosponsored by the atherosclerotic Peripheral Vascular Disease Interdisciplinary Working Group; Cardiovascular Nursing Council; Clinical Cardiology Council; Nutrition, Physical Activity, and Metabolism Council; and the Quality of Care and Outcomes Research Interdisciplinary Working Group: The American Academy of Neurology affirms the value of this guideline. *Stroke*. 2006;37:1583–1633.

107. Kernan WN, Ovbiagele B, Black HR, et al. Guidelines for the prevention of stroke in patients with stroke and transient ischemic attack: a guideline for healthcare professionals from the American Heart Association/American Stroke Association. *Stroke*. 2014;45(7):2160–2236.

CHAPTER 17

Dizziness in the Elderly

MICHAEL S. HARRIS, MD • KAMRAN BARIN, PHD • EDWARD E. DODSON, MD

INTRODUCTION

Dizziness is a broad term used to describe a variety of sensations such as vertigo, unsteadiness, imbalance, light-headedness, and similar symptoms. The prevalence of dizziness increases steadily with age.[1,2] Although debate is still ongoing regarding the underlying causes of this increase in prevalence, there is universal agreement on the devastating consequences and high physical, cognitive, emotional, and financial toll of dizziness and imbalance on the older population.[3–7] Taken together, the impact of dizziness on the quality of life in older patients is profound.[8]

It is estimated that one-fourth to one-third of the population older than 65 years has experienced some form of dizziness.[9–11] This range in the reported prevalence rates reflects differences across the series in the cutoff age of participants, type(s) of symptoms for inclusion, duration and frequency of symptoms, and whether the sample was taken from community-dwelling patients, primary care facilities, or specialty clinics. In the older than 85 years age-group, the number of adults with dizziness increases to about 50%.[1] The prevalence of these symptoms seems to be greater for women.[12,13]

It is important to recognize that older dizzy patients typically present with a different symptom profile compared to their younger counterparts.[14] Younger patients more often complain of true vertigo, nausea, and emesis, whereas older patients more often report symptoms of unsteadiness, imbalance, and disequilibrium.

Older individuals who suffer from dizziness are at a significantly higher risk of accidental falls and consequent injuries.[10,11,15,16] It is estimated that approximately 30% of adults older than 65 years will fall at least once, and roughly 50% of those will fall again.[17,18] The consequences of such falls are devastating. Falls are the leading cause of accidental death in people older than 65 years, and non-fatal falls are the main reason for hospital admissions in this age-group.[6,7] Fall-related injuries can lead to mobility restrictions, loss of independence, and even confinement to nursing facilities.[5,19] In addition to the physical and emotional cost, these injuries also carry a heavy financial burden,

estimated at over $19 billion in direct costs in the year 2000 and rising steadily since.[20,21]

A number of studies have established that for older adults, a history of dizziness or imbalance is an independent risk factor for falling[22–24]; however, the association between the two has not been as strong in other studies.[25,26] This is not surprising as falls are complex phenomena involving neurologic, biomechanical, and other factors; therefore, fall risk factors can be heavily influenced by study design and patient selection methods. Rubenstein and Josephson[24] used a meta-analysis of 12 large studies and found that balance disorders and dizziness were the second and third leading causes of falls in older persons, respectively. Vertigo, unsteadiness, and related symptoms also have an indirect effect on falls. It is well established that these symptoms in older individuals lead to the fear of falling.[27–29] In turn, the fear of falling is considered a strong predictor for those who will suffer one or more actual falls.[24,25]

The general topic of falls is beyond the scope of this chapter. However, the strong association between falls and symptoms of dizziness and imbalance highlights the importance of understanding the causes of these symptoms and devising effective methods for managing them in the older population.

CAUSES OF DIZZINESS AND DISEQUILIBRIUM IN OLDER INDIVIDUALS

A substantial body of research demonstrates that the symptom of dizziness stems from a heterogeneous collection of underlying factors and is often multifactorial. In some studies, no specific etiology could be identified to explain the symptoms of a large subset of the subjects.[30] The term *presbystasis* is used to describe this type of age-related disequilibrium that cannot be attributed to any known pathology. On the other hand, other studies have been able to assign one or more diagnostic categories to the majority of elderly patients suffering from dizziness.[31–33] These discrepancies have led some investigators to suggest that dizziness in the elderly should be viewed as a multifactorial geriatric syndrome involving many different symptoms and originating from many different systems, such as sensory, motor, vestibular, neurologic, cardiovascular, and other systems.[10]

The underlying causes of dizziness and disequilibrium in older adults can be divided into three broad categories:

1. Age-related decline of acuity in sensory and motor pathways as well as deterioration of integration mechanisms within the central nervous system (CNS). Loss of hair cells in the labyrinth is an example of an age-related change in the sensory system. These types of losses are considered a normal part of aging because they are so common in older adults. However, they are most likely caused by subtle pathologies accumulated over a lifetime (e.g., ischemia) that are highly prevalent in the elderly.

2. Pathologies that cause dizziness in any age-group, which become more prevalent in older individuals, either because age-related changes noted earlier make the elderly more susceptible to these pathologies or because the cumulative probability of exposure to these pathologies increases with time. An example of such pathology is benign paroxysmal positional vertigo (BPPV) that can occur at any age but is more common in the elderly, likely because of the ongoing deterioration of the maculae of the otolith organs.

3. An assortment of environmental and lifestyle factors that increases the chance of dizziness and balance problems in the elderly. One such example is polypharmacy in the elderly, with many medications having the common side effect of dizziness (see Chapter 18).

A different type of classification is often used to divide risk factors for falls.[34] This classification involves causes that are intrinsic to the patient versus those that are extrinsic. For dizziness and balance problems, such a classification is more relevant when considering appropriate intervention methods, which will be discussed later in this chapter. Here, each of the aforementioned three categories will be discussed in detail.

Age-Related Deterioration of Sensory and Motor Mechanisms

Human balance function depends on coordinated streams of sensory input from the vestibular, proprioceptive, and visual systems as well as proper integration of those inputs in the CNS. Furthermore, movement control requires the motor centers to accurately process sensory information and transmit the necessary commands to the appropriate muscles. Both structural and functional deteriorations in all of the aforementioned systems are known to occur with advancing age.[35]

Vestibular system

Age-related loss of hair cells has been documented within the cristae ampullares of the semicircular canals and the maculae of the saccule and utricle.[36,37] Earlier studies had indicated greater loss of hair cells in the semicircular canals and saccule and a higher proportion of loss for type I versus type II hair cells.[38] More recent studies have used a counting method that is deemed to be less biased. These studies have confirmed the age-related loss of hair cells in the labyrinth, although the affected sites and type of hair cells have differed somewhat from previous studies.[39]

Structural integrity of the vestibular nerve is also affected by age. The number of primary vestibular neurons within Scarpa's ganglion has been shown to decline by approximately 25% over the life span.[40,41] Similarly, the study of brainstem specimens in different age-groups has demonstrated a decrease in the number of secondary vestibular neurons within the vestibular nuclei.[42]

Age-related degeneration of peripheral and central vestibular structures is similar to that of the auditory system and is most likely caused by subtle changes of blood flow to the inner ear.[42] Microvascular changes with aging have been reported in both human and animal studies.[43-45] Any decrease in blood flow to inner ear structures can have profound effects because inner ear arteries lack anastomotic connections.

Age-related changes of vestibular structures have been objectively confirmed by vestibular function tests. For example, both longitudinal and cross-sectional studies have shown an age-related decrease in vestibulo-ocular reflex (VOR) gain during sinusoidal rotation.[46,47] This finding indicates that, unlike pathologies that usually affect only one labyrinth, age-related changes of vestibular pathways are more likely to mimic bilateral reduction of function. In addition, phase lead for low frequency sinusoidal stimuli and short vestibular time constants for step stimuli have been reported in older subjects.[48] These findings are consistent with deterioration of the velocity storage mechanism within the brainstem. Similar degradation of central vestibular pathways has been demonstrated for otolith-ocular responses during off-vertical axis rotation.[49]

Despite the overwhelming evidence in support of age-related changes of peripheral and central vestibular structures, the relationship between those changes and dizziness or disequilibrium in the elderly is not necessarily linear. Several studies have demonstrated high prevalence of vestibular impairment in elderly individuals.[50,51] However, once patients with specific vestibular pathologies are removed from the sample, the contribution of age-related vestibular decline to balance impairment in the elderly is not as profound.[25,48] Clearly, additional research is needed to examine the association of age-related changes in the vestibular pathways in older adults with symptoms of dizziness and disequilibrium.

Proprioceptive system

Proprioceptive sensors reside in the muscles, joints, and tendons and provide information regarding orientation of one body segment with respect to another. Compared with vestibular and visual inputs, these sensors have lower thresholds for motion detection and operate at significantly higher frequencies.[52,53] Proprioceptive input provides critical information regarding the point of contact with the ground, which can be extrapolated to detect orientation and movement of the body. Proprioceptive cues from the neck also play an important role in detecting head orientation and in providing a stable platform for vestibular and visual receptors.

The proprioceptive system undergoes several age-related changes. Vibration and touch thresholds decline in older individuals, adversely affecting tactile information arising from the feet at their contact point with the ground.[54] Similarly, the ability to detect the position and direction of joint movements declines with age.[55]

A number of studies have demonstrated decreased postural stability when proprioceptive input is altered in such a way that it provides inaccurate information regarding orientation.[56] Horak et al.[57] compared the performance of patients with severe neuropathy with age-matched controls and demonstrated that the performance of the control subjects became similar to that of patients with neuropathy for test conditions in which proprioceptive input was altered. Therefore, it is not surprising that reduction of vibration and tactile sensation at the ankle and knee joints has been associated with an increased risk of falls in the elderly.[58]

Concomitant conditions such as diabetes mellitus or other causes of peripheral neuropathy that can be more common in older patients may have a synergistic effect with age-related decline in lower extremity proprioceptive function. Peripheral neuropathy itself is predictive of falls in patients with bilateral vestibulopathy.[59]

The role of neck proprioception on postural control has been studied using neck muscle vibration.[60–62] Prolonged unilateral vibration of neck muscles during in-place stepping caused subjects to rotate about a vertical axis away from the side of vibration.[60] Using a similar type of neck vibration during locomotion, Deshpande and Patla demonstrated reduced sensitivity of neck

proprioception in older adults.[61] This is an important observation because as noted before, age-related decline of the vestibular system usually involves bilateral reduction of function. In younger patients with bilateral vestibular loss, neck receptors play an important role as substitutes for the vestibular system.[63] This mode of compensation may not be available in the elderly because of reduced neck proprioception.

Visual system

The visual system undergoes significant age-related changes. In addition to visual acuity, several other visual functions, such as depth perception, accommodation, contrast sensitivity, and dark adaptation, decline with age.[64] Deficits in depth perception and contrast sensitivity have been shown to have the largest contributory influence on falls.[65] These impairments affect the ability of older adults to accurately judge distances and to avoid obstacles.

Age-related changes in static visual acuity as measured with stationary subjects and stationary targets have been studied extensively.[64,66] The association between reduced static visual acuity and balance problems in the elderly is still in dispute.[65] Deterioration of dynamic visual acuity, in which either the target or the subject is moving, has also been documented in older individuals.[67] Interestingly, patients with acute unilateral and bilateral vestibular lesions also exhibit impaired dynamic visual acuity and complain of blurred vision during head movements.[68] The coexistence of this impairment in the elderly and in patients with known balance disorders may explain some of the symptoms in older adults.

It has been shown that reliance on visual input increases with age.[69] For example, older subjects exposed to moving visual surrounds were affected more and demonstrated greater postural sway than younger subjects.[70] Although both older and younger subjects were able to adapt to moving visual stimuli, older individuals required significantly more time for adaptation to occur.[71] In addition, postural sway of older subjects who were presented with spatially inaccurate visual stimuli was significantly greater than the response of younger subjects.[72]

Motor system

Sensory information regarding orientation and movement of the body is processed by the motor centers, and appropriate commands are transmitted to a select group of skeletal muscles to preserve balance and maintain upright postural stability. The most notable effect of aging on the motor system relates to changes

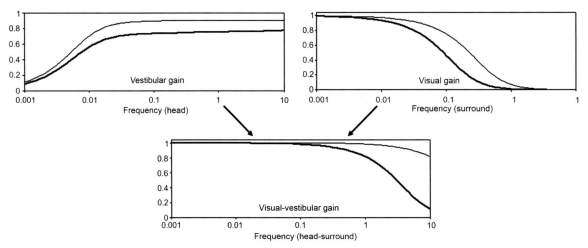

FIG. 17.1 Vestibular gain defined as the ratio of slow-phase eye velocity to head velocity, visual (opto-kinetic) gain defined as the ratio of eye velocity to surround velocity, and visual-vestibular interaction gain defined as the ratio of eye velocity to combined head-visual surround velocity for younger (thin line) and older (thick line) adults. Both the vestibular and visual gains for older individuals represent a subtle decline due to age-related changes. When the visual-vestibular interaction gain is significantly less than 1, visual images will not remain stationary on the retina and will appear blurry. The data are theoretical and do not represent the exact responses. (Adapted from AudiologyOnline presentation by Zapala (2010): http://www.audiologyonline.com/ceus/recordedcoursedetails.asp?class_id=16469.)

in anatomic and physiologic characteristics of the muscles.[73] Muscle strength has been shown to be lowered by 20%–40% in the 70–80 age-group compared to that of young adults. Reduction in muscle strength is related to a decrease in the number and size of muscle fibers as well as changes in the central motor command centers.[74] Similarly, the speed with which muscles can be contracted declines with age.[75] These and other similar age-related changes in skeletal muscles may prevent older individuals from exerting adequate force and reacting quickly to postural disturbances.[72]

Similar changes are observed in extraocular muscles, which can lead to age-related decline of oculomotor function. Fast eye movements or saccades are only modestly affected by aging. Saccade latency has been shown to increase with age, but other saccade parameters, such as peak velocity or accuracy, were not significantly affected.[47] Gain of slow tracking eye movements or smooth pursuit also declined substantially with age, especially for higher-velocity target movements.[76] The ability to suppress vestibular nystagmus by visual fixation accordingly declines, as tracking and fixation mechanisms share many neural pathways.[47] Finally, optokinetic reflex gain is also reduced in older individuals, mainly for high-velocity full-field visual target movement.[47]

Although changes in eye muscles may have an effect on the decline of oculomotor responses, aging of central

structures discussed in the next section seems to have a substantially greater role in age-related control of eye movements.[47] These changes have profound effects on the perception of orientation and balance because they influence the sensory input from the visual system.

Central integration mechanisms

The brainstem, cerebellum, and higher cortical structures within the CNS all suffer from age-related degenerative changes. These changes include decrease in the number of neurons, loss of myelination, decrease in the number of Purkinje cells, and other neuronal changes.[77] Age-related degeneration of central structures is likely to affect the integration of information from different sensory inputs and interfere with accurate perception of orientation and motion.

A few examples of impaired sensory integration have been mentioned previously. Over-reliance on the visual system even when it is providing erroneous spatial information is an example of how prioritization of inputs from different sensory mechanisms can be affected in older individuals.[69,72] Another example is the faulty integration of optokinetic and vestibular inputs that can lead to deterioration of dynamic visual acuity.[67] Fig. 17.1 shows how subtle age-related reduction in the gain of both the VOR and optokinetic reflex can result in images not remaining stationary on the retina, thereby causing blurred vision during head movement. This type of deterioration in visual-vestibular interaction has been documented in older individuals.[47]

One manifestation of impaired sensory integration in the elderly is related to the time required for adaptation after natural changes affect balance control mechanisms. For example, when proprioceptive input was modulated by vibration of different muscles in the lower leg, there were no significant age-related differences in lower-level reflexes; however, older individuals did not adapt to reintroduction of accurate proprioceptive cues as quickly as the younger subjects did.[78] Similar age-related differences in adaptation time were noted when subjects were exposed to moving visual stimuli.[71] These observations have profound and troubling implications for older individuals with regard to recovery and compensation following impairment of the balance system.

Pathologic Causes of Dizziness

Although age-related changes in sensory and motor systems do play a role in the high prevalence of dizziness among the elderly, they are no longer considered the most prominent contributors. In contrast to earlier research, recent studies have identified one or more specific pathologies as the underlying cause(s) of symptoms.[30,33,50,79] None of these pathologies was unique to the elderly: the same diseases are responsible for causing dizziness in both younger and older individuals.[51] These pathologies become more prevalent in older individuals, either because age-related changes detailed earlier make the elderly more susceptible to them, or because the cumulative probability of exposure to them increases with time.

Major causes of dizziness based on primary care encounters (and not including formal assessment of vestibular function) in more than 80% of elderly patients fall into one of the three categories: cardiovascular (including cerebrovascular), peripheral vestibular, and psychiatric diseases.[30,50,51,79] In 8% of patients, no clear cause is identified, and all other causes constitute 11% of patients. Two or more contributing causes are identified in 70% of patients. Adverse medication effects are the leading secondary cause. Dizziness is one of the primary symptoms in over 60 diseases.[80] Thus, a broader differential diagnosis must be maintained when examining an older dizzy patient. Referrals to internal medicine, neurology, and other colleagues must be made, as appropriate, for additional evaluation and definitive management.

Among peripheral vestibular disorders, BPPV is by far the most common. In one study, almost 40% of patients above the age of 70 years were diagnosed with BPPV.[51] While some earlier studies suggest that older patients with BPPV experience a more protracted course and higher rates of recurrence, other more recent prospective reviews show outcomes equivalent to those of younger counterparts.[81] Late-onset Meniere's disease, vestibular neuritis, and other otologic diseases do occur in the elderly but are not as common. Our own clinical experience suggests that some older patients who present with sudden onset of symptoms are experiencing decompensation related to an existing, and sometimes long-standing, condition rather than a new vestibular lesion. These patients may have a history of a previously compensated peripheral vestibular disease, which may have been undiagnosed.

Among non-vestibular causes of dizziness, cardiovascular and cerebrovascular diseases are common in the elderly.[79] Atherosclerotic narrowing of blood vessels can lead to ischemic events and produce symptoms similar to either peripheral vestibular or central lesions depending on the affected sites.[77] Vertebrobasilar insufficiency, which is a common cause of dizziness in the elderly (see Chapter 16), is an example of this type of disorder.[82] Other diseases in this category include those that reduce cardiac output such as arrhythmia and heart valve failure. Orthostatic hypotension is extremely common in the elderly, often associated with dizziness or disequilibrium (see Chapter 15). Vertigo and nystagmus may be present as well.[83]

Some neurologic disorders such Parkinson's disease and Alzheimer's disease are also more prevalent in the elderly, but evidence supporting vestibular dysfunction as a predictor or as a direct result of either condition is limited at this point in time.[84] Unsteady gait associated with Parkinsonism, however, is a strong predictor of falls.[85] Metabolic and endocrine disorders can cause dizziness with similar frequency in both younger and older adults.

Finally, the impact of psychiatric disorders, including cognitive impairment, should be considered in the elderly. Sloane et al.[86] compared the prevalence and characteristics of psychiatric diseases between older patients with chronic dizziness with age- and sex-matched controls. Over 37% in the chronic dizziness group had a psychiatric diagnosis. Although psychiatric diseases rarely were considered the primary cause of dizziness, they were common as a contributing factor to dizziness in the elderly. In this study, anxiety and depression were the most common conditions. This finding is similar to results from other studies that have examined psychogenic aspects of chronic dizziness in patients of all age groups.[87] One psychogenic factor that is specific to the elderly is increased fear of falling. It has been shown that the fear of falling is a risk factor for actual falls.[88,89]

Environmental and Lifestyle Causes of Dizziness

In addition to age-related changes and pathologies that affect balance mechanisms discussed earlier, several lifestyle and environmental factors can contribute to disorientation and the sense of imbalance. The most prominent of these factors is adverse effects of medications. Several studies have linked the use of CNS-acting medications to increased risk of falls in the elderly.[90] Furthermore, adverse medication effects have been considered the leading secondary cause of dizziness.[79] Benzodiazepines, antidepressants, and anticonvulsants have been the most commonly implicated classes of medication.[91] Unlike the well-known ototoxic and vestibulotoxic effects of aminoglycosides or chemotherapeutic agents, adverse drug effects of other classes of medication and their association with dizziness are less clear. There is considerable debate about the methodological efficacy of studying drug effects in at-risk populations. The use of implicated medications may be unavoidable; however, careful review of the necessity, dosage, drug interactions, and possible alternatives can greatly reduce dizziness due to these medications (see Chapter 18).

Another potentially modifiable lifestyle factor relates to vision correction. In general, poor vision contributes to spatial disorientation. Regular eye examinations and use of corrective prescription eyeglasses can greatly improve this deficit. As visual acuity for both distant and near vision decreases with age, more adults are required to wear multifocal lenses for vision correction. The use of these lenses has been associated with disorientation and increased chance of contact with surrounding objects, especially when performing a secondary task.[92] Advising patients to wear single focal lenses during outdoor activities may reduce the chance of falling.[93]

The aforementioned is a partial list of environmental and lifestyle factors that can influence patients' sense of balance. Careful attention to these and other similar factors combined with patient education and simple corrective measures may alleviate or lessen the symptoms and prevent falls, without extensive medical intervention.

DIAGNOSIS OF DIZZINESS IN OLDER INDIVIDUALS

As noted, dizziness in younger and older individuals is generally caused by the same diseases. Therefore, the diagnostic path is essentially the same regardless of age, and includes a careful and detailed history, a thorough physical examination, and targeted laboratory tests, when indicated, all of which are discussed in detail elsewhere in this book. In this section, we will focus only on issues that are specific or particularly relevant to the elderly.

History

As is the case with dizziness in any age group, a case history should include a thorough description of the patient's current and previous medical conditions, medication use, social environment, and fall risk factors. An accurate description of symptoms, their time course, and precipitating events is essential in identifying the underlying cause. These symptoms include vertigo, unsteadiness, imbalance, presyncope, and other less well-defined sensations such as light-headedness.[80] Table 17.1 is a summary of the most common causes of dizziness in the elderly.

Physical Examination

A thorough and efficient physical examination is particularly important in the evaluation of dizziness in the elderly. In some settings such as nursing homes, extensive laboratory tests may not be available or convenient,[94] and every effort should be made to minimize the additional need for travel for medical assessments. A typical physical examination consists of neurologic, neurotologic, and general medical examination.[95] Table 17.2 summarizes different systems evaluated during a typical physical examination for dizziness (see Chapter 2).

The Dix-Hallpike maneuver and its variations are highly useful because of the increased prevalence of BPPV in the elderly (see Chapter 9). Test procedures may be modified if the patient is frail or has neck or back problems. For example, it is not necessary to move the patient vigorously as the displaced otolithic particles are moved by gravity and not by the acceleration of the body. Nor is it necessary to extend the patient's neck excessively as most patients can induce symptoms by simply turning in bed. The safety and comfort of the test can be improved by having additional assistants to help with positioning the patient. Finally, for patients with severe neck or back problems, specialized equipment may be needed to safely perform the procedure.

Another useful test is the head impulse test (HIT),[96] which can easily be performed as a bedside or clinical examination or more quantitatively in an instrumented version—the video head impulse test (vHIT- see Chapter 8). A positive test, characterized by reflexive catch-up saccades following brief, rapid horizontal head impulses

TABLE 17.1
Common Causes of Dizziness in the Elderly for Different Types of Symptoms

Symptom	Subtype	Likely Cause	Comments
Vertigo	Position-induced	BPPV	If nystagmus does not match BPPV, consider central pathologies. If induced by neck rotation, consider cervical vertigo
	Acute-onset, persistent with neurologic signs	Stroke Tumors Degenerative diseases	Acute ischemia involving vestibular structures can mimic vestibular neuritis
	Acute-onset, persistent without neurologic signs	Labyrinthitis Vestibular neuritis	Differential diagnosis is based on the presence of hearing loss
	Recurrent with no neurologic signs	Ménière's disease Migraine	Late-onset Ménière's is possible but not common. Migraines lack progressive auditory symptoms. Transient ischemic attacks should be considered in patients with vascular risk factors
Disequilibrium	Acute or rapidly progressive	Stroke	Autoimmune or post-infectious diseases should also be considered. May include severe oculomotor abnormalities
	Worse in the absence of other sensory inputs	Bilateral vestibular loss	Usually includes history of ototoxicity. Hearing loss or oscillopsia may be present
	Worse in the absence of vision with numbness/weakness	Proprioception and somatosensory loss	Often associated with peripheral neuropathy related to metabolic disorders, diabetes, or renal failure
	With bradykinesia, rigidity, tremor	Parkinson's disease	Frontal lobe or other basal ganglia disorders
	With speech disorder, lack of coordination, intention tremor	Cerebellar lesions	The imbalance is usually the same with or without vision
	Isolated disequilibrium, gait difficulty, light-headedness	Disequilibrium of aging	Often accompanied by borderline diffuse central findings but no other specific complaints
Presyncope	With blood pressure drop on standing	Postural hypotension	Associated with reduced blood volume, autonomic disorders, or chronic use of antihypertensive medications
	Abnormal cardiac examination	Heart valve disease Arrhythmia	When 24-hour electrocardiogram is abnormal, indicates transient arrhythmia
	Induced by fear or anxiety	Vasovagal attacks	Decline in heart rate and blood pressure leads to decrease in cerebral blood flow
Light-headedness, non-specific	Associated with fear, anxiety, and depression	Psychogenic	Often accompanied by autonomic symptoms

BPPV, benign paroxysmal positional vertigo.
Data from Baloh R. Dizziness in older people. *J Am Geriatr Soc*. 1992;40(7):713–721; Kerber K. Dizziness in older people. In: Eggers SD, Zee DS, eds. *Vertigo and imbalance: clinical neurophysiology of the vestibular system*. Elsevier; 2010:9, 491–501.

TABLE 17.2
Common Components of Physical Examination

System	Examination	Comments
Vestibular	Dix-Hallpike	May require special accommodations for patients who are frail or have neck or back problems
	Head impulse	When positive, almost always indicates a peripheral vestibular lesion. When negative, does not rule out peripheral lesions
	Spontaneous nystagmus / pneumatic otoscopy/Valsalva	Use Frenzel lenses to eliminate fixation; look for horizontal nystagmus in perilymph fistula or torsional/vertical nystagmus in superior canal dehiscence
	Hearing	Use tuning forks
Vision	Static visual acuity	Check both monocular and binocular vision
	Dynamic visual acuity	Look for significant drop in visual acuity during head movements
Proprioception	Temperature/pain/vibration	Check for neuropathies
Motor (musculoskeletal)	Muscle tone/strength	Lower extremity weakness is a fall risk factor
	Gait	Check tandem walking for different abnormal patterns
	Postural stability/sensory integration	Romberg test with eyes open and closed while standing on a solid surface or foam
	Coordination	Past-pointing, heel-knee, or similar tests
Oculomotor	Gaze motility/nystagmus	Look for restricted range of motion and nystagmus
	Saccade/tracking	Assess both accuracy and velocity of both slow and fast eye movements
Cardiovascular	Orthostatic drop in blood pressure	Look for drop of greater than 20 mmHg in systolic blood pressure or drop of greater than 10 mmHg in diastolic blood pressure on standing
	Irregular heart rhythm	Can be intermittent
Psychogenic	Cognition	Questionnaire-based assessment such as Mini-Mental State Examination
	Anxiety	Questionnaire-based assessment such as Beck Anxiety Inventory. Hyperventilation test can be helpful
	Depression	Questionnaire-based assessment such as Geriatric Depression Scale
	Handicap	Questionnaire-based assessment such as Dizziness Handicap Inventory

Data from multiple sources including: Kerber K. Dizziness in older people. In: Eggers SD, Zee DS, eds. *Vertigo and imbalance: clinical neurophysiology of the vestibular system*. Vol. 9. Elsevier; 2010:491–501; Jacobson G, McCaslin D, Grantham S, et al. Significant vestibular system impairment is common in a cohort of elderly patients referred for assessment of falls risk. *J Am Acad Audiol*. 2008;19(10):799–807.

or thrusts, almost always indicates peripheral vestibular pathology. The test is also helpful in confirming bilateral vestibular loss when caloric testing is bilaterally weak. Again, the procedure can be modified for elderly patients with neck problems to minimize discomfort or injury by reducing the amplitude of the head thrust while maintaining its relatively high velocity.

Laboratory Tests

Laboratory tests may become necessary after taking a thorough history and performing a complete physical examination. Typical laboratory tests for dizziness include vestibular function tests, auditory tests, imaging tests, cardiovascular tests, and less commonly, endocrinologic tests. It is important to recognize that normal limits for many laboratory tests are ill-defined for older individuals.[95] In fact, it is not clear whether one should consider age-related changes of the balance function a normal phenomenon. Therefore, it is best to use these tests judiciously in the elderly because some perceived abnormal findings may prove to be of little help in the ultimate diagnosis and management of the patient. This section provides a brief review of laboratory test findings that are specific to the elderly.

Vestibular function tests

The most commonly used vestibular function test is videonystagmography (VNG) or electronystagmography. VNG includes tests of oculomotor function (saccade, tracking, and optokinetic), tests of gaze stabilization (gaze, spontaneous nystagmus, and static position), tests of VOR (caloric, rotary chair, vHIT), and specialized tests (Dix-Hallpike test and its variations, pressure/fistula test, Tullio, and vibration).

In the saccade test, saccade latencies increase with age, but other parameters such as accuracy or peak velocities are not significantly affected.[47] Some abnormalities in the saccade test, such as abnormal latencies, may be due to poor visual acuity. This is a particular issue with VNG because patients are usually unable to wear corrective glasses during the test. Most saccade parameters are sensitive to drug effects.

In the tracking test, the gain (defined as the ratio of eye velocities to target velocities) decreases with age, especially for higher frequencies.[76] Similarly, in older adults, slow phase velocity of nystagmus in the optokinetic test decreases for higher-velocity stimuli. Again, effects of poor vision and medications should be considered in the interpretation of results.

In gaze stabilization tests, one should recognize that end-point nystagmus begins at lower off-center gaze positions and is more common in the elderly. End-point nystagmus is a normal occurrence characterized by intermittent low-velocity nystagmus when the eyes are directed at extreme gaze positions and should not be mistaken for abnormal gaze-evoked nystagmus. Also, square-wave jerk nystagmus during visual fixation seems to be common in the elderly and is considered part of normal aging by some investigators[97]; therefore, patient age should be considered carefully when determining the clinical significance of square-wave jerk nystagmus. Unfortunately, age-adjusted normal limits for square waves have not been established.

Bilateral caloric weakness is a common finding in older patients. Although decreased caloric reactivity may represent age-related reduction of vestibular function in some patients, in many others, it is a false-positive finding that reflects poor temperature transfer from the external auditory canal to the labyrinth. The latter group demonstrates normal rotary chair results that indicate normal VOR function.[98] Age-related changes have not been observed in other caloric test parameters.[46]

Issues for the Dix-Hallpike test and its variations performed during laboratory testing are the same as those discussed earlier for bedside testing. That is, safety precautions must be taken with regard to frailty and neck or back problems in the elderly regardless of whether the test is performed as part of the VNG battery or separately.

In rotary chair testing older asymptomatic individuals may show reduced VOR gain and VOR phase lead, mainly in low frequencies. These findings represent age-related decline in vestibular function and loss of the velocity storage mechanism in the vestibular nuclei.[46,48] Rotary chair testing can be helpful in older adults to clarify results of the caloric test as described earlier.

The instrumented correlate to the bedside HIT, the vHIT, has been used increasingly as an indicator of VOR competence (see Chapter 8). Small reductions in VOR gain that would otherwise be considered clinically normal have been found to be associated with compensatory catch-up saccades. Catch-up saccade amplitude has been shown to correlate with aging in healthy older adults, suggesting its utility independent of VOR gain.[99]

Vestibular-evoked myogenic potentials (VEMPs) are based on short-latency muscle responses typically recorded from the sternocleidomastoid muscle (cervical VEMP [cVEMP]) or from infraorbital eye muscles (ocular VEMP [oVEMP]) in response to loud clicks or tone bursts. The use of VEMPs as a test of the saccule and the inferior vestibular nerve is becoming more common. Several studies have demonstrated that both cVEMP and oVEMP parameters are affected by age.[100–105] All of the studies consistently demonstrate that VEMP amplitudes decline while VEMP thresholds increase with age. Response rates also are shown to decrease in older adults. Some studies have described age-related changes in VEMP latencies, whereas others have not.[102–104] One complicating factor in the elderly is the reduced ability to maintain high levels of muscle contraction required, particularly for cVEMP, perhaps due to loss of age-related muscle tone or use of muscle relaxants. This factor can affect VEMP amplitude and threshold and should be considered when interpreting results. As more clinical applications for VEMP are identified in all age groups, the role of this test in evaluating older adults is also emerging.

Dynamic posturography consists of two separate tests: motor coordination test (MCT) in which postural sway is measured in response to sudden translation or rotation of the support base, and sensory organization test (SOT) in which postural sway is measured under different visual and proprioceptive conditions.[46,72] The MCT parameters generally do not change with age except for latency (reaction time), which shows a modest increase with age.[72] In SOT, a significant increase in postural sway is common when visual and proprioceptive inputs are altered.[46] Dynamic posturography is not a diagnostic test, but the results can help identify inappropriate sensory integration and accordingly can provide valuable information for the design of effective exercise programs for the elderly.

Other tests

Magnetic resonance imaging (MRI) and computed tomography imaging are neuroimaging modalities that are used to identify structural abnormalities. Their applications are the same in both younger and older individuals, but there are a few areas of particular interest in the elderly. The imaging studies, MRI in particular, can help with identifying white matter lesions in the brain. Although the significance of small lesions is in doubt, larger white matter enhancements have been associated with a variety of balance-related symptoms in the elderly.[95]

Magnetic resonance angiography and other tests such as Doppler ultrasound can help in identifying a vascular origin of dizziness, which is a common finding in the elderly. Unfortunately, some of the other common causes, such as transient ischemia, may not produce a distinguishable finding in imaging studies.

Tests of cardiovascular function, such as electrocardiography or Holter monitoring, can identify constant or intermittent runs of arrhythmia that would lead to the perception of dizziness. Orthostatic pulse and blood pressure testing can easily be performed in the clinic setting and can document orthostatic hypotension, which is defined as a decrease of 20 mmHg in systolic blood pressure or 10 mmHg in diastolic blood pressure while standing compared to readings taken while sitting. Orthostatic hypotension is a common cause of dizziness in the elderly, especially for those who take antihypertensive medication. Cardiovascular causes of dizziness are also common in the elderly.

MANAGEMENT OF DIZZINESS IN OLDER INDIVIDUALS

Management of dizziness involves a medical, rehabilitative, or in rare cases, surgical approach. Physical therapy either as the primary mode of management or in conjunction with other management modalities seems to be an effective approach in reducing dizziness in older adults (see Chapter 19). This approach is most appropriate when the underlying cause is vestibular-related (vestibular rehabilitation) or when the cause is nonspecific (general gait/balance training and fall prevention strategies).[55] However, physical therapy is a worthwhile option for other causes of dizziness in the elderly too. Exercise therapy may include strength training, fitness training, and other carefully planned exercises. Supervised and customized exercise guided by computer dynamic posturography has been shown to be effective, independent of age, among elderly patients with postural instability.[106] In addition to the traditional outpatient approach to therapy, home-based and group exercise programs can be very effective.[50] As is the case with younger patients, adherence of older patients to balance rehabilitation programs is variable: male sex, older age, and poorer baseline stability based on posturography are all correlated with non-adherence.[107]

If the cause of dizziness is BPPV, simple and effective methods such as canalith repositioning or liberatory maneuvers are available. Again, the same precautions (i.e., neck and spine stability) that are necessary in performing diagnostic maneuvers must be considered when administering therapeutic procedures.

When other specific pathologies are identified, there is usually an established management protocol. For example, the initial treatment for Meniere's disease includes low-salt diet and prescription of diuretics and vestibular suppressants (see Chapter 13). Further treatment may require endolymphatic shunt surgery, vestibular nerve section, or transtympanic gentamicin injections. However, management approaches that rely on central compensation mechanisms for their therapeutic effect, such as vestibular nerve section or gentamicin therapy, must be used cautiously in the elderly. As discussed earlier, compensation mechanisms deteriorate with age and may not provide effective recovery following those procedures.

Management of cerebrovascular and cardiovascular causes of dizziness usually involves controlling the underlying risk factors. Appropriately titrating antihypertensive medication is particularly critical to avoid orthostatic hypotension or adverse drug effects that can result in dizziness.[108] Discussion with the cardiologist or primary care specialist regarding medication adjustment may achieve a better balance of blood pressure control and dizzy symptoms. Similarly, psychogenic causes of dizziness can be addressed by managing the contributing factors such as anxiety or depression. Review of all medications and eliminating, reducing, or adjusting any psychotropic medications may also ameliorate the symptoms of dizziness.

Management of the elderly dizzy patient must also be directed toward fall prevention. Simple interventions including correcting vision, use of a walking stick, turning on a night-light at night, removing area rugs, improving sleep and rest, supervision, and securing railings and banisters in the home may go a long way toward avoiding the most devastating sequela of dizziness in the elderly. Particular attention to bathroom safety is important for older adults. Bathroom injury rates from falls increase with age, with rates exceeding 200 per 100,000 for people aged 85 years and older, and injury to the head or neck occurring in 31% of bathroom falls.[109] Injuries related to toileting are slightly more common than those related to bathing (shower or tub). Minor to moderate injuries (i.e., contusions, sprains) occur at a rate of nearly 160 per 100,000, while fracture rates exceed 165 per 100,000 in older adults. The Centers for Disease Control and Prevention recommends non-skid bathtub mats or strips and grab bars inside and outside of the tub/shower and next to the toilet.

SUMMARY

Dizziness is a common and potentially serious, even life-threatening complaint among the elderly. Left untreated, it can lead to falls and serious injuries. When possible, a multidisciplinary approach with an integrated strategy that includes fall prevention is more effective in the diagnosis and management of dizziness because the underlying causes often span multiple body systems and are not amenable to simple pharmacotherapy.

REFERENCES

1. Jönsson R, Sixt E, Landahl S, Rosenhall U. Prevalence of dizziness and vertigo in an urban elderly population. *J Vestib Res.* 2004;14(1):47–52.
2. Neuhauser H, von Brevern M, Radtke A, et al. Epidemiology of vestibular vertigo: a neurotologic survey of the general population. *Neurology.* 2005;65(6):898–904.
3. Popp P, Wulff M, Finke K, et al. Cognitive deficits in patients with a chronic vestibular failure. *J Neurol.* 2017;264(3):554–563.
4. Mueller M, Strobl R, Jahn K, et al. Burden of disability attributable to vertigo and dizziness in the aged: results from the KORA-Age study. *Eur J Public Health.* 2014;24(5):802–807.
5. Tinetti M, Williams C. Falls, injuries due to falls, and the risk of admission to a nursing home. *N Engl J Med.* 1997;337(18):1279–1284.
6. Kannus P, Parkkari J, Koskinen S, et al. Fall-induced injuries and deaths among older adults. *JAMA.* 1999;281(20):1895–1899.
7. Falls Among Older Adults: An Overview. Found at: http://www.cdc.gov/HomeandRecreationalSafety/Falls/adultfalls.html.
8. Ciorba A, Bianchini C, Scanelli G, et al. The impact of dizziness on quality-of-life in the elderly. *Eur Arch Otorhinolaryngol.* 2017;274(3):1245–1250.
9. Fernández L, Breinbauer HA, Delano PH. Vertigo and dizziness in the elderly. *Front Neurol.* 2015;6:144.
10. Tinetti M, Williams C, Gill T. Dizziness among older adults: a possible geriatric syndrome. *Ann Intern Med.* 2000;132(5):337–344.
11. Sloane P, Baloh R. Persistent dizziness in geriatric patients. *J Am Geriatr Soc.* 1989;37(11):1031–1038.
12. Neuhauser H. Epidemiology of vertigo. *Curr Opin Neurol.* 2007;20(1):40–46.
13. Maarsingh O, Dros J, Schellevis F, et al. Dizziness reported by elderly patients in family practice: prevalence, incidence, and clinical characteristics. *BMC Fam Pract.* 2010;11:2.
14. Piker EG, Jacobson GP. Self-report symptoms differ between younger and older dizzy patients. *Otol Neurotol.* 2014;35(5):873–879.
15. Parry SW, Hill H, Lawson J, et al. A novel approach to proactive primary care-based case finding and multidisciplinary management of falls, syncope, and dizziness in a one-stop service: preliminary results. *J Am Geriatr Soc.* 2016;64(11):2368–2373.
16. Larson LM, Sliter R, Helmer SD, et al. Outcomes in elderly fall victims: what happens after hospital discharge? *Am J Surg.* 2016;212(6):1106–1114.
17. Rubenstein L, Josephson K. The epidemiology of falls and syncope. *Clin Geriatr Med.* 2002;18(2):141–158.
18. King M, Tinetti M. Falls in community-dwelling older persons. *J Am Geriatr Soc.* 1995;43(10):1146–1154.
19. Alexander B, Rivara F, Wolf M. The cost and frequency of hospitalization for fall-related injuries in older adults. *Am J Public Health.* 1992;82(7):1020–1023.
20. Stevens J, Corso P, Finkelstein E, Miller T. The costs of fatal and non-fatal falls among older adults. *Inj Prev.* 2006;12(5):290–295.
21. Costs of Falls Among Older Adults. Found at: http://www.cdc.gov/HomeandRecreationalSafety/Falls/fallcost.html.
22. Graafmans W, Ooms M, Hofstee H, Bezemer P, Bouter L, Lips P. Falls in the elderly: a prospective study of risk factors and risk profiles. *Am J Epidemiol.* 1996;143(11):1129–1136.
23. O'Loughlin J, Boivin J, Robitaille Y, Suissa S. Falls among the elderly: distinguishing indoor and outdoor risk factors in Canada. *J Epidemiol Community Health.* 1994;48(5):488–489.
24. Rubenstein L, Josephson K. Falls and their prevention in elderly people: what does the evidence show? *Med Clin North Am.* 2006;90(5):807–824.

25. Whitney S, Marchetti G, Schade A. The relationship between falls history and computerized dynamic posturography in persons with balance and vestibular disorders. *Arch Phys Med Rehabil.* 2006;87(3):402–407.

26. Moreland J, Richardson J, Goldsmith C, Clase C. Muscle weakness and falls in older adults: a systematic review and meta-analysis. *J Am Geriatr Soc.* 2004;52(7):1121–1129.

27. Burker E, Wong H, Sloane P, et al. Predictors of fear of falling in dizzy and nondizzy elderly. *Psychol Aging.* 1995;10(1):104–110.

28. Perez-Jara J, Enguix A, Fernandez-Quintas J, et al. Fear of falling among elderly patients with dizziness and syncope in a tilt setting. *Can J Aging.* 2009;28(2):157–163.

29. Holmberg J, Karlberg M, Harlacher U, Magnusson M. Experience of handicap and anxiety in phobic postural vertigo. *Acta Otolaryngol.* 2005;125(3):270–275.

30. Belal A, Glorig A. Dysequilibrium of ageing (presbyastasis). *J Laryngol Otol.* 1986;100(9):1037–1041.

31. Lawson J, Fitzgerald J, Birchall J, et al. Diagnosis of geriatric patients with severe dizziness. *J Am Geriatr Soc.* 1999;47(1):12–17.

32. Sloane P. Evaluation and management of dizziness in the older patient. *Clin Geriatr Med.* 1996;12(4):785–801.

33. Katsarkas A. Dizziness in aging: the clinical experience. *Geriatrics.* 2008;63(11):18–20.

34. Bueno-Cavanillas A, Padilla-Ruiz F, Jiménez-Moleón J, et al. Risk factors in falls among the elderly according to extrinsic and intrinsic precipitating causes. *Eur J Epidemiol.* 2000;16(9):849–859.

35. Zalewski CK. Aging of the human vestibular system. *Semin Hear.* 2015;36(3):175–196.

36. Rosenhall U, Rubin W. Degenerative changes in the human vestibular sensory epithelia. *Acta Otolaryngol.* 1975;79(1–2):67–80.

37. Richter E. Quantitative study of human Scarpa's ganglion and vestibular sensory epithelia. *Acta Otolaryngol.* 1980;90(3–4):199–208.

38. Merchant S, Velázquez-Villaseñor L, Tsuji K, Glynn R, Wall C, Rauch S. Temporal bone studies of the human peripheral vestibular system. Normative vestibular hair cell data. *Ann Otol Rhinol Laryngol Suppl.* 2000;181:3–13.

39. Ishiyama G. Imbalance and vertigo: the aging human vestibular periphery. *Semin Neurol.* 2009;29(5):491–499.

40. Ishiyama A, Lopez I, Ishiyama G, Tang Y. Unbiased quantification of the microdissected human Scarpa's ganglion neurons. *Laryngoscope.* 2004;114(8):1496–1499.

41. Lopez I, Ishiyama G, Tang Y, et al. Estimation of the number of nerve fibers in the human vestibular endorgans using unbiased stereology and immunohistochemistry. *J Neurosci Methods.* 2005;145(1–2):37–46.

42. Tang Y, Lopez I, Baloh R. Age-related change of the neuronal number in the human medial vestibular nucleus: a stereological investigation. *J Vestib Res.* 2001–2002;11(6):357–363.

43. Lyon M, Davis J. Age-related blood flow and capillary changes in the rat utricular macula: a quantitative stereological and microsphere study. *J Assoc Res Otolaryngol.* 2002;3(2):167–173.

44. Lyon M, Wanamaker H. Blood flow and assessment of capillaries in the aging rat posterior canal crista. *Hear Res.* 1993;67(1–2):157–165.

45. Johnsson L, Hawkins J. Vascular changes in the human inner ear associated with aging. *Ann Otol Rhinol Laryngol.* 1972;81(3):364–376.

46. Peterka R, Black F, Schoenhoff M. Age-related changes in human vestibulo-ocular reflexes: sinusoidal rotation and caloric tests. *J Vestib Res.* 1990–1991;1(1):49–59.

47. Kerber K, Ishiyama G, Baloh R. A longitudinal study of oculomotor function in normal older people. *Neurobiol Aging.* 2006;27(9):1346–1353.

48. Baloh R, Enrietto J, Jacobson K, Lin A. Age-related changes in vestibular function: a longitudinal study. *Ann N Y Acad Sci.* 2001;942:210–219.

49. Furman J, Redfern M. Effect of aging on the otolith-ocular reflex. *J Vestib Res.* 2001;11(2):91–103.

50. Jacobson G, McCaslin D, Grantham S, Piker E. Significant vestibular system impairment is common in a cohort of elderly patients referred for assessment of falls risk. *J Am Acad Audiol.* 2008;19(10):799–807.

51. Katsarkas A. Dizziness in aging: a retrospective study of 1194 cases. *Otolaryngol Head Neck Surg.* 1994;110(3):296–301.

52. Fitzpatrick R, McCloskey D. Proprioceptive, visual and vestibular thresholds for the perception of sway during standing in humans. *J Physiol.* 1994;478(Pt 1):173–186.

53. Behm D, Bambury A, Cahill F, Power K. Effect of acute static stretching on force, balance, reaction time, and movement time. *Med Sci Sports Exerc.* 2004;36(8):1397–1402.

54. Wiles P, Pearce S, Rice P, Mitchell J. Vibration perception threshold: influence of age, height, sex, and smoking, and calculation of accurate centile values. *Diabet Med.* 1991;8(2):157–161.

55. Sturnieks D, St George R, Lord S. Balance disorders in the elderly. *Neurophysiol Clin.* 2008;38(6):467–478.

56. Peterka R, Black F. Age-related changes in human posture control: sensory organization tests. *J Vestib Res.* 1990–1991;1(1):73–85.

57. Horak F, Dickstein R, Peterka R. Diabetic neuropathy and surface sway-referencing disrupt somatosensory information for postural stability in stance. *Somatosens Mot Res.* 2002;19(4):316–326.

58. Lord S, Clark R, Webster I. Physiological factors associated with falls in an elderly population. *J Am Geriatr Soc.* 1991;39(12):1194–1200.

59. Schniepp R, Schlick C, Schenkel F, et al. Clinical and neurophysiological risk factors for falls in patients with bilateral vestibulopathy. *J Neurol.* 2017;264(2):277–283.

60. Bove M, Courtine G, Schieppati M. Neck muscle vibration and spatial orientation during stepping in place in humans. *J Neurophysiol.* 2002;88(5):2232–2241.

61. Deshpande N, Patla A. Postural responses and spatial orientation to neck proprioceptive and vestibular inputs during locomotion in young and older adults. *Exp Brain Res*. 2005;167(3):468–474.

62. Patel M, Fransson P, Karlberg M, Malmstrom E, Magnusson M. Change of body movement coordination during cervical proprioceptive disturbances with increased age. *Gerontology*. 2010;56(3):284–290.

63. Malmström E, Karlberg M, Fransson P, Lindbladh J, Magnusson M. Cervical proprioception is sufficient for head orientation after bilateral vestibular loss. *Eur J Appl Physiol*. 2009;107(1):73–81.

64. Lord S, Clark R, Webster I. Visual acuity and contrast sensitivity in relation to falls in an elderly population. *Age Ageing*. 1991;20(3):175–181.

65. Lord S. Visual risk factors for falls in older people. *Age Ageing*. 2006;35(suppl 2):ii42–ii45.

66. Haegerstrom-Portnoy G, Morgan MW. Normal age-related vision changes. In: *Rosenbloom & Morgan's Vision and Aging*. St. Louis: Butterworth-Heinemann; 2007:31–48.

67. Ishigaki H, Miyao M. Implications for dynamic visual acuity with changes in aged and sex. *Percept Mot Skills*. 1994;78(2):363–369.

68. Schubert M, Herdman S, Tusa R. Vertical dynamic visual acuity in normal subjects and patients with vestibular hypofunction. *Otol Neurotol*. 2002;23(3):372–377.

69. Poulain I, Giraudet G. Age-related changes of visual contribution in posture control. *Gait Posture*. 2008;27(1):1–7.

70. Borger L, Whitney S, Redfern M, Furman J. The influence of dynamic visual environments on postural sway in the elderly. *J Vestib Res*. 1999;9(3):197–205.

71. O'Connor K, Loughlin P, Redfern M, Sparto P. Postural adaptations to repeated optic flow stimulation in older adults. *Gait Posture*. 2008;28(3):385–391.

72. Peterka R, Black F. Age-related changes in human posture control: motor coordination tests. *J Vestib Res*. 1990-1991;1(1):87–96.

73. Larsson L, Ramamurthy B. Aging-related changes in skeletal muscle. Mechanisms and interventions. *Drugs Aging*. 2000;17(4):303–316.

74. Faulkner J, Larkin L, Claflin D, Brooks S. Age-related changes in the structure and function of skeletal muscles. *Clin Exp Pharmacol Physiol*. 2007;34(11):1091–1096.

75. Roos M, Rice C, Vandervoort A. Age-related changes in motor unit function. *Muscle Nerve*. 1997;20(6):679–690.

76. Moschner C, Baloh R. Age-related changes in visual tracking. *J Gerontol*. 1994;49(5):M235–M238.

77. McPherson D, Whitaker S, Wrobel B. DDX: Disequilibrium of aging. In: *Practical Management of the Dizzy Patient*. Philadelphia: Lippincott Williams & Wilkins; 2008:297–344.

78. Quoniam C, Hay L, Roll J, Harlay F. Age effects on reflex and postural responses to propriomuscular inputs generated by tendon vibration. *J Gerontol A Biol Sci Med Sci*. 1995;50(3):B155–B165.

79. Maarsingh O, Dros J, Schellevis F, et al. Causes of persistent dizziness in elderly patients in primary care. *Ann Fam Med*. 2010;8(3):196–205.

80. Drachman D. A 69-year-old man with chronic dizziness. *JAMA*. 1998;280(24):2111–2118.

81. Yeo SC, Ahn SK, Lee HJ, et al. Idiopathic benign paroxysmal positional vertigo in the elderly: a long-term follow-up study. *Aging Clin Exp Res*. 2017. http://dx.doi.org/10.1007/s40520-017-0763-2.

82. Baloh R. Dizziness in older people. *J Am Geriatr Soc*. 1992;40(7):713–721.

83. Choi JH, Seo JD, Kim MJ, et al. Vertigo and nystagmus in orthostatic hypotension. *Eur J Neurol*. 2015;22(4):648–655.

84. Nakamagoe K, Fujimiya S, Koganezawa T, et al. Vestibular function impairment in Alzheimer's disease. *J Alzheimers Dis*. 2015;47(1):185–196.

85. Bansal S, Hirdes JP, Maxwell CJ, et al. Identifying fallers among home care clients with dementia and Parkinson's disease. *Can J Aging*. 2016;35(3):319–331.

86. Sloane P, Hartman M, Mitchell C. Psychological factors associated with chronic dizziness in patients aged 60 and older. *J Am Geriatr Soc*. 1994;42(8):847–852.

87. Eckhardt-Henn A, Breuer P, Thomalske C, Hoffmann S, Hopf H. Anxiety disorders and other psychiatric subgroups in patients complaining of dizziness. *J Anxiety Disord*. 2003;17(4):369–388.

88. Delbaere K, Crombez G, Vanderstraeten G, Willems T, Cambier D. Fear-related avoidance of activities, falls and physical frailty. A prospective community-based cohort study. *Age Ageing*. 2004;33(4):368–373.

89. Li F, Fisher K, Harmer P, McAuley E, Wilson N. Fear of falling in elderly persons: association with falls, functional ability, and quality of life. *J Gerontol B Psychol Soc Sci*. 2003;58(5):P283–P290.

90. Ganz D, Bao Y, Shekelle P, Rubenstein L. Will my patient fall? *JAMA*. 2007;297(1):77–86.

91. Agostini J, Tinetti M. Drugs and falls: rethinking the approach to medication risk in older adults. *J Am Geriatr Soc*. 2002;50(10):1744–1745.

92. Menant J, St George R, Sandery B, Fitzpatrick R, Lord S. Older people contact more obstacles when wearing multifocal glasses and performing a secondary visual task. *J Am Geriatr Soc*. 2009;57(10):1833–1838.

93. Haran M, Cameron I, Ivers R, et al. Effect on falls of providing single lens distance vision glasses to multifocal glasses wearers: VISIBLE randomised controlled trial. *BMJ*. 2010;340:c2265.

94. Domínguez M, Magro J. Bedside balance testing in elderly people. *Curr Aging Sci*. 2009;2(2):150–157.

95. Kerber K. Dizziness in older people. In: Eggers SD, Zee DS, eds. *Vertigo and Imbalance: Clinical Neurophysiology of the Vestibular System*. vol. 9. Elsevier; 2010:491–501.

96. Aw S, Halmagyi G, Black R, Curthoys I, Yavor R, Todd M. Head impulses reveal loss of individual semicircular canal function. *J Vestib Res*. 1999;9(3):173–180.

97. Square Wave Jerks (SWJ). Found at: http://www.dizziness-and-balance.com/practice/nystagmus/SWJ.htm.

98. Barin K. Interpretation and usefulness of caloric testing. In: Jacobson G, Shepard N, eds. *Balance Function Assessment and Management.* San Diego: Plural Publishing; 2008:229–252.

99. Anson ER, Bigelow RT, Carey JP, et al. Aging increases compensatory saccade amplitude in the video head impulse test. *Front Neurol.* 2016;7:113. http://dx.doi.org/10.3389/fneur.2016.00113.

100. Janky K, Shepard N. Vestibular evoked myogenic potential (VEMP) testing: normative threshold response curves and effects of age. *J Am Acad Audiol.* 2009;20(8):514–522.

101. Tseng C, Chou C, Young Y. Aging effect on the ocular vestibular-evoked myogenic potentials. *Otol Neurotol.* 2010;31(6):959–963.

102. Nguyen K, Welgampola M, Carey J. Test-retest reliability and age-related characteristics of the ocular and cervical vestibular evoked myogenic potential tests. *Otol Neurotol.* 2010;31(5):793–802.

103. Brantberg K, Granath K, Schart N. Age-related changes in vestibular evoked myogenic potentials. *Audiol Neurootol.* 2007;12(4):247–253.

104. Lee S, Cha C, Jung T, Park D, Yeo S. Age-related differences in parameters of vestibular evoked myogenic potentials. *Acta Otolaryngol.* 2008;128(1):66–72.

105. Kumar K, Bhat JS, Sequeira NM, Bhojwani KM. Ageing effect on air-conducted ocular vestibular evoked myogenic potential. *Audiol Res.* 2015;5(2):121. http://dx.doi.org/10.4081/audiores.2015.121.

106. Rossi-Izquierdo M, Gayoso-Diz P, Santos-Pérez S, et al. Short-term effectiveness of vestibular rehabilitation in elderly patients with postural instability: a randomized clinical trial. *Eur Arch Otorhinolaryngol.* 2017;274(6):2395–2403.

107. Soto-Varela A, Faraldo-García A, Del-Río-Valeiras M, et al. Adherence of older people with instability in vestibular rehabilitation programmes: prediction criteria. *J Laryngol Otol.* 2017;131(3):232–238.

108. Pont L, Alhawassi T. Challenges in the management of hypertension in older populations. *Adv Exp Med Biol.* 2016.

109. Centers for Disease Control and Prevention. Non-fatal bathroom injuries among persons > 15 years, United States, 2008. *MMWR.* 2011;60:729–733.

CHAPTER 18

Medication-Related Dizziness in the Older Adult

YAENA MIN, PHD • OSAMA A. SHOAIR, PHD • PATRICIA W. SLATTUM, PHARMD, PHD

KEY POINTS

- Dizziness is highly prevalent among patients aged 65 years and older and may be associated with several common health conditions and the medications used to treat those conditions.
- The consequences of dizziness affect patients' health and quality of life and create an enormous economic burden on the health care system.
- For physicians to manage dizziness appropriately in older adults, it is crucial to assess possible underlying causes of dizziness that will facilitate accurate clinical decision-making.
- Performing a medication history and review are important for adjusting the medication regimen to help prevent or resolve medication-related dizziness.

Clinical Vignette

Mrs. K.J. is a pleasant, articulate 79-year-old woman describing episodic vertigo and chronic lightheadedness that began approximately 2 years ago without antecedent illness or injury. She states that the vertigo occurs without warning, lasts 15–30 minutes at each occurrence, and resolves completely with no residual symptoms. She has noted tightness in her chest, numbness and tingling in her lips and hands, grayed vision, and clammy sweating during these episodes. She denies associated auditory symptoms. She reports that she had four such episodes in the past year. Her symptoms of lightheadedness occur daily and seem slightly worse on transitioning from supine to sitting or sitting to standing position. She feels reasonably well when she first begins her morning routine but reports a foggy, disconnected feeling by midmorning, which persists until evening before gradually improving. She denies falls but reports near-falls two to three times per week. She lives alone following the death of her husband last year and becomes tearful and slightly agitated when expressing concerns for her own future in light of these symptoms. Her medical history is significant for hypertension, peripheral neuropathy affecting her legs below the knees, depression, anxiety, and seasonal allergies. Her medication list includes hydrochlorothiazide, propranolol, diazepam, meclizine, calcium and vitamin D supplements, fish oil, and garlic tablets.

MEDICATION-RELATED DIZZINESS

Dizziness is highly prevalent among adults aged 65 years and older in primary care or family practice settings (see Chapter 17), with estimates of prevalence greater than 30% in community-dwelling older adults and a higher prevalence in women than men.[1-5] A study of emergency department visits (1993–2005) from the National Hospital Ambulatory Medical Care Survey is in agreement with these prevalence rates from studies conducted in single institutions. From a total of 9472 patients presenting to the emergency department with dizziness sampled during this period, the study demonstrated that dizziness is an extremely common emergency department symptom that preferentially affects older adults and a greater proportion of women.[6] From an epidemiologic standpoint, it can be hypothesized that the incidence of dizziness-associated complications is expected to increase in the future based on the increasing US population projections for persons aged 65 years and older. According to the US Census Bureau, it is projected that 20% of Americans will be aged 65 years and older by 2030, and by 2060, this age group is projected to increase to 98 million from 46 million in 2014. Similarly, the 85 years and older population is expected to increase to 20 million by 2060 from 6 million in 2014.[7]

Although dizziness seems to increase with aging, normal aging is not the cause of dizziness, but other factors associated with aging make older adults more susceptible to dizziness.[8] Comorbid conditions, drug-related problems (due in part to altered pharmacokinetics and pharmacodynamics), polypharmacy, larger number of doses of medications per day, low body weight, and a history of adverse drug reactions predispose older adults to dizziness.[9–13]

Pharmacokinetics describes the relationship between the dose of the drug administered and the resulting drug concentrations achieved in the systemic circulation. Aging is generally characterized by changes in all pharmacokinetic processes, including absorption, distribution, metabolism and excretion, although the most clinically important changes are those affecting hepatic and renal drug elimination.[12] Hepatic metabolism may be reduced in older adults, particularly for drugs metabolized primarily by oxidative pathways. Impaired renal function with aging results in reduced renal clearance for drugs eliminated by the kidneys.[12] Altered pharmacokinetics with aging increases the risk of adverse drug events (ADEs), such as dizziness in older adults.

Pharmacodynamics describes the relationship between drug concentrations in the systemic circulation and drug response. Aging also affects pharmacodynamics through several mechanisms including altered concentrations of the drug at the receptor, altered interactions between the drug and its receptor, and changes in homeostatic regulation. Pharmacodynamic changes often result in increased sensitivity to medications, especially for drugs acting on the central nervous system (CNS).[12,14] Altered pharmacodynamics can also contribute to increased risk of ADEs, such as dizziness in older adults.

Polypharmacy refers to the use of multiple medications and/or the administration of more medications than is clinically indicated, representing unnecessary drug use.[15] Polypharmacy is associated with higher risk of ADEs, inappropriate use of medications, non-adherence, geriatric syndromes, and mortality in older adults.[15,16] In addition, ADEs can result from prescriber-related factors, such as therapeutic duplication, that is, prescriptions for one patient initiated by more than one prescriber. Such uncoordinated care further increases the risk of ADEs.[17]

There are a number of serious consequences associated with dizziness, and these may significantly affect the quality of life and health care burden, not only for the individual, but for the family as well.[18–20] For example, Cigolle and colleagues[21] performed a cross-sectional study to examine the prevalence of geriatric conditions (e.g., dizziness) among older adults and the association of these conditions with activities of daily living dependency (e.g., cognitive impairment contributing to dependency for bathing and dressing). In this study, data were obtained from the year 2000 from the Health and Retirement Study, a biennial longitudinal health interview survey of a cohort of adults aged 50 years or older in the United States. The results showed a strong and significant association, suggesting that geriatric conditions are associated with disability.[21]

Considerable progress has been made in the clinical setting to describe and define dizziness and its potential causes. Dizziness is a common symptom reported by older patients during physician visits.[22,23] Dizziness often is a multifactorial symptom associated with various diseases affecting sensory organs, the CNS, or both.[5] It may also be induced by processes outside the CNS or sensory organs, such as cardiovascular diseases, or by medications.[24] Dizziness is a complex subjective complaint.[25] In fact, difficulty diagnosing dizziness in older adults in family practice and specialty practice settings has been reported. The term "dizziness" can describe many different sensations that can be categorized by subtypes. These subtypes include vertigo, presyncope, disequilibrium, and non-specific dizziness.[8] In a medical chart audit study, it was recommended that documentation of selected key quality indicators in the management of dizziness could improve clinical diagnosis.[26]

Medication-related dizziness can be difficult to diagnose, especially in older persons in whom it can masquerade as a geriatric syndrome.[13] Geriatric syndromes are difficult to define, but they are characterized by symptoms with multifactorial causes, which become more common with aging, and are in fact often mistaken for normal aging.[27] Shared risk factors are likely to contribute to geriatric syndromes. The common geriatric syndromes associated with a high degree of morbidity include incontinence, falls, pressure ulcers, delirium, and functional decline.[27] Dizziness is considered by some geriatricians to meet the definition of a geriatric syndrome.[13] ADEs in older patients often present as non-specific symptoms or geriatric syndrome indicators, such as cognitive impairment or falls. Falls may be related to osteoarthritis, poor visual acuity, neurodegenerative disease, altered proprioception (e.g., diabetic peripheral neuropathy), and/or prescription medication affecting balance, cognitive function, and hemodynamics and cardiovascular function; therefore, discovering the underlying cause can be challenging.[28] Similarly, other health issues associated with dizziness are often multifactorial.[29] Involvement of cardiovascular, neurologic, sensory, and psychological domains, as well as medication-related ADEs, suggest that dizziness may be a geriatric syndrome.[26] Results from the emergency department study cited earlier support these associations. The study showed that otovestibular, cerebrovascular, metabolic, and cardiovascular disorders were at least twice as likely among patients presenting with dizziness.[6]

Because dizziness in the elderly may be more serious than in any other age group, accurate diagnosis and appropriate intervention are crucial.[22] A key component in the evaluation and general management of dizziness in older adults is patient history. A complete medication history is considered critical to the evaluation.[8] For this reason, Salles and colleagues[30] suggest that an interdisciplinary treatment approach to minimize contributive causes of dizziness in the elderly should include adjustment of the medication regimen. Medication history should take into account prescription medications, over-the-counter medications, herbal medicines, and nutraceuticals, as well as recreational drugs (including smoking and alcohol).[31] Common drug categories implicated in dizziness in older adults are listed in Table 18.1.[22,23,32-34]

In a report by Karatas examining 13 causes of central vertigo and dizziness, medication-related dizziness was not considered or discussed in detail.[35] Perhaps the omission was because of the paucity of published literature associating medication and dizziness or because medications are simply considered the least consequential factor associated with dizziness. Yet according to the US Food and Drug Administration (FDA) safety information data contained in the Adverse Event Reporting System (AERS) database between the years 2004 and 2009, dizziness was reported to be associated with a wide variety of medications. The authors' preliminary analysis identified more than 70,000 reports.[36] Because AERS reporting is voluntary, it has been suggested that there is a high degree of under-reporting,[37] and thus the actual number of patients with medication-associated dizziness may be considerably higher than previously thought.

In fact, Kroenke and colleagues,[38] in a review of the frequency of various causes of dizziness, categorized medication-related causes as "other causes," accounting for only 16% of the causes of dizziness. Other causes of dizziness included anemia and metabolic sources (e.g., hypoglycemia, hyperglycemia, electrolyte disturbances, thyroid disease).[38] This possible underestimation is not consistent with findings from the most recent cross-sectional diagnostic study assessing the contributory causes of dizziness in older adult patients in a primary care setting.[39] In this study, 417 older adult patients in the Netherlands, aged 65–95 years, who consulted their family physician for persistent dizziness, underwent a comprehensive evaluation by a panel of specialists. It was found that an ADE was considered to be the most common minor contributory cause of dizziness, occurring in 23% of their study sample.[39] In contrast to the results from the study by Kroenke and colleagues,[38] the conclusion drawn from this study was that medications are a significant cause of dizziness in some patients.

This chapter provides an overview of the available literature regarding medication-related dizziness in adults aged 65 years and older.

LITERATURE SEARCH STRATEGY

We searched MEDLINE/PubMed to identify potential studies of drug-induced dizziness in older adults for inclusion in this review. The search strategy included all articles published between January 1996 and April 2017 and used various MeSH terms, including dizziness, combined with one of the following search terms at a time: pharmaceutical preparations, psychotropic drugs, histamine antagonists, benzodiazepines, cholinergic antagonists, antihypertensive agents, anticonvulsants, hypnotics and sedatives, and polypharmacy. Additional articles were also obtained by searching databases such as CINAHL and PsycINFO and by manually reviewing the bibliographies of retrieved articles. Relevant English-language articles that studied adults aged 65 years and older were included. All studies were required to have medications as a predictor variable and dizziness as an outcome variable. Articles in foreign languages, including Chinese and German, were excluded. Relevant articles were selected by reviewing the abstracts to ensure that inclusion and exclusion criteria were met.

The following were excluded: studies that focused on relationships between dizziness and other outcomes not related to the objective of this article, case studies and case series, studies only assessing efficacy of drugs and not their safety or tolerability, studies of investigational drugs, studies of drug assays and pharmacokinetic evaluation, Phase 1 clinical studies, and studies focusing on drug use (rather than dizziness) as a predictor for falls and fractures. After applying these criteria, a total of 12 unique original research studies and systematic reviews were found to be suitable for conducting this review, which we organized by the class of medication: antihypertensives, benzodiazepines, hypnotics, anxiolytics, and antiepileptics.

TABLE 18.1
Medications That often Cause Dizziness in Older Adults

Class of Medication	Possible Mechanism
α_1-Adrenergic antagonists	Orthostatic hypotension
Alcohol	Hypotension, osmotic effects
Aminoglycosides	Ototoxicity
Anticonvulsants	Orthostatic hypotension, cerebellar dysfunction
Antidepressants	Orthostatic hypotension
Anti-Parkinson medication	Orthostatic hypotension
Antipsychotics	Orthostatic hypotension
β-Blockers	Hypotension or bradycardia
Calcium channel blockers	Hypotension, vasodilation
Class 1a antiarrhythmics	Torsades de pointes
Digitalis glycosides	Hypotension
Diuretics	Volume contraction, vasodilation
Narcotics	CNS depression, Torsades de pointes
Oral sulfonylurea	Hypoglycemia
Vasodilators	Hypotension, vasodilation
Anticoagulants	Bleeding complications
Antidementia agents	Bradycardia, syncope
Antihistamines: sedating	Torsades de pointes
Antirheumatic agents	Vestibular disturbance
Antiinfectives: antiinfluenza agents antifungals (oral), quinolones	Torsades de pointes
Antithyroid agents	Bone marrow toxicity
Anxiolytics	CNS depression
Attention-deficit/hyperactivity disorder agents	Cardiac arrhythmias
Cholesterol-lowering agents	Hypotension
Bronchodilators	Hypotension
Skeletal muscle relaxants	Central anticholinergic effects
Urinary and gastrointestinal antispasmodics	Central anticholinergic effects
Analgesics	Torsades de pointes
Chemotherapeutic agents	Torsades de pointes

Data from Sloane PD, Coeytaux RR, Beck RS, Dallara J. Dizziness: state of the science. *Ann Intern Med*. 2001;134(9 Pt 2):823–832; Jahn K, Kressig RW, Bridenbaugh SA, Brandt T, Schniepp R. Dizziness and unstable gait in old age: etiology, diagnosis and treatment. *Dtsch Arztebl Int*. 2015;112(23):387–393; *Lexi-Drugs*. Lexi-Comp, Inc. Available at: http://online.lexi.com/crlsql/servlet/crlonline; CredibleMeds. Available at: https://www.crediblemeds.org; Lempert T. Recurrent spontaneous attacks of dizziness. *Continuum (Minneap Minn)*. 2012;18(5 Neuro-otology): 1086–1101.

ANTIHYPERTENSIVE DRUGS

Antihypertensive drug use among older adults is common.[40,41] According to one study, the proportion of persons in 2003 reporting treatment of hypertension increased with age and was highest (49.6%) among those aged 65 years and older. Generally, women were more likely than men to report treatment of hypertension.[40] Box 18.1 provides a list of all FDA-approved antihypertensive medications available at present.[42] Of the adverse effects associated with antihypertensives, dizziness is more frequent among users than non-users of these drugs.[22] Information from the FDA[42] indicates that dizziness is a common side effect associated with the classes of medications listed in Box 18.1, except for calcium channel blockers and renin inhibitors.

Several other studies investigated in detail the potential association between antihypertensive medication use and dizziness in older adults. Hale and colleagues[43] performed a prospective study to evaluate CNS effects in older subjects using antihypertensive drugs. In this study, older adult participants were first screened on an annual basis for undetected medical disorders, and those in whom medical disorders were detected were referred to private physicians for 2 years of follow-up care. Findings from this study showed that dizziness was identified significantly more often in women than in men, and an association with antihypertensive medication dose was noted. This trend was particularly observed among women using propranolol, diuretics alone, and diuretics in combination with another antihypertensive agent, such as hydralazine, reserpine, or clonidine. Clearly, this information seems to suggest that the use of multiple medications (polypharmacy) contributes to the incidence of dizziness observed among women.[43] This finding is in agreement with results from a study by Hussain and colleagues,[44] which showed that the occurrence of adverse drug reactions to antihypertensive drugs was high among

women and was further increased among those on combination therapy compared with monotherapy. However, for men, propranolol was the only antihypertensive drug associated with a significant increase in episodes of dizziness.[43]

Cleophas and colleagues[45] examined whether using the combination of a β-blocker with a negative chronotropic calcium channel blocker (amlodipine, diltiazem, or mibefradil) would cause intolerable side effects in 335 patients (aged 18–75 years) with chronic stable angina pectoris. This study was a 10-week, double-blind, parallel-group comparison of amlodipine (5 and 10 mg), diltiazem (200 and 300 mg), and mibefradil (50 and 100 mg) treatment added to stable (i.e., baseline) β-blocker treatment. Serious symptoms of dizziness occurred in 14% of patients, resulting in their withdrawal from therapy: 19 patients were taking mibefradil (8 on low dose, 11 on high dose); 4 patients were taking diltiazem (1 on low dose, 3 on high dose); and 9 patients were taking amlodipine (4 on low dose, 5 on high dose).[45] Doses of diltiazem in this trial were low compared with doses used in standard practice in the United States. It was observed that low-dose diltiazem caused fewer symptoms of dizziness, and fewer patient withdrawals were observed among low-dose mibefradil users. Therefore, these data suggest that patients in the United States (with higher dose standards) might experience more pronounced symptoms or a higher incidence of dizziness with this combination of medications and dosage.

On the other hand, Ko and colleagues[46] studied adverse cardiovascular effects of β-blockers individually (carvedilol, metoprolol, bisoprolol, and bucindolol) in comparison with placebo. In this study, the investigators analyzed randomized trials on β-blockers in patients with heart failure and systolic dysfunction. The analysis included nine trials involving 14,594 patients, with follow-up periods ranging from 6 to 24 months. Results showed that β-blocker use was associated with a significant relative increase in reported dizziness (relative risk, 1.37; 95% confidence interval [CI], 1.09–1.71) and an absolute increase with a risk of 57 per 1000 cases (95% CI, 11–104). Results further indicated that the increased risk of dizziness was accompanied by hypotension because β-blockers lower blood pressure using various mechanisms. In addition, the study assessed withdrawal from therapy due to dizziness in 7789 patients from four trials. Overall, the investigators concluded that most patients in this study did not experience cardiovascular adverse effects (including dizziness) because the trials that were reviewed enrolled healthier and relatively fewer female and older adult patients.[46]

Angiotensin-converting enzyme (ACE) inhibitors have also been associated with dizziness.[42] Blakley and Gulati[47] illustrated the use of a practical new technique that may be useful in identifying groups of medications associated with dizziness. The patient group for this study included those who had electronystagmography at the Health Sciences Centre, Winnipeg, Canada. The mean age of the study group of 102 dizzy patients was 60 (±16) years, and these patients were taking a total of 173 drugs in 22 categories. ACE inhibitors were shown to be associated with dizziness.

A similar association was not found with other antihypertensive agents. In general, results indicate that antihypertensive drug use is more common in dizzy patients, and that the pattern of drug use in dizzy patients is different from that of non-dizzy patients. In other words, dizzy patients take more medications, and the dizziness they experience may be attributed to polypharmacy.[47]

Ensrud and colleagues[48] performed a cross-sectional examination of the prevalence and correlates of postural hypotension, postural dizziness, and associated risk factors, including medical conditions, medications, and physical findings in 9704 patients. The patients were non-black, ambulatory women, aged 65 years and older, living in a general community setting, participating in the multicenter Study of Osteoporotic Fractures. Of the risks identified, use of medications, specifically diuretics (odds ratio [OR], 1.15; 95% CI, 1.03–1.28), was associated with postural dizziness. However, these associations were only age-adjusted and might have been confounded by other covariates or risk factors.[48]

Finally, in an Oslo Health Study by Tamber and Bruusgaard,[49] a multipurpose health survey was conducted to explore the association between dizziness and factors such as self-reported diseases and medicines used. Results from the self-administered questionnaire showed increased likelihood of faintness or dizziness with the use (weekly or more frequent use) of blood pressure medications (OR, 1.27; 95% CI, 1.11–1.45). However, the investigators did not provide the details of the type of high blood pressure medication used, making it unclear which particular class or classes of antihypertensives are directly associated with dizziness.

BENZODIAZEPINES AND RELATED DRUGS

Benzodiazepines and related drugs (BZDs/RDs) are another group of medications commonly used in persons aged 65 years or older.[50,51] The likelihood of BZDs/RDs causing adverse events is high, and caution is advised.[51] Of particular interest, dizziness has been reported from a non-randomized clinical study by Puustinen and colleagues.[52] The primary objective of the study was to

describe the relationship between long-term use of BZDs/RDs and health, functional abilities and cognitive function in patients aged 65 years and older who were admitted to two acute care hospitals in Finland. The association between BZDs/RDs and dizziness was established after adjusting for the confounding variables of gender and the number of medications with CNS effects. Moreover, these findings were observed following long-term use of these agents, and the effect of dizziness tended to be related to the number of BZDs/RDs used. Unfortunately, the investigators did not report detailed data supporting these observations. Furthermore, the investigators noted that the use of BZDs/RDs, even concomitantly with other BZDs/RDs, was common and long-standing in this frail population under study, suggesting that the side effects experienced are likely to be attributed to polypharmacy. In addition, a study by Ensrud and colleagues evaluating the risk of falls measured self-reported dizziness and found 35% of benzodiazepine users (N = 626) had trouble with dizziness compared with 25% of non-users of benzodiazepine, antidepressant, anticonvulsant, and narcotics (N = 6720).[53]

SEDATIVE HYPNOTICS AND OTHER DRUGS

There is a paucity of data regarding drug-related dizziness caused by sedative hypnotics; only two studies were identified in the literature. In one study, medications other than antihypertensives were considered by Tamber and Bruusgaard.[49] This study showed an increased likelihood of faintness or dizziness with the use (weekly or more frequent) of sedatives (adjusted OR, 1.60; 95% CI, 1.34–1.92), tranquilizers (OR, 1.61; 95% CI, 1.26–2.04), and other medications or prescriptions (OR, 1.35; 95% CI, 1.23–1.49). In this study, women reported faintness or dizziness more often than men in age-adjusted multivariate analyses. For cutoff points of dizziness (i.e., any trouble, a little trouble, quite a lot of trouble, and extreme trouble), an increasing number of medications used (1–6) was associated with an increasing likelihood of faintness or dizziness. Again, polypharmacy seems to play a role in causing dizziness. Surprisingly and in contrast to other reports, prevalence of dizziness was not observed to increase with age. In fact, on multivariate analysis there was no difference in cutoff points of dizziness between participants aged 75 or 76 years and those aged 30 years. However, the investigators noted that because the study was based on self-reports, recall bias may have influenced patients' self-reports, thereby affecting interpretation of results.[49]

The second study is a meta-analysis to quantify and compare potential benefits and risks of short-term treatment with sedative hypnotics in older people with insomnia, who are otherwise free of psychiatric or psychologic disorders.[54] The meta-analysis included randomized, double-blind, controlled trials of any pharmacologic treatment of insomnia (including agents such as antihistamines, benzodiazepines, zolpidem, zopiclone, and zaleplon) for at least five consecutive nights; 24 studies (involving 2417 participants) with extractable data met inclusion and exclusion criteria. Results showed that of the adverse effects identified, psychomotor-type side effects, such as dizziness or loss of balance, were reported in 13 studies (1016 participants) and were more common after treatment with a sedative than placebo, although the results were not statistically significant (OR, 2.25; 95% CI, 0.93–5.41; $p = 0.07$).[43] Investigators noted, however, that interpretation of the data must take into account that all sedatives or all benzodiazepines were grouped together for analysis, irrespective of differences in half-life, potency, or dose, and that a potential source of variability exists because participants in the studies were from different settings (i.e., community-dwelling vs. inpatient/skilled nursing facility). Although modest clinical benefits were observed with the use of sedative hypnotics, the added risk of adverse events may not justify these benefits, particularly in the vulnerable older adult population.[54]

ANXIOLYTIC DRUGS

Although there is also a paucity of data regarding anxiolytic medications and dizziness, available evidence suggests that anxiolytic agents are associated with dizziness in older adult patients. Hale and colleagues[55] conducted a study to determine if the use of antianxiety agents is associated with more frequent complaints of CNS symptoms of dizziness, fainting, and blackout spells in an ambulatory older adult population. These participants were enrolled in the Dunedin Program (Dunedin, Florida). Results showed that three benzodiazepines (chlordiazepoxide, diazepam, and flurazepam) accounted for 87.2% and 79.8% of all anxiolytic drugs used by men and women, respectively. For women, statistically significant increases in reports of dizziness were observed in users of anxiolytic drugs compared with controls, although not observed in men. When reports of CNS symptoms were analyzed by individual drugs, few significant associations were found. Only users of diazepam reported a higher prevalence of dizziness than controls, probably because of the pharmacokinetic characteristics of diazepam in older adults taking multiple doses.[55] Diazepam accumulation is extensive and its washout is slow, with active compounds present 2 weeks after the last dose.[56] However, the observed association of anxiety-related

dizziness should be interpreted with caution. Dizziness may be a manifestation of anxiety itself, and therefore the symptom may simply reflect the underlying condition being treated rather than medication side effect.[55]

Additional investigations from the study by Ensrud and colleagues found that anxiety and/or sleeping medications taken at least once weekly were also associated with postural dizziness (OR, 1.43; 95% CI, 1.26–1.62).[48] However, the association was only age-adjusted, and thus the strength of association obtained might be confounded by other possible risk factors of postural dizziness.

ANTIEPILEPTIC DRUGS

Epilepsy among older persons in the United States is common, requiring frequent use of antiepileptic drugs.[57,58] In addition, these drugs are commonly used off-label to treat conditions such as neuropathic pain and diabetic neuropathy, neuromuscular disorders, and behavioral disturbances in Alzheimer's disease and other psychiatric disorders.[59–61] In fact, it has been reported that the frequency of antiepileptic drug use is even greater in patients residing in long-term care facilities, ranging from 10% to 12% of patients in skilled nursing facilities.[62] Dizziness is one of the most common adverse effects reported in clinical trials of antiepileptic medications and may occur even at therapeutic doses.[63,64] A summary of side effects of commonly prescribed antiepileptic drugs is shown in Table 18.2. In particular, barbiturates, carbamazepine, felbamate, gabapentin, lamotrigine, levetiracetam, phenytoin, tiagabine, topiramate, valproic acid, zonisamide, and oxcarbazepine are reported to be associated with dizziness in older adults; furthermore, the dizziness is dose-dependent.[61] This list agrees with a recent study performed by the Agency for Healthcare Research and Quality (AHRQ) regarding the Effective Health Care Program for Epilepsy. This study examined untoward side effects (including dizziness) associated with antiepileptic drugs.[65] Although the AHRQ report was general and included patients of all ages, dose-dependent side effects are also demonstrated in a study by Thompson and colleagues,[66] in which dose reduction for older adults was recommended for valproic acid, gabapentin, and pregabalin.

Older adults may be particularly vulnerable to medications that compromise balance because of a variety of factors, such as polypharmacy and pharmacodynamic changes.[63,67,68] Pharmacodynamic changes at the organ system level involve age-related impairment of homeostatic mechanisms resulting in an exaggerated response to a drug.[68] Fife and Sirven[63] summarized findings of

TABLE 18.2
Side Effects of Antiepileptic Drugs

Drug (Brand Name)	Side Effects
Phenytoin (Dilantin, Phenytek)	Dizziness, ataxia, diplopia, slurred speech, decreased coordination, confusion, gum hyperplasia
Carbamazepine (Carbatrol Equetro, Tegretol, Tegretol XR)	Dizziness, diplopia, ataxia, vertigo
Valproic acid (Depakene, Stavzor)	Dizziness, nausea, diarrhea, vomiting, dyspepsia weight gain, tremor, drowsiness, ataxia
Gabapentin (Neurontin)	Somnolence, dizziness, ataxia, weight gain, peripheral edema, fatigue, sedation
Pregabalin (Lyrica)	Somnolence, dizziness, ataxia, dry mouth, confusion, diarrhea, diplopia, blurred vision
Lamotrigine (Lamictal)	Somnolence, dizziness, ataxia, confusion, nausea, diplopia, sedation, headache
Topiramate (Topamax)	Somnolence, dizziness, ataxia, psychomotor slowing, anemia
Zonisamide (Zonegran)	Somnolence, dizziness, anorexia, nausea, irritability, sedation, confusion, headache, psychosis
Oxcarbazepine (Trileptal)	Somnolence, dizziness, diplopia, fatigue, nausea, vomiting, ataxia, abnormal vision, abdominal pain, tremor, dyspepsia, abnormal gait
Levetiracetam (Keppra, Keppra XR)	Somnolence, asthenia, infection, dizziness
Tiagabine (Gabitril)	Dizziness, asthenia, somnolence, nausea, nervousness/irritability, tremor, abdominal pain, impaired attention
Primidone (Mysoline)	Dizziness, sedation, ataxia, confusion, depression
Felbamate (Felbatol)	Insomnia, dizziness, sedation, headache
Rufinamide (Banzel)	Headache, dizziness, fatigue, somnolence, convulsion, diplopia, tremor, nystagmus
Lacosamide (Vimpat)	Headache, dizziness, diplopia, ataxia, fatigue, tremor, somnolence, blurred vision

Data from Lackner TE. Strategies for optimizing antiepileptic drug therapy in elderly people. *Pharmacotherapy*. 2002;22(3):329–64; Fife TD, Sirven J. Antiepileptic drugs and their impact on balance. *Aging Health*. 2005;1:147–55.

primarily randomized controlled trials on the incidence of dizziness, gait imbalance, or ataxia in patients taking antiepileptic drugs compared with those taking placebo. In contrast to the study by Thompson and colleagues,[66] primidone was included and was significantly associated with dizziness. According to Fife and Sirven, primidone and phenytoin are more likely to cause dizziness or imbalance than other antiepileptic drugs. In the study by Ensrud and colleagues, antiepileptic medication use was also associated with postural dizziness (OR, 1.25; 95% CI, 1.03–1.53).[48] Investigators noted, however, that the direct effects of antiepileptic drugs on balance are seriously understudied, and they suggested that prospective trials are needed to better understand these effects.[66]

CONCLUSIONS AND RECOMMENDATIONS

Evidence from the available literature clearly implicates medications as a risk factor for dizziness in the older adult population. Use of three or more medications (polypharmacy) for all classes considered is associated with an increased risk of dizziness. The association between polypharmacy and dizziness is also suggested in a cross-sectional diagnostic study of community-dwelling older adult patients.[39] This study found that the use of drugs in older adults was high: 33% of the dizzy patients used more than five drugs.[39] Kao and colleagues[29] made similar observations. Additionally, Runganga and colleagues found that older adults who took 5–9 medications and those who took 10 or more medications show more symptoms of dizziness than those who took fewer than 5 medications.[69]

This review found that there is a paucity of available literature reporting detailed studies on medication-related dizziness. In fact, most studies have focused on cardiovascular and CNS agents, and there is insufficient or a complete lack of studies on other classes of medications. Alarmingly, in 2012, the top five therapeutic classes of prescribed drugs purchased by Medicare beneficiaries aged 65 years and older (ranked by total expense) were metabolic, cardiovascular, CNS, respiratory, and gastrointestinal agents.[70,71] Of these top five therapeutic classes, metabolic and gastrointestinal agents are also associated with dizziness and are presented in Table 18.1. On this basis, the risk of medication-related dizziness may be underestimated. In fact, this limitation has been noted by Maarsingh and colleagues,[39] who suggest that the varying rates in reports of medication-related dizziness can possibly be explained by the fact that previous investigators may have underestimated the contribution of drugs as a cause of dizziness in older adults, because most of these reports studied only a small selection of all drugs potentially causing dizziness.[39]

It is crucial for physicians in clinical practice to have as much information as possible to make appropriate clinical decisions in the management of dizziness in the older adult population. Effective and safe patient care is challenging, especially for the vulnerable older population. As Salles and colleagues suggest, one goal for successfully managing dizziness in older adults is to identify and reduce the risk factors of chronic dizziness to minimize physical, psychologic, and social morbidity.[30] Dizziness must be carefully investigated to establish the possible cause and hence the appropriate intervention. To this end, the most important tools available to help the physician reach a diagnosis are patient history, clinical examination, and follow-up care.[22] Patients should be asked about details of their medication history; medical history, specifically systemic disorders that interfere with cerebral blood supply (such as vasculitis), which may produce vertigo because of either focal brainstem involvement or diffuse cerebral ischemia (see Chapter 16); description of the nature of the dizziness, including sensation, frequency, and duration; and any associated symptoms such as hearing loss, tinnitus, nausea and vomiting, and cranial nerve deficits. It is also important to determine the relationship between dizziness and position and motion.[8,30] Eleven instruments available to quantify functional effects of dizziness are listed in Table 18.3. These tools have been validated for use in older adults

for detecting patient burden due to dizziness.[4,77,85] Discontinuation of medications in older adults who are on complex drug regimens to manage multiple chronic diseases can be challenging, particularly when multiple prescribers are involved. Centrally acting medications generally require slow tapering rather than an abrupt discontinuation to avoid withdrawal symptoms. This requirement is also true with β-blockers. Determining a specific medication-related cause for dizziness can therefore take time, because changes are made to the medication regimen and symptoms are followed over time. Interestingly, most medication discontinuations or reductions do not result in adverse outcomes for older patients.[86]

Pharmacologic treatment with drugs such as meclizine (Antivert) is often recommended to manage dizziness in older adults.[87] Caution is advised, however, when prescribing meclizine for older adults. Meclizine is problematic because it is an antihistamine medication with anticholinergic properties.[88,89] Anticholinergic medications may contribute to adverse effects, including dizziness, confusion, memory impairment, falls, dry mouth, dry eyes, urinary incontinence, and constipation.[89,90] Because the anticholinergic adverse effects of meclizine include dizziness, the cumulative anticholinergic burden needs to be considered when deciding whether to prescribe this medication, as older adults may also be taking medications that are highly anticholinergic for treatment of incontinence and other conditions. Moreover, changes in sensitivity to anticholinergic medications have been associated with aging.[89] Because meclizine is available over the counter (Bonine), it is important to provide older patients with appropriate counseling regarding dose and frequency of use.

In particular, prescribing cascades involving anticholinergic drugs should be avoided. A prescribing cascade occurs when a medication is prescribed to treat the side effects of another medication.[91] Using meclizine to treat medication-related dizziness is an example of a prescribing cascade. Alternatives to the medication possibly contributing to dizziness should be considered before adding other medications. When anticholinergic medications such as meclizine are determined to be necessary, the minimum dose possible for the shortest duration of time should be prescribed. Dose reduction may sometimes ameliorate the anticholinergic effects.[92] Overall, the management of a medication regimen requires careful risk-benefit assessment.

In conclusion, medication-related dizziness is an important consideration in older adults. Attention should be paid to older adult patients who are particularly prone to ADEs caused by polypharmacy,

TABLE 18.3
Standardized Instruments for Evaluating the Severity and Effect of Dizziness on Quality of Life

Instrument or Tool	Domains	Items (n)	Scalability
Dizziness Handicap Inventory[72]	Activities that bring on or worsen dizziness, effect of symptoms on daily activities, emotional effect of dizziness (isolation, depression, fear)	25	One overall scale (range, 0–50) and three subscales (functional, emotional, and physical)
Dizziness Handicap Inventory Short Form[73]	Activities that bring on or worsen dizziness, effect of symptoms on daily activities, emotional effect of dizziness (isolation, depression, fear)	13	One scale (range, 0–13)
UCLA Dizziness Questionnaire[74]	Frequency and severity of dizziness, effect on daily activities and quality of life, fear of becoming dizzy	5	Scale range of 5 (least severe) to 25 (most severe)[75]
Vertigo-Dizziness-Imbalance Questionnaire[76]	Characterization of dizziness and associated symptoms, effect on quality of life	36	Two scales: symptoms (range, 0–100) and health-related quality of life (range, 0–100)
Dizziness Needs Assessment[77]	Identify the priorities of older adults with dizziness, evaluate psychometric properties of dizziness	18 quantitative items; one presumed etiology	Likert scale 1–6, yes/sometimes/no, other predefined answers
Vestibular Disorders of Daily Living Scale[78]	Effects of vertigo and balance disorders on independence and on routine activities of daily living	28	Four scales: total scale (range, 1–8), functional subscale (range, 1–5), ambulation subscale (range, 1–8), and instrumental subscale (range, 1–10)
Activities-specific Balance Confidence[79]	Assess balance confidence in daily activities	16	0–100 response continuum
Vertigo Handicap Questionnaire[80]	Handicap of restriction activity, social anxieties, fears about vertigo, severity of vertigo attacks	22	5-point Likert verbal scale (range, 0–4)
Dizzy Factor Inventory[81]	Symptom factors, obvious responses of significant others to the dizzy activity level	44	5-point Likert verbal scale (range, 0–5)
Vertigo Symptom Scale[82]	Acute attack of vertigo scale, vertigo of short duration, somatization scale, autonomic symptom scale	27	6-point Likert verbal scale (range, 0–5)
Vertigo Visual Analogue Scale[83,84]	Symptoms related to dizziness, vertigo, and imbalance	9	Using a 100 mm closed visual analogue scale—0 mm (no dizziness) to 100 mm (extreme dizziness)

changes in pharmacokinetics and pharmacodynamics, and the burden of comorbid conditions. However, more detailed investigations are needed to confidently assess the effects of specific medications on dizziness. Current evidence provides prescribers with some guidance on managing the potential effect of medications for patients presenting with dizziness. It is anticipated that the number of older adult patients presenting with conditions such as dizziness, possibly related to medication or polypharmacy, will likely increase in the future as medication use increases in the expanding older adult population.

REFERENCES

1. Colledge NR, Wilson JA, Macintyre CC, MacLennan WJ. The prevalence and characteristics of dizziness in an elderly community. *Age Ageing.* 1994;23(2):117–120.
2. Stevens KN, Lang IA, Guralnik JM, Melzer D. Epidemiology of balance and dizziness in a national population: findings from the English longitudinal study of ageing. *Age Ageing.* 2008;37(3):300–305.
3. Maarsingh OR, Dros J, Schellevis FG, van Weert HC, Bindels PJ, Horst HE. Dizziness reported by elderly patients in family practice: prevalence, incidence, and clinical characteristics. *BMC Fam Pract.* 2010;11:2.
4. Fong E, Li C, Aslakson R, Agrawal Y. Systematic review of patient-reported outcome measures in clinical vestibular research. *Arch Phys Med Rehabil.* 2015;96(2):357–365.
5. Barin K, Dodson EE. Dizziness in the elderly. *Otolaryngol Clin North Am.* 2011;44(2):437–454.
6. Newman-Toker DE, Hsieh YH, Camargo Jr CA, Pelletier AJ, Butchy GT, Edlow JA. Spectrum of dizziness visits to US emergency departments: cross-sectional analysis from a nationally representative sample. *Mayo Clin Proc.* 2008;83(7):765–775.
7. U.S. Census Bureau. *2014 National Population Projections;* 2014. Available at: http://www.census.gov/population/www/projections/data/national/2014.html.
8. Eaton DA, Roland PS. Dizziness in the older adult, part 1. Evaluation and general treatment strategies. *Geriatrics.* 2003;58(4): 28–30, 33–36.
9. Hayes BD, Klein-Schwartz W, Barrueto Jr F. Polypharmacy and the geriatric patient. *Clin Geriatr Med.* 2007;23(2):371–390, vii.
10. Catania PN. Risk factors for drug-related problems in elderly ambulatory patients. *Home Care Provid.* 1998;3(1): 20–21, 24.
11. Hanlon JT, Lindblad CI, Hajjar ER, McCarthy TC. Update on drug-related problems in the elderly. *Am J Geriatr Pharmacother.* 2003;1(1):38–43.
12. Corsonello A, Pedone C, Incalzi RA. Age-related pharmacokinetic and pharmacodynamic changes and related risk of adverse drug reactions. *Curr Med Chem.* 2010;17(6):571–584.
13. Tinetti ME, Williams CS, Gill TM. Dizziness among older adults: a possible geriatric syndrome. *Ann Intern Med.* 2000;132(5):337–344.
14. Hilmer SN, McLachlan AJ, Le Couteur DG. Clinical pharmacology in the geriatric patient. *Fundam Clin Pharmacol.* 2007;21(3):217–230.
15. Hajjar ER, Cafiero AC, Hanlon JT. Polypharmacy in elderly patients. *Am J Geriatr Pharmacother.* 2007;5(4): 345–351.
16. Hohl CM, Dankoff J, Colacone A, Afilalo M. Polypharmacy, adverse drug-related events, and potential adverse drug interactions in elderly patients presenting to an emergency department. *Ann Emerg Med.* 2001;38(6):666–671.
17. Vinks TH, de Koning FH, de Lange TM, Egberts TC. Identification of potential drug-related problems in the elderly: the role of the community pharmacist. *Pharm World Sci.* 2006;28(1):33–38.
18. Neuhauser HK, Radtke A, von Brevern M, Lezius F, Feldmann M, Lempert T. Burden of dizziness and vertigo in the community. *Arch Intern Med.* 2008;168(19):2118–2124.
19. Tinetti ME, Williams CS, Gill TM. Health, functional, and psychological outcomes among older persons with chronic dizziness. *J Am Geriatr Soc.* 2000;48(4):417–421.
20. Stam H, van der Wouden JC, van der Horst HE, Maarsingh OR. Impairment reduction in older dizzy people in primary care: study protocol for a cluster randomised controlled trial. *Trials.* 2015;16:313.
21. Cigolle CT, Langa KM, Kabeto MU, Tian Z, Blaum CS. Geriatric conditions and disability: the health and retirement study. *Ann Intern Med.* 2007;147(3):156–164.
22. Sloane PD, Coeytaux RR, Beck RS, Dallara J. Dizziness: state of the science. *Ann Intern Med.* 2001;134(9 Pt 2): 823–832.
23. Jahn K, Kressig RW, Bridenbaugh SA, Brandt T, Schniepp R. Dizziness and unstable gait in old age: etiology, diagnosis and treatment. *Dtsch Arztebl Int.* 2015;112(23): 387–393.
24. Katsarkas A. Dizziness in aging: the clinical experience. *Geriatrics.* 2008;63(11):18–20.
25. Kroenke K, Lucas CA, Rosenberg ML, et al. Causes of persistent dizziness. A prospective study of 100 patients in ambulatory care. *Ann Intern Med.* 1992;117(11):898–904.
26. Kwong EC, Pimlott NJ. Assessment of dizziness among older patients at a family practice clinic: a chart audit study. *BMC Fam Pract.* 2005;6(1):2.
27. Inouye SK, Studenski S, Tinetti ME, Kuchel GA. Geriatric syndromes: clinical, research, and policy implications of a core geriatric concept. *J Am Geriatr Soc.* 2007;55(5):780–791.
28. Hamilton HJ, Gallagher PF, O'Mahony D. Inappropriate prescribing and adverse drug events in older people. *BMC Geriatr.* 2009;9:5.
29. Kao AC, Nanda A, Williams CS, Tinetti ME. Validation of dizziness as a possible geriatric syndrome. *J Am Geriatr Soc.* 2001;49(1):72–75.
30. Salles N, Kressig RW, Michel JP. Management of chronic dizziness in elderly people. *Z Gerontol Geriatr.* 2003; 36(1):10–15.
31. Samy HM, Hamid MA. *Dizziness, Vertigo, and Imbalance. Emedicine Neuro-otology;* 2010. Available at: http://www.emedicine.medscape.com.
32. *Lexi-Drugs.* Lexi-Comp, Inc. Available at: http://online.lexi.com/crlsql/servlet/crlonline.
33. CredibleMeds. Available at: https://www.crediblemeds.org.
34. Lempert T. Recurrent spontaneous attacks of dizziness. *Continuum (Minneap Minn).* 2012;18(5 Neuro-otology):1086–1101.
35. Karatas M. Central vertigo and dizziness: epidemiology, differential diagnosis, and common causes. *Neurologist.* 2008;14(6):355–364.
36. U.S. Food and Drug Administration. *Adverse Event Reporting System (AERS).* Available at: http://www.fda.gov/Drugs/GuidanceComplianceRegulatoryInformation/Surveillance/AdverseDrugEffects/default.htm.

37. U.S. Food and Drug Administration. *MedWatch: The FDA Safety Information and Adverse Event Reporting Program.* Available at: http://www.fda.gov/Safety/MedWatch/default.htm.

38. Kroenke K, Hoffman RM, Einstadter D. How common are various causes of dizziness? A critical review. *South Med J.* 2000;93(2):160–167. [quiz: 168].

39. Maarsingh OR, Dros J, Schellevis FG, et al. Causes of persistent dizziness in elderly patients in primary care. *Ann Fam Med.* 2010;8(3):196–205.

40. Miller GE, Zodet M. *Trends in the Pharmaceutical Treatment of Hypertension, 1997 to 2003* Research findings No. 25 Rockville, MD: Agency for Healthcare Research and Quality; 2006. Available at: http://meps.ahrq.gov/mepsweb/data_files/publications/rf25/rf25.pdf.

41. Centers for Disease Control and Prevention. *Health, United States, 2015: With Special Feature on Racial and Ethnic Health Disparities*Hyattsville, Maryland; 2016. https://www.cdc.gov/nchs/data/hus/hus15.pdf.

42. U.S. Food and Drug Administration, Office of Women's Health. *High Blood Pressure Medicines to Help You.* Available at: http://www.fda.gov/forconsumers/byaudience/forwomen/ucm118594.htm.

43. Hale WE, Stewart RB, Marks RG. Central nervous system symptoms of elderly subjects using antihypertensive drugs. *J Am Geriatr Soc.* 1984;32(1):5–10.

44. Hussain A, Aqil M, Alam MS, Khan MR, Kapur P, Pillai KK. A pharmacovigilance study of antihypertensive medicines at a South Delhi hospital. *Indian J Pharm Sci.* 2009;71(3):338–341.

45. Cleophas TJ, van der Sluijs J, van der Vring JA, et al. Combination of calcium channel blockers and beta-blockers for patients with exercise-induced angina pectoris: beneficial effect of calcium channel blockers largely determined by their effect on heart rate. *J Clin Pharmacol.* 1999;39(7):738–746.

46. Ko DT, Hebert PR, Coffey CS, et al. Adverse effects of beta-blocker therapy for patients with heart failure: a quantitative overview of randomized trials. *Arch Intern Med.* 2004;164(13):1389–1394.

47. Blakley BW, Gulati H. Identifying drugs that cause dizziness. *J Otolaryngol Head Neck Surg.* 2008;37(1):11–15.

48. Ensrud KE, Nevitt MC, Yunis C, Hulley SB, Grimm RH, Cummings SR. Postural hypotension and postural dizziness in elderly women. The study of osteoporotic fractures. The Study of Osteoporotic Fractures Research Group. *Arch Intern Med.* 1992;152(5):1058–1064.

49. Tamber AL, Bruusgaard D. Self-reported faintness or dizziness – comorbidity and use of medicines. An epidemiological study. *Scand J Public Health.* 2009;37(6):613–620.

50. Bartlett G, Abrahamowicz M, Tamblyn R, Grad R, Capek R, du Berger R. Longitudinal patterns of new benzodiazepine use in the elderly. *Pharmacoepidemiol Drug Saf.* 2004;13(10):669–682.

51. Bogunovic OJ, Greenfield SF. Practical geriatrics: use of benzodiazepines among elderly patients. *Psychiatr Serv.* 2004;55(3):233–235.

52. Puustinen J, Nurminen J, Kukola M, Vahlberg T, Laiane K, Kivela SL. Associations between use of benzodiazepines or related drugs and health, physical abilities and cognitive function: a non-randomised clinical study in the elderly. *Drugs Aging.* 2007;24(12):1045–1059.

53. Ensrud KE, Blackwell TL, Mangione CM, et al. Central nervous system-active medications and risk for falls in older women. *J Am Geriatr Soc.* 2002;50(10):1629–1637.

54. Glass J, Lanctot KL, Herrmann N, Sproule BA, Busto UE. Sedative hypnotics in older people with insomnia: meta-analysis of risks and benefits. *BMJ.* 2005;331(7526):1169.

55. Hale WE, Stewart RB, Marks RG. Antianxiety drugs and central nervous system symptoms in an ambulatory elderly population. *Drug Intell Clin Pharm.* 1985;19(1):37–40.

56. Salzman C, Shader RI, Greenblatt DJ, Harmatz JS. Long v short half-life benzodiazepines in the elderly. Kinetics and clinical effects of diazepam and oxazepam. *Arch Gen Psychiatry.* 1983;40(3):293–297.

57. Leppik IE, Birnbaum A. Epilepsy in the elderly. *Semin Neurol.* 2002;22(3):309–320.

58. Choi H, Pack A, Elkind MS, Longstreth Jr WT, Ton TG, Onchiri F. Predictors of incident epilepsy in older adults: the cardiovascular health study. *Neurology.* 2017;88(9):870–877.

59. Rogawski MA, Loscher W. The neurobiology of antiepileptic drugs for the treatment of nonepileptic conditions. *Nat Med.* 2004;10(7):685–692.

60. Roane DM, Feinberg TE, Meckler L, Miner CR, Scicutella A, Rosenthal RN. Treatment of dementia-associated agitation with gabapentin. *J Neuropsychiatry Clin Neurosci.* 2000;12(1):40–43.

61. Lackner TE. Strategies for optimizing antiepileptic drug therapy in elderly people. *Pharmacotherapy.* 2002;22(3):329–364.

62. Cloyd JC, Lackner TE, Leppik IE. Antiepileptics in the elderly. Pharmacoepidemiology and pharmacokinetics. *Arch Fam Med.* 1994;3(7):589–598.

63. Fife TD, Sirven J. Antiepileptic drugs and their impact on balance. *Aging Health.* 2005;1:147–155.

64. Zaccara G, Giovannelli F, Cincotta M, Loiacono G, Verrotti A. Adverse events of placebo-treated, drug-resistant, focal epileptic patients in randomized controlled trials: a systematic review. *J Neurol.* 2015;262(3):501–515.

65. Agency for Healthcare Research and Quality (AHRQ), Effective Health Care Program. *Evaluation of Effectiveness and Safety of Antiepileptic Medications in Patients with Epilepsy.* Available at: http://www.effectivehealthcare.ahrq.gov/ehc/products/159/868/Epilepsy_FinalReport_20120802.pdf.

66. Thompson D, Takeshita J, Thompson T, Mulligan M. Selecting antiepileptic drugs for symptomatic patients with brain tumors. *J Support Oncol.* 2006;4(8):411–416.

67. Agostini JV, Han L, Tinetti ME. The relationship between number of medications and weight loss or impaired balance in older adults. *J Am Geriatr Soc.* 2004;52(10):1719–1723.

68. Jackson SH. Pharmacodynamics in the elderly. *J R Soc Med.* 1994;87(suppl 23):5–7.

69. Runganga M, Peel NM, Hubbard RE. Multiple medication use in older patients in post-acute transitional care: a prospective cohort study. *Clin Interv Aging.* 2014;9:1453–1462.

70. Marc R. *Expenditures for the Top Five Therapeutic Classes of Outpatient Prescription Drugs, Medicare Beneficiaries, Age 65 and Older*U.S. Civilian Noninstitutionalized Population, 2012. Statistical brief #469 Rockville, MD: Agency for Healthcare Research and Quality; 2015. Available at: http://www.meps.ahrq.gov/data_file/publications/st469.pdf.

71. Ruckenstein MJ, Staab JP. The basic symptom inventory-53 and its use in the management of patients with psychogenic dizziness. *Otolaryngol Head Neck Surg.* 2001;125(5):533–536.

72. Jacobson GP, Newman CW. The development of the dizziness handicap inventory. *Arch Otolaryngol Head Neck Surg.* 1990;116(4):424–427.

73. Tesio L, Alpini D, Cesarani A, Perucca L. Short form of the dizziness handicap inventory: construction and validation through Rasch analysis. *Am J Phys Med Rehabil.* 1999;78(3):233–241.

74. Honrubia V, Bell TS, Harris MR, Baloh RW, Fisher LM. Quantitative evaluation of dizziness characteristics and impact on quality of life. *Am J Otol.* 1996;17(4):595–602.

75. Treleaven J, Peterson G, Ludvigsson ML, Kammerlind AS, Peolsson A. Balance, dizziness and proprioception in patients with chronic whiplash associated disorders complaining of dizziness: a prospective randomized study comparing three exercise programs. *Man Ther.* 2016;22:122–130.

76. Prieto L, Santed R, Cobo E, Alonso J. A new measure for assessing the health-related quality of life of patients with vertigo, dizziness or imbalance: the VDI questionnaire. *Qual Life Res.* 1999;8(1–2):131–139.

77. Kruschinski C, Klaassen A, Breull A, Broll A, Hummers-Pradier E. Priorities of elderly dizzy patients in general practice: findings and psychometric properties of the "Dizziness Needs Assessment" (DiNA). *Z Gerontol Geriatr.* 2010;43(5):317–323.

78. Cohen HS, Kimball KT. Development of the vestibular disorders activities of daily living scale. *Arch Otolaryngol Head Neck Surg.* 2000;126(7):881–887.

79. Powell LE, Myers AM. The activities-specific balance confidence (ABC) scale. *J Gerontol A Biol Sci Med Sci.* 1995;50(1):M28–M34.

80. Yardley L, Putman J. Quantitative analysis of factors contributing to handicap and distress in vertiginous patients: a questionnaire study. *Clin Otolaryngol Allied Sci.* 1992;17(3):231–236.

81. Hazlett RL, Tusa RJ, Waranch HR. Development of an inventory for dizziness and related factors. *J Behav Med.* 1996;19(1):73–85.

82. Yardley L, Masson E, Verschuur C, Haacke N, Luxon L. Symptoms, anxiety and handicap in dizzy patients: development of the vertigo symptom scale. *J Psychosom Res.* 1992;36(8):731–741.

83. Dannenbaum E, Chilingaryan G, Fung J. Visual vertigo analogue scale: an assessment questionnaire for visual vertigo. *J Vestib Res.* 2011;21(3):153–159.

84. Kammerlind AS, Håkansson JK, Skogsberg MC. Effects of balance training in elderly people with nonperipheral vertigo and unsteadiness. *Clin Rehabil.* 2001;15(5):463–470.

85. Duracinsky M, Mosnier I, Bouccara D, Sterkers O, Chassany O, Working Group of the Societe Francaise d'Oto-Rhino-Laryngologie (ORL). Literature review of questionnaires assessing vertigo and dizziness, and their impact on patients' quality of life. *Value Health.* 2007;10(4):273–284.

86. Iyer S, Naganathan V, McLachlan AJ, Le Couter DG. Medication withdrawal trials in people aged 65 years and older: a systematic review. *Drugs Aging.* 2008;25:1021–1031.

87. Eaton DA, Roland PS. Dizziness in the older adult, part 2. Treatments for causes of the four most common symptoms. *Geriatrics.* 2003;58(4)(46):49–52.

88. Rudd KM, Raehl CL, Bond CA, Abbruscato TJ, Stenhouse AC. Methods for assessing drug-related anticholinergic activity. *Pharmacotherapy.* 2005;25(11):1592–1601.

89. Rudolph JL, Salow MJ, Angelini MC, McGlinchey RE. The anticholinergic risk scale and anti- cholinergic adverse effects in older persons. *Arch Intern Med.* 2008;168(5):508–513.

90. Mintzer J, Burns A. Anticholinergic side-effects of drugs in elderly people. *J R Soc Med.* 2000;93(9):457–462.

91. Gill SS, Mamdani M, Naglie G, et al. A prescribing cascade involving cholinesterase inhibitors and anticholinergic drugs. *Arch Intern Med.* 2005;165(7):808–813.

92. Lieberman 3rd JA. Managing anticholinergic side effects. *Prim Care Companion J Clin Psychiatry.* 2004;6(suppl 2):20–23.

CHAPTER 19

Older Adults With Dizziness: Rehabilitation Strategies and Novel Interventions

MUHAMMAD ALRWAILY, PT, MS, PHD • SUSAN L. WHITNEY, DPT, PHD

INTRODUCTION

Dizziness is a common problem in the elderly (65 years and older),[1] with a prevalence between 13% and 38% depending on the population studied.[2-4] Dizziness affects the lives of older adults and is associated with restrictions in activities of daily living,[5] worsening of cognitive status,[6] fear of falling,[7] and an increased risk of falling.[8] Dizziness and its relationship to falls are of particular concern because falls pose a serious threat for older adults.[8] Of older adults who fall, 10% sustain a major injury, including head injury, hip fractures, or dislocation.[9] Of those who fracture their hip, 20% die within 1 year.[10] Such consequences not only suggest the disabling nature of dizziness and imbalance but also demonstrate the detrimental repercussions of dizziness in older adults.

Dizziness is an imprecise term used by patients to describe symptoms of vertigo, syncope, lightheadedness, disequilibrium, and other non-specific sensations.[11] Each of these terms is defined and linked to a host of diagnoses listed in Table 19.1. Dizziness may stem from central disorders and/or peripheral vestibular disorders. Central disorders that give rise to dizziness include cerebrovascular disease/vertebrobasilar insufficiency,[12] multiple sclerosis (MS),[13] Parkinson disease (PD),[14] tumors,[15] normal-pressure hydrocephalus, and global atrophy. Although central disorders appear in only 8% of patients with dizziness,[16] they are strong predictors of falls, with more than 50% of patients with central disorders falling more than twice a year.[17] Of patients with central disorders and history of frequent falls, 12%–42% sustain head injury or hip fracture.[17]

Dizziness may also stem from peripheral vestibular disorders. In contrast to central disorders, peripheral disorders are considered the principle cause of dizziness, appearing in 40%–50% of patients with dizziness.[8] Peripheral vestibular disorders constitute a host of diagnoses (Table 19.1), with benign paroxysmal positional vertigo (BPPV) being the most common.[16]

Peripheral disorders result in recurrent falls in approximately 25% of patients, and up to 10% of these patients sustain serious injuries.[17]

It is worth noting that dizziness can stem from a combination of peripheral and central disorders in 20%–40% of patients.[17] In addition, dizziness may occur from causes unrelated to the vestibular system, such as cardiovascular disorders,[18] medication and polypharmacy,[19] age-related structural deterioration of the vestibular system,[20-22] and psychogenic disorders.[11]

Many types of dizziness, when assessed appropriately, can be managed with vestibular rehabilitation exercises (VREs). VREs may be blended with novel technologies such as virtual reality or the Nintendo Wii system.[23,24] VREs have been shown to improve dizziness, quality of life, and postural control and reduce the risk of falling.

In the next sections, the role of rehabilitation providers in screening, assessing risk of falling, assessing quality of life, and managing patients with dizziness is illustrated. Also, VREs and theories related to functional recovery of certain conditions of dizziness are discussed. In addition, novel rehabilitation technologies for older adults with dizziness are described.

THE ROLE OF THE REHABILITATION PROVIDER IN EVALUATING PATIENTS WITH DIZZINESS

The evaluation of older adults with dizziness by rehabilitation providers generally includes screening, assessment of fall risk, and assessment of quality of life.

Screening

Because dizziness stems from many causes, rehabilitation providers need to work with physicians and other healthcare providers to determine the cause and recommend the optimal treatment strategy. To do that, rehabilitation providers can screen patients with dizziness using

TABLE 19.1
Dizziness Terms, Description of Symptoms, and Common Diseases Associated With Each Description[a]

Symptom	Description of Symptom	Associated Pathologies
Vertigo	Illusion of movement of the body or spinning of the environment Cause: peripheral or central vestibular disorder	**Peripheral vestibular disorders:** • Benign paroxysmal positional vertigo • Meniere disease • Acute peripheral vestibulopathy • Otosclerosis • Acoustic neuroma • Infection of the acoustic nerve • Perilymphatic fistula • Autoimmune disease of the inner ear • Toxic vestibulopathy **Central vestibular disorders:** • Wernicke encephalopathy • Cerebellar infection • Cerebellar degeneration • Spinocerebellar degeneration • Hypothyroidism • Migraine • Wilson disease • Creutzfeldt-Jakob disease • Posterior fossa tumors • Chiari malformation • Familial paroxysmal ataxia • Ataxia-telangiectasia
Syncope	Loss of consciousness that is not associated with illusion of movement Cause: vascular disorder	**Pancerebral hypoperfusion:** • Vasovagal presyncope • Cardiovascular presyncope • Takayasu disease • Carotid sinus syndrome • Orthostatic hypotension • Hyperventilation • Cough-related syncope • Micturition syncope • Glossopharyngeal neuralgia • Hypoglycemia **Brainstem hypoperfusion:** • Vertebrobasilar insufficiency • Vertebrobasilar infarction • Vertebrobasilar migraine • Subclavian steal syndrome
Disequilibrium	Sensation of imbalance without illusion of movement or loss of consciousness Cause: visual/somatosensory impairment	**Visual impairment** **Somatosensory impairment**
Other nonspecific forms	Vague floating sensation that does not follow the description of any other form. Cause: not particular to a specific system	**Musculoskeletal:** • Cervicogenic dizziness • Temporomandibular joint dizziness **Psychogenic:** • Panic disorder • Depression • Anxiety disorder

[a]People with complete bilateral vestibular lesion do not complain of dizziness. Their chief complaint is "oscillopsia," which is often described as visual jumping or environment moving.

TABLE 19.2
Symptoms, Symptom Behavior, and Signs that Indicate Serious Pathology (Red Flags)

Symptoms in patients with dizziness that may indicate the presence of serious pathology
- Slurred speech
- Hearing loss that occurs suddenly, gradually, or unilaterally
- Double vision (diplopia)
- Visual field loss
- Color vision loss
- Bilateral paresthesia or numbness
- Nondermatomal pattern paresthesia or numbness
- Paresthesia or numbness in the face
- Weakness of the face
- Difficulty swallowing
- Memory loss
- Unexplained weight loss
- Increasing and expanding severe pain

Symptom behavior in patients with dizziness that may indicate the presence of serious pathology
- Constant
- Triggered only with change in body position (e.g., sit to stand)
- Presence of prodromal symptoms[a]

Signs in patients with dizziness that may indicate the presence of serious pathology
- Eye movement abnormalities:
  - Persistent spontaneous nystagmus
  - Persistent upbeating, downbeating, or torsional nystagmus with or without a change of head position
  - Seesaw nystagmus
  - Periodic alternating nystagmus
  - Skew deviation
  - Horner syndrome (ptosis, meiosis)
- The finding of negative head-thrust test, direction-changing nystagmus in eccentric gaze, and skew deviation with new onset of dizziness
- Weakness
- Ataxic gait
- Positive Babinski/increased deep tendon reflexes
- Facial weakness

Patients with red flags are not appropriate for vestibular rehabilitation unless a physician has already cleared them. These signs and symptoms when found during the clinical examination indicate that the patient should be referred to other healthcare providers.
[a]Symptoms that occur in the period between the triggering factor and the onset of dizziness and include lightheadedness, pallor, salivation, blurred vision, or increased heart rate.

a classification system that places the patients into three groups: red flags, yellow flags, and green flags.[11] Red flag screening involves assessing patients with dizziness for signs, symptoms, or symptom behavior indicative of serious pathologies (Table 19.2). Yellow flag screening involves assessing patients for the presence of behavioral or nonbehavioral disorders. Behavioral disorders that may be associated with dizziness include panic disorders, phobic disorders, and depression. Nonbehavioral disorders include PD, stroke, head injuries, MS, migraine (not common among older adults with dizziness),[16] and musculoskeletal disorders. Green flags indicate patients whose dizziness stems from primarily peripheral vestibular disorders, and the assessment involves determining whether the patient has BPPV, unilateral vestibular hypofunction, or bilateral vestibular loss.

This screening process of dizziness can aid the rehabilitation provider and the physician in determining the best management strategy. For red flags, patients are less likely to benefit from VREs; these patients require specialized, often urgent medical attention that could involve medication or surgery. For yellow flags, patients may benefit from VREs; however, the effect of VREs may be lessened or delayed because of the presence of concomitant disorders, vestibular/ocular motor impairment,[25] or catastrophic emotional reaction to dizziness.[26] As such, the concomitant disorders or impairments should be treated as the patient is receiving VREs, which would likely improve the results of VREs.[27] For green flags, patients are more likely to benefit from VREs, and as such, rehabilitation providers may treat these patients independently. If an acute vestibular hypofunction is identified (within 4 weeks), a medical referral for consideration of steroids is advised.[28]

Assessment of Falling Risk and Quality of Life in Older Adults

The rehabilitation provider uses a multidimensional assessment of fall risk and quality of life. The assessment starts with history taking to identify frequent fallers (i.e., more than twice a year), use of medication(s) associated with increased fall risk, fear of falling, and functional limitations in daily living activities. The assessment continues by identifying physical factors related to falls, such as visual acuity, cognitive status, need for an assistive device, balance, orthostatic vital signs, sensation, and fallers' vital signs. Fallers' vital signs include gait speed, gait variability, the stop walking when talking test, and the Timed Up and Go (TUG) test.[29-31]

Similar to measuring blood pressure and body temperature to screen for general health status, gait speed can also be used to assess general health status and disability in older adults.[32] Age-appropriate gait speed is reflective of health status because gait requires body support, muscle power, coordination, and timing. Thus the interaction of these factors to produce an adequate gait speed can be viewed as a proxy for effective interaction of the musculoskeletal, nervous, and cardiopulmonary systems.[33]

When testing gait speed, it is important to specifically attend to gait fluctuations during slow walking; such fluctuations are predictive of falls.[34] Also, it is important to observe whether a patient stops walking when talking because such behavior is linked to fall-related anxiety.[35] Gait speed is a suitable measure to assess fall risk and quality of life because it provides quick, inexpensive, and reliable information regarding quality of life and risk of falling. Therefore improvement in gait speed has been shown to be a good indicator of treatment effectiveness, and slowing of gait speed can indicate a worsening medical condition.[36]

The TUG test is often used to assess a person's ability to rise from a chair, ambulate, and turn, which can be difficult for individuals with central and/or peripheral vestibular disorders.[37] The time (in seconds) required to perform the test is strongly correlated with functional mobility.[30] People who can complete the TUG within 20 seconds are found to be independent in transfer tasks such as moving from the wheelchair to a bed, and have sufficient gait speed (0.5 meters/second) for limited community mobility.[30] Podsiadlo and Richardson reported that people who walk very slowly (0.5 meters/second) were not able to ambulate freely in the community.[30] Older adults who took 13.5 seconds or longer to perform the TUG test were classified as frequent fallers, with an overall correct prediction rate of 90%.[37] Also, people who required more than 13.5 seconds to perform the TUG were 3.7 times more likely to have reported a fall in the previous 6 months.[38] The sensitivity of the TUG test for fall prediction in persons with vestibular disorders is 80%, and the specificity is 56% for those who score greater than 11.1 seconds on the test.[38] Generally, slow completion of the TUG test is associated with an increased impairment of function and warrants referral for rehabilitation, particularly if symptoms listed in Table 19.3 are present.

THE ROLE OF THE REHABILITATION PROVIDER IN TREATING PATIENTS WITH DIZZINESS

Dysfunction in the vestibular system can result in dizziness, postural imbalance, increased risk of falling, and ultimately a lower quality of life.[39] To rehabilitate the vestibular system, VREs are commonly recommended (Table 19.4).[40] Currently, VREs are utilized by various practitioners but mainly physical therapists specializing in vestibular physical therapy.

TABLE 19.3
Older Adults Should Be Referred to Rehabilitation If They Have One or More of the Following Signs
Positive Dix-Hallpike test
Positive Romberg test
Dizziness with movement of the head
Dizziness associated with neck pain
Slow gait
History of falling two or more times within the past 6 months
Inability to rise from a chair without using arm support
Fear of falling that prohibits the person from participating in activities of interest
Arrhythmic gait

Improvements in a variety of areas after VREs have been reported regardless of patient age.[39] VREs were found to be effective in patients with vestibular disorders (even with a history of symptoms lasting over 20 years),[27,41] patients with PD,[42] patients with anxiety and depression,[43] and in postsurgical patients, such as after removal of an acoustic neuroma.[44]

After VREs, patients show dramatic improvements in their perception of dizziness,[39,45] ability to perform activities of daily living,[39,45] emotional status,[46] and improved static and dynamic balance.[39,47] Positive effects of VREs are reported to occur as early as 3 weeks after initiation of therapy; for those who do not receive VREs, improvement may take as long as 3 months.[47] This suggests that VREs expedite improvement.

The effect of VREs on gait and balance may be significantly enhanced if the performance of VREs is closely monitored[48]; if VREs are combined with flexibility, cognition, sensory interaction, and muscle strength exercises[27]; or if VREs are combined with canalith repositioning maneuvers when appropriate.[49,50] Combining VREs with other interventions might be preferred when a patient has a concomitant disorder or a poorer baseline status; this combination can be achieved without increasing the number of treatment visits.[51]

THE EFFECT OF VESTIBULAR REHABILITATION ON VARIOUS CONDITIONS

Table 19.5 summarizes conditions that improve with vestibular rehabilitation and positive outcomes that were found with each condition. Theories that underlie why vestibular rehabilitation may be effective are described in Table 19.6.

TABLE 19.4
Exercises Commonly Used in Vestibular Physical Therapy Management

Type of the Exercise	Reason for the Exercise	Description
Vestibulo-ocular reflex (VOR) adaptation exercises	Help the central nervous system to adapt to a change or loss in the vestibular system input	VOR × 1: The patient moves the head to both sides (yawing or pitching) while keeping his eyes fixed on a stationary target (Fig. 19.1) VOR × 2: The head and the hand holding the target are moving in opposite directions with the eyes fixated on the target
Habituation exercises	Involves repeated exposure to a provoking stimulus or movement so the pathologic response to the stimulus is reduced	The therapist selects movements that provoke the patient's symptoms, and the patient repeats these motions until the patient no longer reacts adversely to the stimuli
Substitution exercises	Help patients improve one channel of sensory input (vision, somatosensory, proprioception) by blocking sensory inputs from the other two channels	To challenge proprioception, the patient closes the eyes and tries to maintain balance while standing
Optokinetic stimulation	Can help to desensitize people who are very sensitive to motion in the periphery and also who are motion sensitive	Example: Have the patient sitting and spin an umbrella about 1 m away from them in a circle while they look at the center of the umbrella

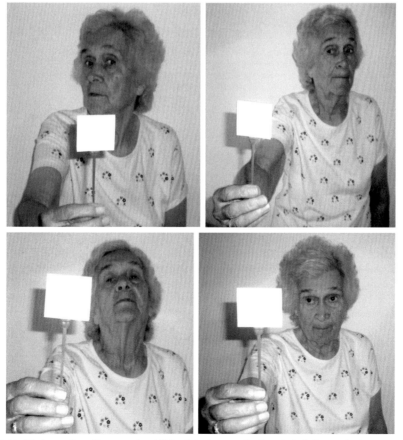

FIG. 19.1 Vestibulo-ocular reflex exercise (VOR × 1) in the yaw (top) and pitch (bottom) planes. An older woman performing VOR × 1 adaptation exercises. The patient holds the target in her hand and moves the head in the yaw plane (right and left) or in the pitch plane (up and down) while fixating the eyes on the target.

TABLE 19.5
Conditions That Improve With Vestibular Rehabilitation

Patient Diagnosis	Noted Improvement With Vestibular Physical Therapy
Benign paroxysmal positional vertigo	Subjective report of vertigo,[49,52–57] nystagmus,[49,53] quality of life[52]
Unilateral vestibular disorders	Fall risk,[58,59] vision,[59–61] balance,[62,63] quality of life[64]
Chronic peripheral vestibular dysfunction	Vestibulo-ocular reflex gain and dizziness,[65,66] standing balance,[64,67,68] emotional status (i.e., anxiety)[43]
Bilateral vestibular dysfunction	Postural control,[69–71] gait speed,[69,70] dizziness,[69–71] vision[72]
Vestibular neuritis	Ocular torsion (i.e., nystagmus),[73] postural control,[44,73] ambulation skills and gait[74]
Post-acoustic neuroma resection	Postural control,[44,75,76] dizziness,[77] motion sensitivity[44]
Meniere's disease	Self-report of symptoms,[78] balance,[78] dizziness, motion sensitivity[79]
Anxiety associated with vestibular disorder	Anxiety,[80] subjective report,[81] postural control,[80] presence of nystagmus, and ability to cope with dizziness[46]
Cervical vertigo	Postural stability,[82] decreased neck pain,[83] intensity of dizziness,[82,83] postural sway[82]
Head injury	Gait improved,[84] postural stability,[84,85] less dizziness,[86] gaze stability[87]
Cerebellar disease and dysfunction	Self-perception of symptoms,[88,89] postural control,[88,89] gait,[89] decreased risk of falling[88,89]
Multiple sclerosis	Subjective report of dizziness and postural control[90,91]
Parkinson's disease	Subjective complaint of vertigo[42]

Peripheral Vestibular Disorders

Benign paroxysmal positional vertigo

Even though dizziness is very common among older adults, it seems that BPPV is underestimated in this population[92], possibly because the majority of older adults (61%) do not report dizziness unless they are asked.[93] This is concerning because older adults with BPPV have a higher prevalence of falls compared to those without BPPV.[93] These findings suggest that older adults should be screened for dizziness even if they do not report it as a symptom.

Clinically, BPPV can be easily identified by provoking symptoms using the Dix-Hallpike test (see Chapter 9). If BPPV is noted, patient referral to clinicians who are trained in canalith repositioning procedures (CRPs) is warranted. Based on strong evidence, CRPs are reported to be very effective in treating symptoms of BPPV[94,95] and improving the perception of verticality.[96] Shepard and Telian reported complete resolution of symptoms in 100% of their population after performing CRPs.[97] If CRPs do not resolve patients' symptoms, it is likely that another type of VRE would improve symptoms; a combination of the CRPs and VREs may also improve outcomes.[49,50]

Special consideration must be taken into account when testing or treating older adults with BPPV. Because skilled or self-administered repositioning maneuvers typically require approximately 30 degrees of neck extension and 45 degrees of neck rotation,[95,98] patients with spine conditions must be addressed cautiously. Patients with neck or low back pain should have cervical or lumbar support during CRP because limited neck or trunk mobility can be affected by quick and unanticipated movements, which might reproduce the patient's pain. Patients with osteoporosis or Paget's disease are at risk for pathologic fractures. Most importantly, patients with severe rheumatoid arthritis must be treated with great care because ligamentous laxity, especially within the upper cervical spine, is very common, and moving the neck beyond normal limits may cause serious injury or a lesion to the spinal cord. Thus it is important to screen patients with BPPV for these conditions before beginning testing or intervening.

Chronic unilateral vestibular dysfunction

Patients with chronic unilateral vestibular dysfunction are good candidates for VREs and have a good prognosis.

TABLE 19.6
Theories Underlying Vestibular Rehabilitation

Theory	Brief Description	Function	Malfunction	Exercises
Vestibulo-ocular reflex (VOR) adaptation	A reflex mediated by a three-neuron arc: 1. Vestibular afferent 2. Vestibular efferent 3. Ocular motor neuron	Enables stabilization of a visual image on the retina during head movement Produces an eye movement of equal velocity to head movement but in the opposite direction. When the head moves to the right, the eyes instantaneously move to the left at the same speed of the head. This ratio of eye movement velocity opposite to head movement velocity is referred to as VOR gain	The eyes are not moving in the opposite direction of the head with the same speed as the head. The image stabilization on the retina during head movement is affected resulting in corrective eye movements	VOR × 1 and VOR × 2 (Fig. 19.1). It is believed that these exercises decrease symptoms of dizziness and improve function in elderly patients with vestibular hypofunction
Cervicoocular reflex (COR)	Eye movement induced by neck stimulation during trunk rotation while the head is stationary	Interacts with the VOR to drive eye movement based on input from cervical proprioceptors	The COR may be adaptable in some but not all people with vestibular hypofunction. This response is called for when needed, although not all patients have the ability to utilize the COR	Body moving with the head stable
Vestibulo-spinal reflex (VSR)	Input regarding body position is sent from semicircular canals and vestibular nuclei to medial and lateral vestibulospinal tracts	Stabilize the body via increasing extensor muscle activity on the side to which the head is turned with concomitant flexion activity on the other side	Inability to maintain balance	Balance training and gait exercises
Sensory reweighting	Sensory reweighting consists of: 1. Somatosensation 2. Vision 3. Vestibular function	There are three sensory modalities through which the body maintains balance or controls posture	When somatosensation, vision, or vestibular function is lost or impaired, the central nervous system readjusts to become more reliant on the remaining intact modalities	During vestibular rehabilitation the patient is repeatedly exposed to various sensory information so the brain can optimize postural responses to maintain balance

Ninety percent of patients dramatically improve or completely recover postural control and disability status after rehabilitation, provided that the patient has no central disorders.[97] Improvements in these patients were reported in dizziness symptoms, postural control, as well as physical and emotional status after VREs.

Improvements after VREs are correlated with plasticity and compensation mechanisms in the central nervous system (CNS).[67] This correlation between VREs and plasticity is expressed as changes in the vestibulo-ocular reflex (VOR), enhanced balance and reduced "retinal slip" or apparent motion of visual images.[67] Improvements in dizziness, postural control, and quality of life have been reported in patients with chronic vestibular disorders after receiving a combination of VREs and visual stimuli by digital images.[99] Based on strong evidence, using VREs for patients with unilateral or bilateral vestibular hypofunction is suggested in a recent practice guideline.[100]

Bilateral vestibular dysfunction

Although full recovery of symptoms does not occur in patients with bilateral vestibular dysfunction, patients can benefit from VREs.[60,69,101] Improvements in these patients have been reported in gait speed, stair negotiation, and postural stability.[70,102] Patients with bilateral vestibular loss fall more frequently than others with vestibular loss and age-matched controls.[103] As a result, exercise programs are designed to decrease the likelihood of falling and to minimize the risk of injury from falling. Patients with bilateral vestibular loss should also receive specific instruction regarding how to get up off the floor after a fall.

Vestibular neuritis

VREs can assist the patient with vestibular neuritis to recover functional abilities after an episode. The aim of VREs is to promote neural plasticity in the CNS and to accelerate central compensation via adaptation of the VOR and through enhancement of vestibulospinal reflexes and distal somatosensory optimization (Table 19.4).[73,104]

After administration of VREs for patients with vestibular neuritis, Strupp et al. reported faster recovery of postural stability in stance, vestibulospinal compensation, and earlier resumption of normal daily activities (e.g., playing tennis or returning to work) compared with a control group.[73] Also, early VREs seem to produce satisfactory outcomes in performing daily functions within 2 months on average.[104]

Meniere's disease

Patients with Meniere's disease may benefit from referral to vestibular rehabilitation providers during the inactive phase of the disease to receive support and education about the disease process. The rehabilitation provider assesses the patient's current balance abilities and strength and provides advice regarding how to prevent falls during an active attack of the disease.[105] Patients with Meniere's disease and vertigo receiving medical therapy or minimally invasive techniques may benefit from VREs to improve balance and dizziness symptoms associated with the disease and its effects on the involved vestibular system. Exercises such as gaze stabilization, visual acuity, and static and dynamic postural exercises were found to have some positive effect on balance function and gait.[78,106]

Functional dizziness (functional movement disorder)

Functional dizziness refers to changes in the functioning of the organ system rather than structural defects.[107] Functional dizziness includes phobic postural vertigo disorder, chronic subjective dizziness, and persistent postural-perceptual dizziness.[107] In neurotology clinics, functional dizziness is reported in 10% of patients with vestibular symptoms.[107] Functional dizziness is not the same as psychogenic comorbidities (e.g., anxiety and depression) that may occur concomitantly with structural defects of the vestibular system. Compared with functional dizziness, the prevalence of psychogenic comorbidities is reported to be higher among patients with BPPV (51%), bilateral vestibular loss (24%), and vestibular neuritis (37%).[108]

Whether the patient has functional dizziness or a vestibular defect with associated psychogenic comorbidities, treatment should include a combination of VREs, psychological therapy, and possibly antidepressant medication.[107,109,110] This combination of interventions has been shown to improve self-reported dizziness symptoms and postural control.[111]

Postsurgical conditions

The use of VREs aids in optimizing results both before and after ablative vestibular surgery and acoustic neuroma resection.[112,113] A rehabilitation program is recommended especially if reduction of dizziness-related symptoms (e.g., vertigo or postural instability) after the surgery does not match the surgeon's expectations. After surgery, dizziness can be the result of incomplete or delayed postoperative compensation. Instead of proceeding to additional surgery, a trial of VREs is advised when incomplete compensation is suspected.[97] Receiving VREs after surgery has been shown to reduce self-reported dizziness, nystagmus, disequilibrium, and motion sensitivity and improve postural and dynamic stability.[44,77,79] These improvements can occur as early as 1–3 weeks after the postsurgical VREs.[114]

A few reports have suggested that preoperative VREs may hasten patients' recovery after ablative surgery.[112,113,115] Preoperative VREs that include movement of the head help patients avoid postoperative vertigo and symptoms of acute vestibular loss.[113] A preoperative VRE program starts 14 days before the surgery and continues into the first weeks after surgery. Preoperative VREs can improve postural stability for up to 6 months after ablative surgery.[115]

Central Vestibular Disorders

Patients who complain of dizziness due to central disorders or mixed central and peripheral disorders are harder to treat with VREs than those with only peripheral disorders.[84,116]

Parkinson's disease

Falls are reported in 38%–68% of patients with PD.[117–119] In 12% of patients with PD, the cause of a fall is attributed to dizziness.[120] Thirteen percent of patients living with PD who fall sustain a fracture.[121] The risk of a fall and the report of dizziness in patients with PD can be significantly reduced by VREs.[42,122] Vestibular exercises are believed to play a key role in plasticity and compensation mechanisms within the central vestibular system.[67] Vestibular rehabilitation for patients with PD seems to be effective in improving self-reported dizziness, activities of daily living, gait speed, balance, and, most importantly, the risk of falling.[123] Such improvements seem to persist at least 1 year after the rehabilitation program.[122]

Falls in patients with PD can be caused by impairments other than dizziness, such as tremor, freezing, retropulsion, and rigidity.[120] Loss of postural reflexes is a cardinal manifestation of PD and likely represents complex interruption of signals within and between several body systems. In any case, falls in patients with PD should be assessed and addressed, and in addition to consideration of personal safety issues, management should include balance and muscle strengthening exercises,[124] which may be combined with vestibular rehabilitation if necessary.

Multiple sclerosis

Dizziness is a common complaint of patients with MS.[125] Vertigo is the initial symptom in approximately 5% of patients with MS; 50% of patients with MS experience dizziness at some time during the disease course.[125] After rehabilitation, improvements in self-reported dizziness, the TUG test, gait speed, and postural and dynamic balance have been reported in patients with MS.[90,91,126]

However, dizziness is not the only important clinical manifestation in patients with MS. Other symptoms such as fatigue, muscle weakness, sensory abnormalities, visual impairment, and depression occur in patients with MS.[127] Consideration of these symptoms along with dizziness is likely to improve treatment outcomes.

Head injuries

Head injuries are commonly associated with reports of dizziness or vertigo, especially in older adults.[128,129] Dizziness may result from hemorrhage of the brainstem or the brain if trauma is severe.[129] If trauma is mild and there are no fractures or hemorrhage, dizziness may be caused by damage to the inner ear or vestibular nerve[128] or may be attributed to concussion, posttraumatic BPPV, or perilymphatic fistula.[130] Dizziness related to

head injuries can persist for 6 months or more after the event.[105,131]

Dizziness after head injury is predictive of delayed recovery,[132] particularly if the patient has vestibulo-ocular dysfunction.[133] This could be due to injury of the CNS, which can impair compensatory mechanisms in the central vestibular system.[134] Dizziness caused by head injuries can be effectively treated with vestibular rehabilitation.[135] After head injury, patients who developed unilateral vestibular dysfunction had improved self-reported dizziness and postural stability after participation in a vestibular rehabilitation program.[86] However, careful consideration of comorbid symptoms (e.g., muscle tone abnormalities, lack of coordination, cognitive impairment, concussive symptoms of fatigue, fogginess, headache) optimizes the results of an exercise program.[128]

IMPORTANT CONSIDERATIONS WITH VESTIBULAR REHABILITATION

Vestibular rehabilitation is not limited to the conditions discussed earlier, although this review presents common examples of central disorders affecting vestibular system function that can be improved with vestibular rehabilitation. Conditions such as cerebellar disorders,[88] cervical vertigo,[82,136] vertebrobasilar artery insufficiency, and stroke can all result in dizziness and can benefit from vestibular rehabilitation.[89,116,136,137]

Although improvements after rehabilitation are established,[47,58,138] there are several other variables that affect the outcome of rehabilitation. As noted, people with bilateral vestibular dysfunction, despite the reported benefit after therapy,[70] do not respond as quickly and favorably to exercises as those with unilateral vestibular dysfunction.[139,140] Similarly, patients with central or mixed central and peripheral vestibular disorders show less successful rehabilitation outcomes as compared to patients with a peripheral vestibular lesion.[141] However, patients with posttraumatic head injury do report improvement in symptoms.[135,141] Vestibular suppressant medications, such as meclizine, have been found to reduce or delay improvements and are generally not recommended.[62,142] Anxiety, depression, visual dependence, and autonomic arousal have also been linked to protracted recovery in persons with vestibular neuritis.[143]

Customized or supervised exercises seem to be superior to generic or home-based exercises.[46,67,100,144,145] Customized exercise programs allow rehabilitation providers to assess progress of their patients regularly and to provide feedback to the patient about the correct way of performing the exercises.[145] Although elderly males with limited balance and stability are more likely to abandon vestibular rehabilitation programs,[146] it seems that customized exercises with remote telephone support improve patient compliance.[147]

Compensation mechanisms can be effectively induced by exercises that provide sensory feedback appropriate for behavioral changes to promote sensory-motor reorganization. However, variables that may delay compensation include fear of falling, anxiety, multiple vestibular dysfunction, late physical therapy intervention,[148] and impaired sensation (e.g., peripheral neuropathy).[149]

NOVEL INTERVENTIONS IN TREATING OLDER ADULTS WITH VESTIBULAR DISORDERS

In addition to exercises to assist patients with vestibular disorders, there are promising new technologies and novel interventions in the field of vestibular rehabilitation.

Virtual Reality

Virtual reality has long been used in the treatment of motor or psychological dysfunction.[150] This human-computer interaction-based technology (Fig. 19.2)

allows patients to actively participate in a real-time three-dimensional virtual world. Virtual reality uses images and graphics that are generated by the computer, making the patients sense that they are immersed in a real environment (e.g., supermarket), while in the clinic.[24,151]

Virtual reality technology use for vestibular rehabilitation may promote adaptation and compensation by causing retinal slip. Induction of retinal slip produces optokinetic eye movements, which in turn stimulates adaptation mechanisms, and has been shown to improve balance in patients with uncompensated peripheral vestibular lesions.[67] Rehabilitation involving conflicting visual environments may be more effective than traditional exercises.[144] Virtual reality allows rehabilitation providers to dose the exercise in a very safe environment with the ability to control the stimulation that provokes the patient's symptoms.

Virtual reality may be used to provoke stimuli repetitively and quickly. Repeated exposure to provoking stimuli is known as habituation exercise and is suggested to promote compensation and adaptation in patients with vestibular dysfunction.[152] Places with repeated and robust visual sensory stimulation, such as supermarkets or shopping malls, induce symptoms of dizziness and postural sway[153]; however, it is impractical for a rehabilitation provider to monitor a patient's

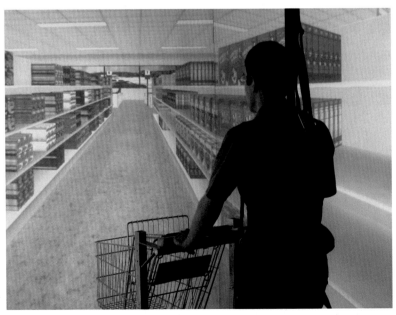

FIG. 19.2 Virtual reality grocery store. The patient is pushing the grocery cart at the self-selected gait speed, and the scene moves at the same velocity.

performance in these real-life situations. Therefore virtual reality provides a suitable alternative for rehabilitation providers to immerse the patient in a real-life environment, improving the patients' visual vertigo and/or space and motion discomfort in the safety of the clinic.[154]

Because maintenance of balance relies on sensory inputs coming from vision, proprioception, and vestibular function, virtual reality can work to reprioritize these senses when one or more is compromised. Virtual-reality-aided exercises can increase the patient's ability to maintain balance by using both visual and proprioceptive inputs instead of relying on only the sensory system.[151] Virtual reality has been used to treat older patients with balance problems and those at risk for falling; such patients showed less trunk sway and better postural responses after virtual reality exposures.[155] Virtual reality has been shown to result in no difference in gait speed, balance, visual acuity, and anxiety or depression levels compared with traditional vestibular rehabilitation; however, virtual reality was judged to be more exciting and less tiring for the patients.[156]

Balance-Enhancing Insoles

Reduction or loss of distal sensation in the lower extremities has been associated with aging.[157–159] Loss of distal sensation is correlated with gait abnormalities, impaired balance, and increased risk of falling.[160–162] Enhancement of distal sensation may occur via stimulating mechanoreceptors in the sole of the foot using a balance-enhancing insole (Fig. 19.3). One type of footwear insole has a raised ridge around the perimeter to increase stimulation of the receptors in the vicinity of the outer ridge.

Perry et al. studied the effects of these insoles on medial-lateral balance control during gait and whether long-term benefits were achieved.[163] They found that use of insoles influenced the ability to

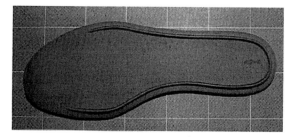

FIG. 19.3 Balance-enhancing insoles. The balance enhancing insole is placed inside the shoe. The outer edge provides "feedback" to the patient regarding postural stability. (Courtesy of Dr. Stephen Perry; with permission.)

control body motion when walking over uneven surfaces. Positive effects occurred during the most unstable phase of gait (single support). Improved balance control persisted even after 12 weeks of use, indicating that the brain did not habituate to the cutaneous stimulation produced by the insole. Footwear insoles may play an essential role in maintaining dynamic balance and enhancing stability for older adults in the future.

Tai Chi

Tai Chi is a traditional Chinese martial art that uses slow movements, breathing exercises, and meditation. Breathing is coordinated with slow movement to achieve mind tranquility. It is practiced in a semisquat position with adjustable intensities by increasing or decreasing the knee angle. Older adults tend to remain in the high-squat position.

Evidence in the literature supports the use of Tai Chi in people with vestibular pathology.[164] Tai Chi intervention resulted in improved gait speed and postural stability in people with vestibular pathology[165,166]; however, improvement in gaze stability was not evident after Tai Chi. These findings advocate the use of Tai Chi along with VREs.[165,166]

Tai Chi has also been shown to reduce the number of falls in older adults.[167] After Tai Chi training, improvements have been shown in balance ability,[168] plantar sensory function, muscle strength, gait, lower extremity flexibility, and general mobility.[169,170]

Telerehabilitation technology using Tai Chi has been utilized to exercise older adults.[171] Using telerehabilitation increases compliance, and using Tai Chi resulted in a reduction in the risk of falling and improvements in balance. Although further investigation is needed, these studies provide preliminary evidence of a promising intervention technique for older adults with vestibular disorders who are at risk of falling.

Vibrotactile Feedback Devices

Vibrotactile feedback devices (Fig. 19.4) are prosthetic devices that are being developed to restore loss of self-motion information caused by disease, injuries, and aging.[172] These prosthetic devices have been shown to influence postural control in standing as well as during gait and to reduce the risk of falling in older adults.[173] In patients with vestibular pathologies, vibrotactile feedback improved anteroposterior trunk tilt, trunk sway,[174] as well as gait and sway during tandem walking.[173,175] Although vibrotactile feedback might not be as effective in improving trunk sway and balance control when used in combination with a cognitive

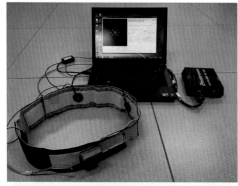

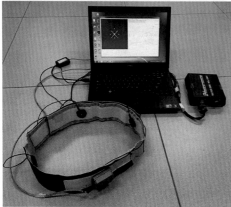

FIG. 19.4 Vibrotactile device. The vibrotactile device fits around the waist and provides augmented feedback regarding body tilt position. (Courtesy of Conrad Wall III; with permission.)

task (e.g., counting backward),[176] vibrotactile biofeedback may be helpful in the future with older adults to improve balance.

Optokinetic Stimulation

Visual vertigo is seen in some patients with vestibular dysfunction in whom symptoms are provoked by complex sensory stimuli (e.g., supermarkets).[153] Habituation exercises aim to desensitize patients through continuous exposure to stimuli that provoke the patient's symptoms. These exercises require the patient to maintain balance when one or more sensory inputs are disturbed. Habituation exercises can improve patient symptoms when combined with optokinetic stimulation. Pavlou et al. concluded that customized vestibular rehabilitation utilizing optokinetic stimuli is more beneficial than vestibular rehabilitation without optokinetic stimulation in persons with chronic unilateral vestibular dysfunction.[153]

The Nintendo Wii

Although no controlled trials have been published to support the use of the Nintendo Wii in patients with vestibular and/or balance disorders, some reports have demonstrated improvements in patients with balance and standing posture.[177,178] The Wii Balance Board is a valid tool for assessing standing balance.[179] The Wii is convenient and easy to move compared to other laboratory equipment (i.e., force platforms) used to assess balance. The Wii system is handy to use in clinics or at home and has been shown to hasten recovery in patients with vestibular neuritis (improved balance, reduced dizziness, shorter in-patient stay, quicker resolution of nystagmus).[23] The Wii is a promising technology that needs further statistically powered studies in patients with vestibular and balance dysfunction.

SUMMARY

Most patients with vestibular dysfunction can be helped with the variety of vestibular rehabilitation programs available. Vestibular rehabilitation has demonstrated effectiveness in the treatment of older persons with peripheral and central vestibular disorders, yet there is less evidence for the effectiveness of vestibular rehabilitation in older adults with central vestibular disorders. Dizziness reduction and enhanced postural stability are typical outcomes of a rehabilitation program. Improved quality of life and lower levels of anxiety have been shown after vestibular rehabilitation. Improvement in gait speed and marked reduction in risk of falling have also been reported. There is strong evidence that supports the use of canalith repositioning maneuvers in older adults with BPPV. Innovative technologies in vestibular rehabilitation are promising new interventions that may enhance treatment effectiveness for older adults with balance and vestibular disorders.

REFERENCES

1. Fernández L, Breinbauer HA, Delano PH. Vertigo and dizziness in the elderly. *Front Neurol.* 2015;6:144.
2. Sloane P, Blazer D, George LK. Dizziness in a community elderly population. *J Am Geriatr Soc.* 1989;37(2):101–108.
3. Colledge NR, Wilson JA, Macintyre CC, MacLennan WJ. The prevalence and characteristics of dizziness in an elderly community. *Age Ageing.* 1994;23(2):117–120.
4. Boult C, Murphy J, Sloane P, Mor V, Drone C. The relation of dizziness to functional decline. *J Am Geriatr Soc.* 1991;39(9):858–861.
5. Lasisi AO, Gureje O. Disability and quality of life among community elderly with dizziness: report from the Ibadan Study of Ageing. *J Laryngol Otol.* 2010:1–6.

6. Popp P, Wulff M, Finke K, Rühl M, Brandt T, Dieterich M. Cognitive deficits in patients with a chronic vestibular failure. *J Neurol.* 2017:1–10.

7. Olmos Zapata P, Abad Mateos MA, Perez-Jara J. Fear of falling in the elderly with recurrent dizziness: a descriptive study. *Rev Esp Geriatr Gerontol.* 2010;45(5).

8. Agrawal Y, Carey JP, Della Santina CC, Schubert MC, Minor LB. Disorders of balance and vestibular function in US adults: data from the National Health and Nutrition Examination Survey, 2001–2004. *Arch Int Med.* 2009;169(10):938–944.

9. Tinetti ME, Speechley M, Ginter SF. Risk factors for falls among elderly persons living in the community. *New Engl J Med.* 1988;319(26):1701–1707.

10. Todd CJ, Freeman CJ, Camilleri-Ferrante C, et al. Differences in mortality after fracture of hip: the east Anglian audit. *BMJ.* 1995;310(6984):904–908.

11. Alrwaily M, Whitney S, Holmberg J. A physical therapist classification system for persons with complaints of dizziness and balance dysfunction. *Phys Ther Rev.* 2015;20(2):110–121.

12. Baloh RW. Differentiating between peripheral and central causes of vertigo. *J Neurol Sci.* 2004;221(1–2):3.

13. Herrera WG. Vestibular and other balance disorders in multiple sclerosis. Differential diagnosis of disequilibrium and topognostic localization. *Neurol Clin.* 1990;8(2):407–420.

14. Pastor MA, Day BL, Marsden CD. Vestibular induced postural responses in Parkinson's disease. *Brain A J Neurol.* 1993;116(Pt 5):1177–1190.

15. Stucken EZ, Brown K, Selesnick SH. Clinical and diagnostic evaluation of acoustic neuromas. *Otolaryngol Clin North Am.* 2012;45(2):269–284, vii.

16. Bath AP, Walsh RM, Ranalli P, et al. Experience from a multidisciplinary "dizzy" clinic. *Am J Otol.* 2000;21(1):92–97.

17. Schlick C, Schniepp R, Loidl V, Wuehr M, Hesselbarth K, Jahn K. Falls and fear of falling in vertigo and balance disorders: a controlled cross-sectional study. *J Vestib Res.* 2015;25(5–6):241–251.

18. Maarsingh OR, Dros J, Schellevis FG, et al. Causes of persistent dizziness in elderly patients in primary care. *Ann Family Med.* 2010;8(3):196–205.

19. Tinetti ME, Williams CS, Gill TM. Dizziness among older adults: a possible geriatric syndrome. *Ann Int Med.* 2000;132(5):337–344.

20. Matheson AJ, Darlington CL, Smith PF. Further evidence for age-related deficits in human postural function. *J Vestib Res Equilib Orientat.* 1999;9(4):261–264.

21. Paige GD. Senescence of human visual-vestibular interactions. 1. Vestibulo-ocular reflex and adaptive plasticity with aging. *J Vestib Res Equilib Orientat.* 1992;2(2):133–151.

22. Furman JM, Raz Y, Whitney SL. Geriatric vestibulopathy assessment and management. *Curr Opin Otolaryngol Head Neck Surg.* 2010;18(5).

23. Sparrer I, Duong Dinh TA, Ilgner J, Westhofen M. Vestibular rehabilitation using the Nintendo® Wii Balance Board–a user-friendly alternative for central nervous compensation. *Acta Otolaryngol.* 2013;133(3):239–245.

24. Whitney SL, Sparto PJ, Brown KE, Furman JM, Jacobson JL, Redfern MS. The potential use of virtual reality in vestibular rehabilitation: preliminary findings with the BNAVE. *J Neurol Phys Ther.* 2002;26(2):72–78.

25. Anzalone AJ, Blueitt D, Case T, et al. A positive vestibular/ocular motor screening (VOMS) is associated with increased recovery time after sports-related concussion in youth and adolescent athletes. *Am J Sports Med.* 2016. http://dx.doi.org/0363546516668624.

26. Goto F, Nomura K, Taka F, Arai M, Sugaya N. Analysis of factors affecting the outcomes of in-hospitalized vestibular rehabilitation in patients with intractable dizziness. *Otol Neurotol.* 2017;38(3).

27. Ricci NA, Aratani MC, Caovilla HH, Ganança FF. Effects of vestibular rehabilitation on balance control in older people with chronic dizziness: a randomized clinical trial. *Am J Phys Med Rehabil.* 2016;95(4):256–269.

28. Strupp M, Zingler VC, Arbusow V, et al. Methylprednisolone, valacyclovir, or the combination for vestibular neuritis. *New Engl J Med.* 2004;351(4):354–361.

29. Studenski S, Perera S, Patel K, et al. Gait speed and survival in older adults. *JAMA.* 2011;305(1):50–58.

30. Podsiadlo D, Richardson S. The timed "up & go": a test of basic functional mobility for frail elderly persons. *J Am Geriatr Soc.* 1991;39(2):142–148.

31. Verghese J, Kuslansky G, Holtzer R, et al. Walking while talking: effect of task prioritization in the elderly. *Arch Phys Med Rehabil.* 2007;88(1):50–53.

32. Mantello EB, Moriguti JC, Rodrigues-Junior AL, Ferrioli E. Vestibular rehabilitation's effect over the quality of life of geriatric patients with labyrinth disease. *Braz J Otorhinolaryngol.* 2008;74(2):172–180.

33. Guralnik JM, Ferrucci L, Pieper CF, et al. Lower extremity function and subsequent disability: consistency across studies, predictive models, and value of gait speed alone compared with the short physical performance battery. *J Gerontol A Biol Sci Med Sci.* 2000;55(4):M221–M231.

34. Schniepp R, Schlick C, Schenkel F, et al. Clinical and neurophysiological risk factors for falls in patients with bilateral vestibulopathy. *J Neurol.* 2016:1–7.

35. Young WR, Olonilua M, Masters RS, Dimitriadis S, Williams AM. Examining links between anxiety, reinvestment and walking when talking by older adults during adaptive gait. *Exp Brain Res.* 2016;234(1):161–172.

36. Studenski S. Bradypedia: is gait speed ready for clinical use? *J Nutr Health Aging.* 2009;13(10):878–880.

37. Shumway-Cook A, Brauer S, Woollacott M. Predicting the probability for falls in community-dwelling older adults using the timed up & go test. *Phys Ther.* 2000;80(9):896–903.

38. Whitney SL, Marchetti GF, Schade A, Wrisley DM. The sensitivity and specificity of the timed "up & go" and the dynamic gait index for self-reported falls in persons with vestibular disorders. *J Vestib Res Equilib Orientat.* 2004;14(5):397–409.

39. Ricci NA, Aratani MC, Doná F, Macedo C, Caovilla HH, Ganança FF. A systematic review about the effects of the vestibular rehabilitation in middle-age and older adults. *Braz J Phys Ther.* 2010;14(5):361–371.

40. Cawthorne T. Vestibular injuries. *Proc R Soc Med.* 1946;39(5):270–273.

41. Cowand JL, Wrisley DM, Walker M, Strasnick B, Jacobson JT. Efficacy of vestibular rehabilitation. *Otolaryngol Head Neck Surg.* 1998;118(1):49–54.

42. Zeigelboim BS, Klagenberg KF, Teive HA, Munhoz RP, Martins-Bassetto J. Vestibular rehabilitation: clinical benefits to patients with Parkinson's disease. *Arq Neuropsiquiatr.* 2009;67(2A):219–223.

43. Meli A, Zimatore G, Badaracco C, De Angelis E, Tufarelli D. Effects of vestibular rehabilitation therapy on emotional aspects in chronic vestibular patients. *J Psychosom Res.* 2007;63(2):185–190.

44. Herdman SJ, Clendaniel RA, Mattox DE, Holliday MJ, Niparko JK. Vestibular adaptation exercises and recovery: acute stage after acoustic neuroma resection. *Otolaryngol Head Neck Surg.* 1995;113(1):77–87.

45. Telian SA, Shepard NT, Smith-Wheelock M, Kemink JL. Habituation therapy for chronic vestibular dysfunction: preliminary results. *Otolaryngol Head Neck Surg.* 1990;103(1):89–95.

46. Yardley L, Beech S, Zander L, Evans T, Weinman J. A randomized controlled trial of exercise therapy for dizziness and vertigo in primary care. *Br J Gen Pract.* 1998;48(429):1136–1140.

47. Jung JY, Kim JS, Chung PS, Woo SH, Rhee CK. Effect of vestibular rehabilitation on dizziness in the elderly. *Am J Otolaryngol.* 2009;30(5):295–299.

48. Itani M, Koaik Y, Sabri A. The value of close monitoring in vestibular rehabilitation therapy. *J Laryngol Otol.* 2017;131(3):227.

49. Angeli SI, Hawley R, Gomez O. Systematic approach to benign paroxysmal positional vertigo in the elderly. *Otolaryngol Head Neck Surg.* 2003;128(5):719–725.

50. McDonnell MN, Hillier SL. Vestibular rehabilitation for unilateral peripheral vestibular dysfunction. *Cochrane Libr.* 2015;(1):CD005397. http://dx.doi.org/10.1002/14651858.CD005397.pub4.

51. Macias JD, Massingale S, Gerkin RD. Efficacy of vestibular rehabilitation therapy in reducing falls. *Otolaryngol Head Neck Surg.* 2005;133(3):323–325.

52. Salvinelli F, Casale M, Trivelli M, et al. Benign paroxysmal positional vertigo: a comparative prospective study on the efficacy of Semont's maneuver and no treatment strategy. *Clin Ter.* 2003;154(1):7–11.

53. Cohen HS, Kimball KT. Effectiveness of treatments for benign paroxysmal positional vertigo of the posterior canal. *Otol Neurotol.* 2005;26(5):1034–1040.

54. Munoz JE, Miklea JT, Howard M, Springate R, Kaczorowski J. Canalith repositioning maneuver for benign paroxysmal positional vertigo: randomized controlled trial in family practice. *Can Fam Physician.* 2007;53(6): 1049–1053, 1048.

55. Richard W, Bruintjes TD, Oostenbrink P, van Leeuwen RB. Efficacy of the Epley maneuver for posterior canal BPPV: a long-term, controlled study of 81 patients. *Ear Nose Throat J.* 2005;84(1):22–25.

56. von Brevern M, Seelig T, Radtke A, Tiel-Wilck K, Neuhauser H, Lempert T. Short-term efficacy of Epley's manoeuvre: a double-blind randomised trial. *J Neurol Neurosurg Psychiatry.* 2006;77(8):980–982.

57. Simhadri S, Panda N, Raghunathan M. Efficacy of particle repositioning maneuver in BPPV: a prospective study. *Am J Otolaryngol.* 2003;24(6):355–360.

58. Hall CD, Schubert MC, Herdman SJ. Prediction of fall risk reduction as measured by dynamic gait index in individuals with unilateral vestibular hypofunction. *Otol Neurotol.* 2004;25(5):746–751.

59. Hall CD, Heusel-Gillig L, Tusa RJ, Herdman SJ. Efficacy of gaze stability exercises in older adults with dizziness. *J Neurol Phys Ther.* 2010;34(2):64–69.

60. Telian SA, Shepard NT, Smith-Wheelock M, Hoberg M. Bilateral vestibular paresis: diagnosis and treatment. *Otolaryngol Head Neck Surg.* 1991;104(1):67–71.

61. Herdman SJ, Schubert MC, Das VE, Tusa RJ. Recovery of dynamic visual acuity in unilateral vestibular hypofunction. *Arch Otolaryngol Head Neck Surg.* 2003;129(8): 819–824.

62. Horak FB, Jones-Rycewicz C, Black FO, Shumway-Cook A. Effects of vestibular rehabilitation on dizziness and imbalance. *Otolaryngol Head Neck Surg.* 1992;106(2): 175–180.

63. Corna S, Nardone A, Prestinari A, Galante M, Grasso M, Schieppati M. Comparison of Cawthorne-Cooksey exercises and sinusoidal support surface translations to improve balance in patients with unilateral vestibular deficit. *Arch Phys Med Rehabil.* 2003;84(8):1173–1184.

64. Meli A, Zimatore G, Badaracco C, De Angelis E, Tufarelli D. Vestibular rehabilitation and 6-month follow-up using objective and subjective measures. *Acta Otolaryngol.* 2006;126(3):259–266.

65. Topuz O, Topuz B, Ardic FN, Sarhus M, Ogmen G, Ardic F. Efficacy of vestibular rehabilitation on chronic unilateral vestibular dysfunction. *Clin Rehabil.* 2004;18(1):76–83.

66. Cohen HS, Kimball KT. Increased independence and decreased vertigo after vestibular rehabilitation. *Otolaryngol Head Neck Surg.* 2003;128(1):60–70.

67. Szturm T, Ireland DJ, Lessing-Turner M. Comparison of different exercise programs in the rehabilitation of patients with chronic peripheral vestibular dysfunction. *J Vestib Res Equilib Orientat.* 1994;4(6):461–479.

68. Giray M, Kirazli Y, Karapolat H, Celebisoy N, Bilgen C, Kirazli T. Short-term effects of vestibular rehabilitation in patients with chronic unilateral vestibular dysfunction: a randomized controlled study. *Arch Phys Med Rehabil.* 2009;90(8):1325–1331.

69. Brown KE, Whitney SL, Wrisley DM, Furman JM. Physical therapy outcomes for persons with bilateral vestibular loss. *Laryngoscope.* 2001;111(10):1812–1817.

70. Krebs DE, Gill-Body KM, Riley PO, Parker SW. Double-blind, placebo-controlled trial of rehabilitation for bilateral vestibular hypofunction: preliminary report. *Otolaryngol Head Neck Surg.* 1993;109(4):735–741.

71. Asai M, Watanabe Y, Shimizu K. Effects of vestibular rehabilitation on postural control. *Acta Otolaryngol Suppl.* 1997;528:116–120.

72. Herdman SJ, Hall CD, Schubert MC, Das VE, Tusa RJ. Recovery of dynamic visual acuity in bilateral vestibular hypofunction. *Arch Otolaryngol Head Neck Surg.* 2007;133(4):383–389.

73. Strupp M, Arbusow V, Maag KP, Gall C, Brandt T. Vestibular exercises improve central vestibulospinal compensation after vestibular neuritis. *Neurology.* 1998;51(3):838–844.

74. Cohen HS, Kimball KT. Decreased ataxia and improved balance after vestibular rehabilitation. *Otolaryngol Head Neck Surg.* 2004;130(4):418–425.

75. Cakrt O, Chovanec M, Funda T, et al. Exercise with visual feedback improves postural stability after vestibular schwannoma surgery. *Eur Arch Otorhinolaryngol.* 2010;267(9).

76. Levo H, Blomstedt G, Pyykko I. Postural stability after vestibular schwannoma surgery. *Ann Otol Rhinol Laryngol.* 2004;113(12):994–999.

77. Enticott JC, O'Leary SJ, Briggs RJ. Effects of vestibulo-ocular reflex exercises on vestibular compensation after vestibular schwannoma surgery. *Otol Neurotol.* 2005;26(2):265–269.

78. Gottshall KR, Hoffer ME, Moore RJ, Balough BJ. The role of vestibular rehabilitation in the treatment of Meniere's disease. *Otolaryngol Head Neck Surg.* 2005;133(3):326–328.

79. Mruzek M, Barin K, Nichols DS, Burnett CN, Welling DB. Effects of vestibular rehabilitation and social reinforcement on recovery following ablative vestibular surgery. *Laryngoscope.* 1995;105(7 Pt 1):686–692.

80. Gurr B, Moffat N. Psychological consequences of vertigo and the effectiveness of vestibular rehabilitation for brain injury patients. *Brain Inj.* 2001;15(5):387–400.

81. Jacob RG, Whitney SL, Detweiler-Shostak G, Furman JM. Vestibular rehabilitation for patients with agoraphobia and vestibular dysfunction: a pilot study. *J Anxiety Disord.* 2001;15(1–2):131–146.

82. Karlberg M, Magnusson M, Malmstrom EM, Melander A, Moritz U. Postural and symptomatic improvement after physiotherapy in patients with dizziness of suspected cervical origin. *Arch Phys Med Rehabil.* 1996;77(9):874–882.

83. Wrisley DM, Sparto PJ, Whitney SL, Furman JM. Cervicogenic dizziness: a review of diagnosis and treatment. *J Orthop Sports Phys Ther.* 2000;30(12):755–766.

84. Gizzi M. The efficacy of vestibular rehabilitation for patients with head trauma. *J Head Trauma Rehabil.* 1995;10(6):60–77.

85. Telian SA, Shepard NT. Update on vestibular rehabilitation therapy. *Otolaryngol Clin North Am.* 1996;29(2):359–371.

86. Herdman SJ. Treatment of vestibular disorders in traumatically brain-injured patients. *J Head Trauma Rehabil.* 1990;5(4):63–76.

87. Gottshall KR, Hoffer ME. Tracking recovery of vestibular function in individuals with blast-induced head trauma using vestibular-visual-cognitive interaction tests. *J Neurol Phys Ther.* 2010;34(2):94–97.

88. Gill-Body KM, Popat RA, Parker SW, Krebs DE. Rehabilitation of balance in two patients with cerebellar dysfunction. *Phys Ther.* 1997;77(5):534–552.

89. Gill-Body KM, Krebs DE, Parker SW, Riley PO. Physical therapy management of peripheral vestibular dysfunction: two clinical case reports. *Phys Ther.* 1994;74(2):129–142.

90. Pavan K, Marangoni BE, Schmidt KB, et al. Vestibular rehabilitation in patients with relapsing-remitting multiple sclerosis. *Arq Neuropsiquiatr.* 2007;65(2A):332–335.

91. Zeigelboim BS, Arruda WO, Mangabeira-Albernaz PL, et al. Vestibular findings in relapsing, remitting multiple sclerosis: a study of thirty patients. *Int Tinnitus J.* 2008;14(2):139–145.

92. Ekvall Hansson E, Mansson NO, Hakansson A. Benign paroxysmal positional vertigo among elderly patients in primary health care. *Gerontology.* 2005;51(6):386–389.

93. Oghalai JS, Manolidis S, Barth JL, Stewart MG, Jenkins HA. Unrecognized benign paroxysmal positional vertigo in elderly patients. *Otolaryngol Head Neck Surg.* 2000;122(5):630–634.

94. Helminski JO, Zee DS, Janssen I, Hain TC. Effectiveness of particle repositioning maneuvers in the treatment of benign paroxysmal positional vertigo: a systematic review. *Phys Ther.* 2010;90(5):663–678.

95. Bhattacharyya N, Gubbels SP, Schwartz SR, et al. Clinical practice guideline: benign paroxysmal positional vertigo (update) executive summary. *Otolaryngol Head Neck Surg.* 2017;156(3):403–416.

96. Ferreira MM, Ganança MM, Caovilla HH. Subjective visual vertical after treatment of benign paroxysmal positional vertigo. *Braz J Otorhinolaryngol.* 2017;83:659–664.

97. Shepard NT, Telian SA. Programmatic vestibular rehabilitation. *Otolaryngol Head Neck Surg.* 1995;112(1):173–182.

98. Obrist D, Nienhaus A, Zamaro E, Kalla R, Mantokoudis G, Strupp M. Determinants for a successful sémont Maneuver: an in vitro study with a semicircular canal Model. *Front Neurol.* 2016;7.

99. Manso A, Ganança MM, Caovilla HH. Vestibular rehabilitation with visual stimuli in peripheral vestibular disorders. *Braz J Otorhinolaryngol.* 2016;82(2):232–241.

100. Hall CD, Herdman SJ, Whitney SL, et al. Vestibular rehabilitation for peripheral vestibular hypofunction: an evidence-based clinical practice guideline: from the American physical therapy association neurology section. *J Neurol Phys Ther.* 2016;40(2):124–155.

101. Minor LB. Gentamicin-induced bilateral vestibular hypofunction. *JAMA.* 1998;279(7):541–544.

102. Smith-Wheelock M, Shepard NT, Telian SA. Physical therapy program for vestibular rehabilitation. *Am J Otol.* 1991;12(3):218-225.

103. Herdman SJ, Clendaniel RA. Assessment and intervention for the patient with complete vestibular loss. In: Herdman SJ, ed. *Vestibular Rehabilitation.* 3rd ed. Philadelphia: F. A. Davis Company; 2007:338-359.

104. Komazec Z, Lemajic S. Specific vestibular exercises in the treatment of vestibular neuritis. *Med Pregl.* 2004;57(5-6): 269-274.

105. Whitney SL, Rossi MM. Efficacy of vestibular rehabilitation. *Otolaryngol Clin North Am.* 2000;33(3):659-672.

106. Clendaniel RA, Tucci DL. Vestibular rehabilitation strategies in Meniere's disease. *Otolaryngol Clin North Am.* 1997;30(6):1145-1158.

107. Dieterich M, Staab JP. Functional dizziness: from phobic postural vertigo and chronic subjective dizziness to persistent postural-perceptual dizziness. *Curr Opin Neurol.* 2017;30(1):107-113.

108. Lahmann C, Henningsen P, Brandt T, et al. Psychiatric comorbidity and psychosocial impairment among patients with vertigo and dizziness. *J Neurol Neurosurg Psychiatry.* 2014. http://dx.doi.org/10.1136/jnnp-2014-307601.

109. Walker A, Kantaris X, Chambers M. Understanding therapeutic approaches to anxiety in vestibular rehabilitation: a qualitative study of specialist physiotherapists in the UK. *Disabil Rehabil.* 2017:1-10.

110. Staab JP, Ruckenstein MJ, Amsterdam JD. A prospective trial of sertraline for chronic subjective dizziness. *Laryngoscope.* 2004;114(9):1637-1641.

111. Tschan R, Eckhardt-Henn A, Scheurich V, Best C, Dieterich M, Beutel M. Steadfast–effectiveness of a cognitive-behavioral self-management program for patients with somatoform vertigo and dizziness. *Psychother Psychosom Med Psychol.* 2011;62(3-4):111-119.

112. Magnusson M, Kahlon B, Karlberg M, Lindberg S, Siesjo P. Preoperative vestibular ablation with gentamicin and vestibular 'prehab' enhance postoperative recovery after surgery for pontine angle tumours–first report. *Acta Otolaryngol.* 2007;127(12):1236-1240.

113. Magnusson M, Kahlon B, Karlberg M, Lindberg S, Siesjo P, Tjernstrom F. Vestibular "PREHAB". *Ann N Y Acad Sci.* 2009;1164:257-262.

114. El-Kashlan HK, Shepard NT, Arts HA, Telian SA. Disability from vestibular symptoms after acoustic neuroma resection. *Am J Otol.* 1998;19(1):104-111.

115. Tjernstrom F, Fransson PA, Kahlon B, et al. Vestibular PREHAB and gentamicin before schwannoma surgery may improve long-term postural function. *J Neurol Neurosurg Psychiatry.* 2009;80(11):1254-1260.

116. Furman JM, Whitney SL. Central causes of dizziness. *Phys Ther.* 2000;80(2):179-187.

117. Bloem BR, Grimbergen YA, Cramer M, Willemsen M, Zwinderman AH. Prospective assessment of falls in Parkinson's disease. *J Neurol.* 2001;248(11):950-958.

118. Wielinski CL, Erickson-Davis C, Wichmann R, Walde-Douglas M, Parashos SA. Falls and injuries resulting from falls among patients with Parkinson's disease and other parkinsonian syndromes. *Mov Disord.* 2005;20(4): 410-415.

119. Wood BH, Bilclough JA, Bowron A, Walker RW. Incidence and prediction of falls in Parkinson's disease: a prospective multidisciplinary study. *J Neurol Neurosurg Psychiatry.* 2002;72(6):721-725.

120. Rudzinska M, Bukowczan S, Stozek J, et al. Causes and consequences of falls in Parkinson disease patients in a prospective study. *Neurol Neurochir Pol.* 2013;47(5): 423-430.

121. Koller WC, Glatt S, Vetere-Overfield B, Hassanein R. Falls and Parkinson's disease. *Clin Neuropharmacol.* 1989;12(2):98-105.

122. Rossi-Izquierdo M, Soto-Varela A, Santos-Perez S, Sesar-Ignacio A, Labella-Caballero T. Vestibular rehabilitation with computerised dynamic posturography in patients with Parkinson's disease: improving balance impairment. *Disabil Rehabil.* 2009;31(23):1907-1916.

123. Acarer A, Karapolat H, Celebisoy N, Ozgen G, Colakoglu Z. Is customized vestibular rehabilitation effective in patients with Parkinson's? *NeuroRehabilitation.* 2015;37(2):255-262.

124. Hirsch MA, Toole T, Maitland CG, Rider RA. The effects of balance training and high-intensity resistance training on persons with idiopathic Parkinson's disease. *Arch Phys Med Rehabil.* 2003;84(8):1109-1117.

125. Karatas M. Central vertigo and dizziness: epidemiology, differential diagnosis, and common causes. *Neurologist.* 2008;14(6):355-364.

126. Ozgen G, Karapolat H, Akkoc Y, Yuceyar N. Is customized vestibular rehabilitation effective in patients with multiple sclerosis? A randomized controlled trial. *Eur J Phys Rehabil Med.* 2016;52(4):466-478.

127. Calabresi PA. Diagnosis and management of multiple sclerosis. *Am Fam Physician.* 2004;70(10):1935-1944.

128. Collins MW, Kontos AP, Reynolds E, Murawski CD, Fu FH. A comprehensive, targeted approach to the clinical care of athletes following sport-related concussion. *Knee Surg Sports Traumatol Arthrosc.* 2014;22(2):235-246.

129. Shumway-Cook A. Assessment and management of the patient with traumatic brain injury and vestibular dysfunction. *Vestib Rehabil.* 2007:444-445.

130. Davies RA, Luxon LM. Dizziness following head injury: a neuro-otological study. *J Neurol.* 1995;242(4):222-230.

131. Tuohimaa P. Vestibular disturbances after acute mild head injury. *Acta Otolaryngol Suppl.* 1978;359:3-67.

132. Lau BC, Kontos AP, Collins MW, Mucha A, Lovell MR. Which on-field signs/symptoms predict protracted recovery from sport-related concussion among high school football players? *Am J Sports Med.* 2011;39(11):2311-2318.

133. Ellis MJ, Cordingley D, Vis S, Reimer K, Leiter J, Russell K. Vestibulo-ocular dysfunction in pediatric sports-related concussion. *J Neurosurg Pediatr.* 2015;16(3):248-255.

134. Furman JM, Balaban CD, Pollack IF. Vestibular compensation in a patient with a cerebellar infarction. *Neurology.* 1997;48(4):916–920.

135. Alsalaheen BA, Mucha A, Morris LO, et al. Vestibular rehabilitation for dizziness and balance disorders after concussion. *J Neurol Phys Ther.* 2010;34(2):87–93.

136. Revel M, Andre-Deshays C, Minguet M. Cervicocephalic kinesthetic sensibility in patients with cervical pain. *Arch Phys Med Rehabil.* 1991;72(5):288–291.

137. Cass SP, Borello-France D, Furman JM. Functional outcome of vestibular rehabilitation in patients with abnormal sensory-organization testing. *Am J Otol.* 1996;17(4):581–594.

138. Whitney SL, Wrisley DM, Marchetti GF, Furman JM. The effect of age on vestibular rehabilitation outcomes. *Laryngoscope.* 2002;112(10):1785–1790.

139. Macias JD, Lambert KM, Massingale S, Ellensohn A, Fritz JA. Variables affecting treatment in benign paroxysmal positional vertigo. *Laryngoscope.* 2000;110(11):1921–1924.

140. Whitney SL, France DB. Bilateral vestibular disease: an overview. *J Neurol Phys Ther.* 1996;20(3):41–45.

141. Shepard NT, Telian SA, Smith-Wheelock M, Raj A. Vestibular and balance rehabilitation therapy. *Ann Otol Rhinol Laryngol.* 1993;102(3 Pt 1):198–205.

142. Konrad HR, Tomlinson D, Stockwell CW, et al. Rehabilitation therapy for patients with disequilibrium and balance disorders. *Otolaryngol Head Neck Surg.* 1992;107(1):105–108.

143. Cousins S, Kaski D, Cutfield N, et al. Predictors of clinical recovery from vestibular neuritis: a prospective study. *Ann Clin Transl Neurol.* 2017;4(5).

144. Pavlou M, Lingeswaran A, Davies RA, Gresty MA, Bronstein AM. Simulator based rehabilitation in refractory dizziness. *J Neurol.* 2004;251(8):983–995.

145. Black FO, Angel CR, Pesznecker SC, Gianna C. Outcome analysis of individualized vestibular rehabilitation protocols. *Am J Otol.* 2000;21(4):543–551.

146. Soto-Varela A, Faraldo-Garcia A, Del-Rio-Valeiras M, et al. Adherence of older people with instability in vestibular rehabilitation programmes: prediction criteria. *J Laryngol Otol.* 2017;131(3):232–238.

147. Muller I, Kirby S, Yardley L. Understanding patient experiences of self-managing chronic dizziness: a qualitative study of booklet-based vestibular rehabilitation, with or without remote support. *BMJ Open.* 2015;5(5):e007680.

148. Bamiou DE, Davies RA, McKee M, Luxon LM. Symptoms, disability and handicap in unilateral peripheral vestibular disorders. Effects of early presentation and initiation of balance exercises. *Scand Audiol.* 2000;29(4):238–244.

149. Vrancken AF, Franssen H, Wokke JH, Teunissen LL, Notermans NC. Chronic idiopathic axonal polyneuropathy and successful aging of the peripheral nervous system in elderly people. *Arch Neurol.* 2002;59(4):533–540.

150. Rothbaum BO, Hodges LF. The use of virtual reality exposure in the treatment of anxiety disorders. *Behav Modif.* 1999;23(4):507–525.

151. Virk S, McConville KM. Virtual reality applications in improving postural control and minimizing falls. *Conf Proc IEEE Eng Med Biol Soc.* 2006;1:2694–2697.

152. Norre ME, De Weerdt W. Treatment of vertigo based on habituation. 2. Technique and results of habituation training. *J Laryngol Otol.* 1980;94(9):971–977.

153. Bronstein AM. Visual vertigo syndrome: clinical and posturography findings. *J Neurol Neurosurg Psychiatry.* 1995;59(5):472–476.

154. Whitney SL, Sparto PJ, Hodges LF, Babu SV, Furman JM, Redfern MS. Responses to a virtual reality grocery store in persons with and without vestibular dysfunction. *Cyberpsychol Behav.* 2006;9(2):152–156.

155. Suarez H, Suarez A, Lavinsky L. Postural adaptation in elderly patients with instability and risk of falling after balance training using a virtual-reality system. *Int Tinnitus J.* 2006;12(1):41–44.

156. Meldrum D, Herdman S, Vance R, et al. Effectiveness of conventional versus virtual reality-based balance exercises in vestibular rehabilitation for unilateral peripheral vestibular loss: results of a randomized controlled trial. *Arch Phys Med Rehabil.* 2015;96(7):1319–1328.e1311.

157. Gescheider GA, Edwards RR, Lackner EA, Bolanowski SJ, Verrillo RT. The effects of aging on information-processing channels in the sense of touch: III. Differential sensitivity to changes in stimulus intensity. *Somatosens Mot Res.* 1996;13(1):73–80.

158. Gescheider GA, Beiles EJ, Checkosky CM, Bolanowski SJ, Verrillo RT. The effects of aging on information-processing channels in the sense of touch: II. Temporal summation in the P channel. *Somatosens Mot Res.* 1994;11(4):359–365.

159. Verrillo RT, Gescheider GA, Bolanowski SJ, Hoffman KE. When feeling is failing – the effects of aging on the sense of touch (Vol 93, Pg 2360, 1993). *J Acoust Soc Am.* 1993;94(6):3518.

160. Richardson JK, Hurvitz EA. Peripheral neuropathy: a true risk factor for falls. *J Gerontol A Biol Sci Med Sci.* 1995;50(4):M211–M215.

161. Lord SR, Menz HB, Tiedemann A. A physiological profile approach to falls risk assessment and prevention. *Phys Ther.* 2003;83(3):237–252.

162. Resnick HE, Vinik AI, Schwartz AV, et al. Independent effects of peripheral nerve dysfunction on lower-extremity physical function in old age: the Women's Health and Aging Study. *Diabetes Care.* 2000;23(11):1642–1647.

163. Perry SD, Radtke A, McIlroy WE, Fernie GR, Maki BE. Efficacy and effectiveness of a balance-enhancing insole. *J Gerontol A Biol Sci Med Sci.* 2008;63(6):595–602.

164. Wayne PM, Krebs DE, Wolf SL, et al. Can Tai Chi improve vestibulopathic postural control? *Arch Phys Med Rehabil.* 2004;85(1):142–152.

165. McGibbon CA, Krebs DE, Parker SW, Scarborough DM, Wayne PM, Wolf SL. Tai Chi and vestibular rehabilitation improve vestibulopathic gait via different neuromuscular mechanisms: preliminary report. *BMC Neurol.* 2005; 5(1):3.

166. McGibbon CA, Krebs DE, Wolf SL, Wayne PM, Scarborough DM, Parker SW. Tai Chi and vestibular rehabilitation effects on gaze and whole-body stability. *J Vestib Res Equilib Orientat.* 2004;14(6):467–478.

167. Richerson S, Rosendale K. Does Tai Chi improve plantar sensory ability? A pilot study. *Diabetes Technol Ther.* 2007;9(3):276–286.

168. Tsang WW, Hui-Chan CW. Effect of 4- and 8-wk intensive Tai Chi Training on balance control in the elderly. *Med Sci Sports Exerc.* 2004;36(4):648–657.

169. Choi JH, Moon JS, Song R. Effects of Sun-style Tai Chi exercise on physical fitness and fall prevention in fall-prone older adults. *J Adv Nurs.* 2005;51(2):150–157.

170. Lin MR, Hwang HF, Wang YW, Chang SH, Wolf SL. Community-based tai chi and its effect on injurious falls, balance, gait, and fear of falling in older people. *Phys Ther.* 2006;86(9):1189–1201.

171. Wu G, Keyes L, Callas P, Ren X, Bookchin B. Comparison of telecommunication, community, and home-based Tai Chi exercise programs on compliance and effectiveness in elders at risk for falls. *Arch Phys Med Rehabil.* 2010;91(6):849–856.

172. Sienko K, Whitney S, Carender W, Wall III C. The role of sensory augmentation for people with vestibular deficits: real-time balance aid and/or rehabilitation device? *J Vestib Res.* 2017;27(1):63–76.

173. Wall CI. Application of vibrotactile feedback of body motion to improve rehabilitation in individuals with imbalance. *J Neurol Phys Ther.* 2010;34(2):98–104. http://dx.doi.org/10.1097/NPT.0b013e3181dde6f0.

174. Wall C 3rd, Kentala E. Control of sway using vibrotactile feedback of body tilt in patients with moderate and severe postural control deficits. *J Vestib Res Equilib Orientat.* 2005;15(5–6):313–325.

175. Dozza M, Wall C 3rd, Peterka RJ, Chiari L, Horak FB. Effects of practicing tandem gait with and without vibrotactile biofeedback in subjects with unilateral vestibular loss. *J Vestib Res.* 2007;17(4):195–204.

176. Verhoeff LL, Horlings CG, Janssen LJ, Bridenbaugh SA, Allum JH. Effects of biofeedback on trunk sway during dual tasking in the healthy young and elderly. *Gait Posture.* 2009;30(1):76–81.

177. Shih CH, Shih CT, Chiang MS. A new standing posture detector to enable people with multiple disabilities to control environmental stimulation by changing their standing posture through a commercial Wii Balance Board. *Res Dev Disabil.* 2010;31(1):281–286.

178. Shih CH, Shih CT, Chu CL. Assisting people with multiple disabilities actively correct abnormal standing posture with a Nintendo Wii balance board through controlling environmental stimulation. *Res Dev Disabil.* 2010;31(4):936–942.

179. Clark RA, Bryant AL, Pua Y, McCrory P, Bennell K, Hunt M. Validity and reliability of the Nintendo Wii balance board for assessment of standing balance. *Gait Posture.* 2010;31(3):307–310.

Index

Note: Page numbers followed by "f" indicate figures, "t" indicate tables and "b" indicate boxes.

Printed in the United States
By Bookmasters